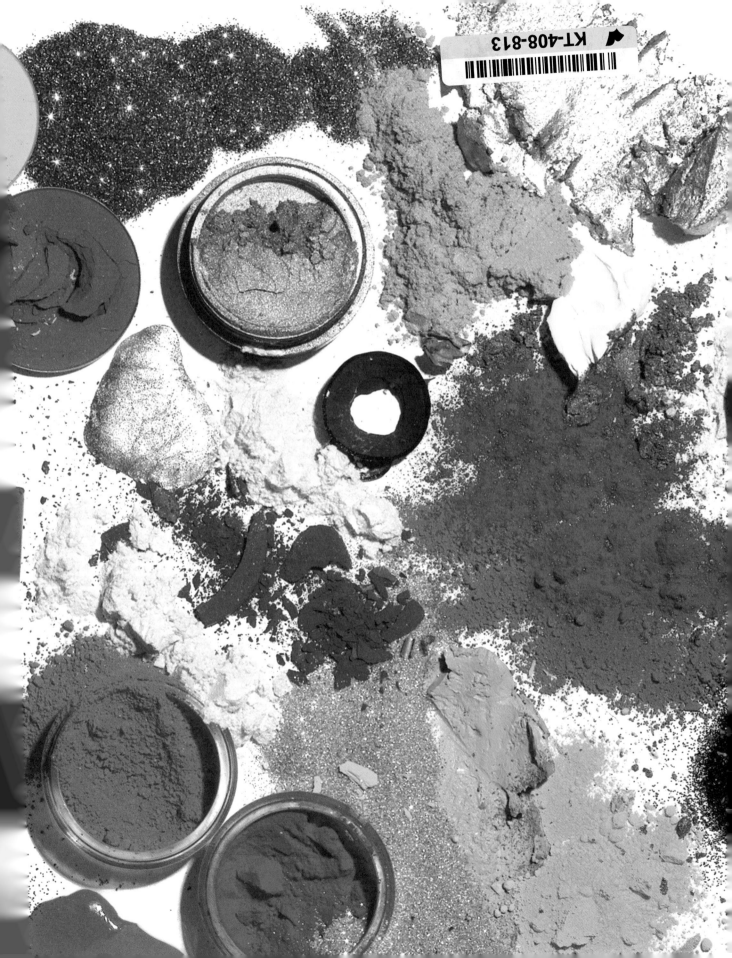

BOBBI BROWN MAKEUP MANUAL

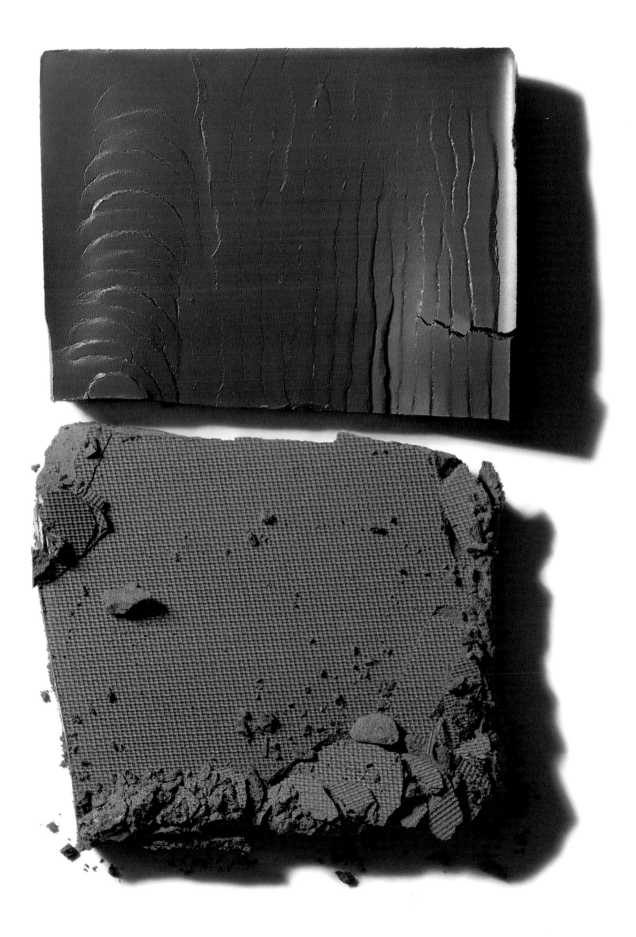

For Everyone from
Beginner to Pro

BOBBI BROWN MAKEUP MANUAL

Bobbi Brown

with Debra Bergsma Otte and Sally Wadyka

with photographs by Henry Leutwyler

headline
springboard

Photography credits and permissions information on p. 221.

First published in 2008 by Springboard Press.
Springboard Press is an imprint of Grand Central
Publishing. The Springboard Press name and logo
are trademarks of Hachette Book Group, Inc.

First published in Great Britain in 2008 by
Headline Springboard. An imprint of
HEADLINE PUBLISHING GROUP

Design by Ruba Abu-Nimah & Eleanor Rogers

Cataloging-in-Publication Data
ISBN 978 0 7553 1847 6

Printed and bound in the UK by Butler Tanner and Dennis Ltd, Frome

HEADLINE PUBLISHING GROUP
An Hachette Livre UK Company
338 Euston Road
London NW1 3BH
www.headline.co.uk
www.hachettelivre.co.uk

This book is dedicated to makeup artists everywhere — from the ones that taught me to the ones that I now teach.

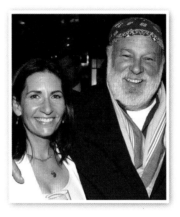

And to Bruce Weber, who taught me how to see the natural tones in people's faces — and that you can be both talented and famous, humble and nice.

And, always, to the boys/men in my life who make my heart sing.

Bobbi Brown

CONTENTS

I BASICS

II ARTISTRY

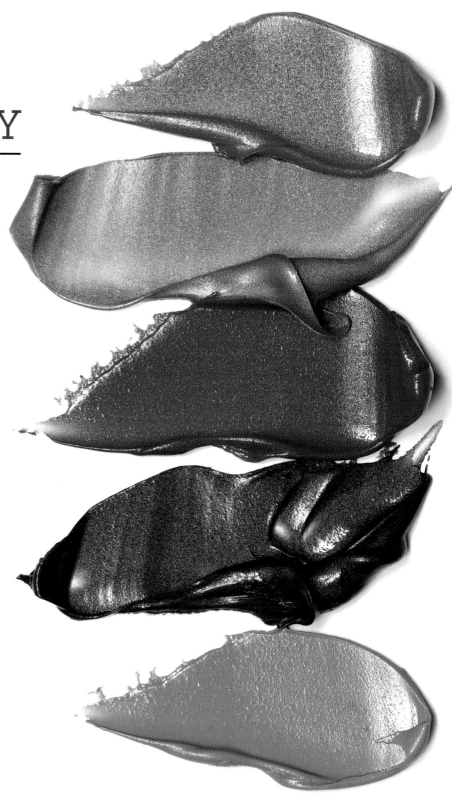

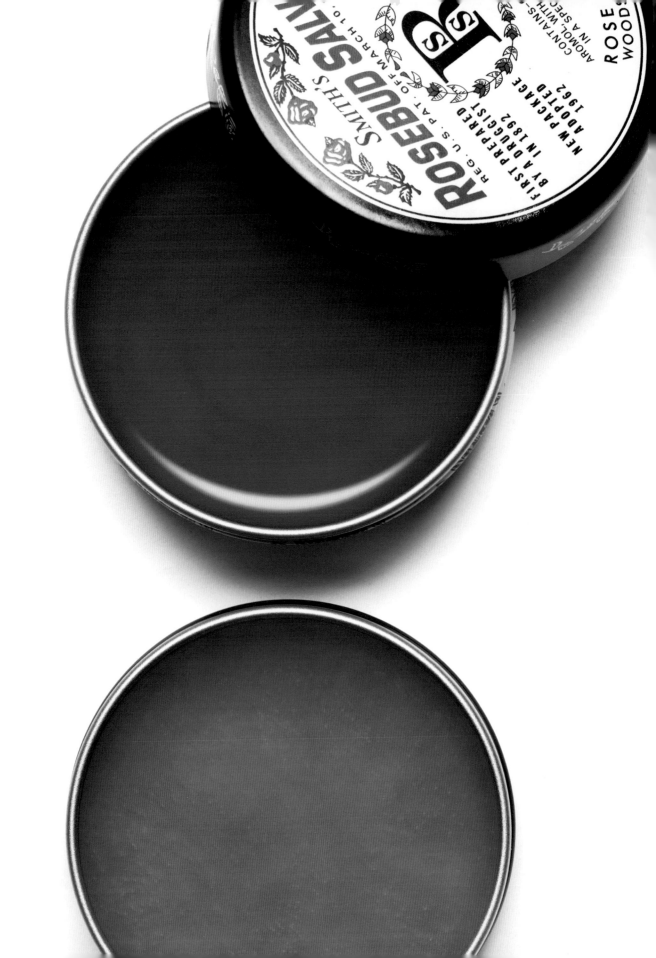

PART I: BASICS

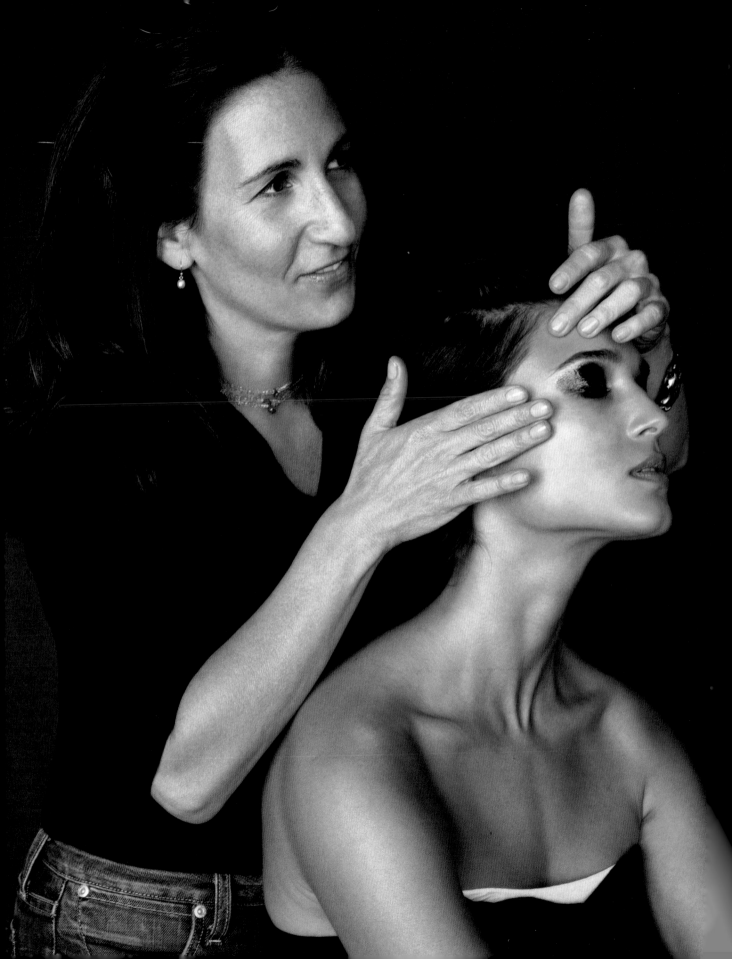

Chapter 1

MAKEUP ARTISTRY

I've set out to write the **simplest, most comprehensive makeup lesson you will ever have.** I've written this book for everyone: my artists, students, friends, and every woman who ever wanted to put on makeup like a professional.

When I first started working as a freelance makeup artist, it was almost impossible to find books dedicated to makeup artistry. This situation has improved over the years, but there is still a noticeable lack of good and accessible resources on makeup artistry. After scouring countless bookstores in search of the perfect makeup reference, I finally decided to write my own guide. My vision for this book is simple. I wanted it to be filled with complete step-by-step lessons, industry tips, and beautiful pictures. I wanted this book to serve as a complete reference guide for everyone who wants to know about beauty and makeup.

I have found that women are either intrigued with or mystified by cosmetics, but most are interested in learning more about makeup and how it can transform a face. All women really want the same thing: to look like themselves, only prettier and more confident. That desire is what actually inspired me, at twelve years old, to create the "natural look" for which I'm known. In seventh grade, the coolest thing was to hear how tan you were. So I used my mother's bronzer, put it on my cheeks, forehead, nose, and chin—until it looked like a real tan. I put on her lipstick and then rubbed it off. I wanted people to say I looked pretty—and not notice the makeup.

Years later, when I worked as a makeup artist, I learned from many of the leading professionals. My early work was a mixture of the natural look with risky bolts of color. I worked with George Newell, who did beautiful pale skin, very 80s red lips, bronze cheeks, and dark eyes. His style was not mine, but he was a great talent who taught me things I could not have learned elsewhere. I also studied under Linda Mason, the artist known for her abstract uses of color on the face. She taught me to go beyond my comfort zone and push myself to the unexpected. Then I met my mentor, Bonnie Maller. I first saw her work in a magazine profile. She did all the makeup for Bruce Weber and all the ads for Perry Ellis, Calvin Klein,

and Ralph Lauren. Her style was outdoorsy, as you can imagine. She had the same aesthetic as I did, and perfected the look. It changed my life. Her makeup was most instrumental in helping my style emerge. It was clean, natural, and always beautiful.

In the early days, I was like a sponge, learning from others, and then experimenting to see what I liked. I now look back on this time as graduate school. I read and studied every fashion spread. I loved the way light hit the colors on the face, and tried to recreate the looks. I began assisting makeup artists and eventually, with that experience, started to lead my own team.

When you are hired to do a show, you meet with the designer, and sometimes the stylist, to discuss the desired look and to possibly try the makeup on a model. The makeup has to be beautiful and work with the clothes. I used to experiment with concealer on lips to make a pale lip color statement while doing Brigitte Bardot–inspired, dark, smoky eyes or the brightest red and pink lips with very little on the eyes. I also remember using brown eye pencil on lips, which started the whole brown lip look.

By the time I started Bobbi Brown Cosmetics, I already had a group of artists who helped me do fashion shows. Early in my career, I couldn't pay them much, so I hired the ones who were eager to do the work for the experience and training. I started by inviting them to assist me—even if they just held brushes or observed. I watched them do makeup. I watched them watch me do makeup.

I love working with people who soak up information. Everyone has potential. I've never met anyone who could not master the skills needed, but many who lacked the confidence. I do believe that there is always more to learn, and I love the process.

I also believe every woman would gain confidence if she understood more about applying her makeup, using the right tools, finding the colors that work for her and perfecting the basic techniques.

I've written this book for everyone: my artists, students, friends, and every woman who ever wanted professional instruction. I've gone into more detail than ever before and photographed hundreds of step-by-step photos to show you as much detail as possible. I've also put the entire "class" into the sequence that I believe works best. Understanding the skin is the best way to start, and then building from foundation and concealer to color, lips, eyes, and everything in between. I believe this will be the most comprehensive makeup lesson you will ever have.

For the makeup artist or those who aspire to be one, I've written a section for professionals in the second part of the book. In this section, you'll find important information from how to pack a professional makeup kit to how to work with photographers.

The best artists continually want to learn. Artists who think they know everything don't grow. Professional makeup artists must love makeup. They need to be obsessed with the art and the business and cannot be afraid of hard work. Artists have to be able to see, evaluate their work, and take criticism as an

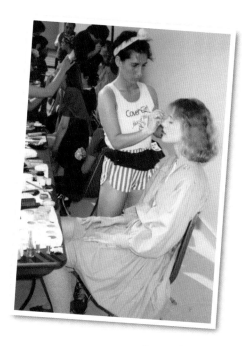

opportunity to grow. In makeup that means learning to recognize skin condition and texture, evaluate and effectively use color, and determine when formulation and application choices work and what to do when they don't.

This book is a true labor of love. It was written with the help of my team of makeup artists, friends, and customers—who have all contributed questions, concerns, and tips about makeup. Even though I've been in the makeup industry for over twenty years, I continue to learn.

The beauty industry is constantly changing, so it is important to stay open to new ideas, to acknowledge when techniques or styles don't work anymore, and to try new approaches and solutions. The goal is always to help women look and feel beautiful.

I expect that aspiring makeup artists will want to read every word of this book. Others may pick and choose to read those sections that apply to their concerns. Makeup artistry is incredibly gratifying. So be open, have fun, and never stop learning.

Bobbi Brown

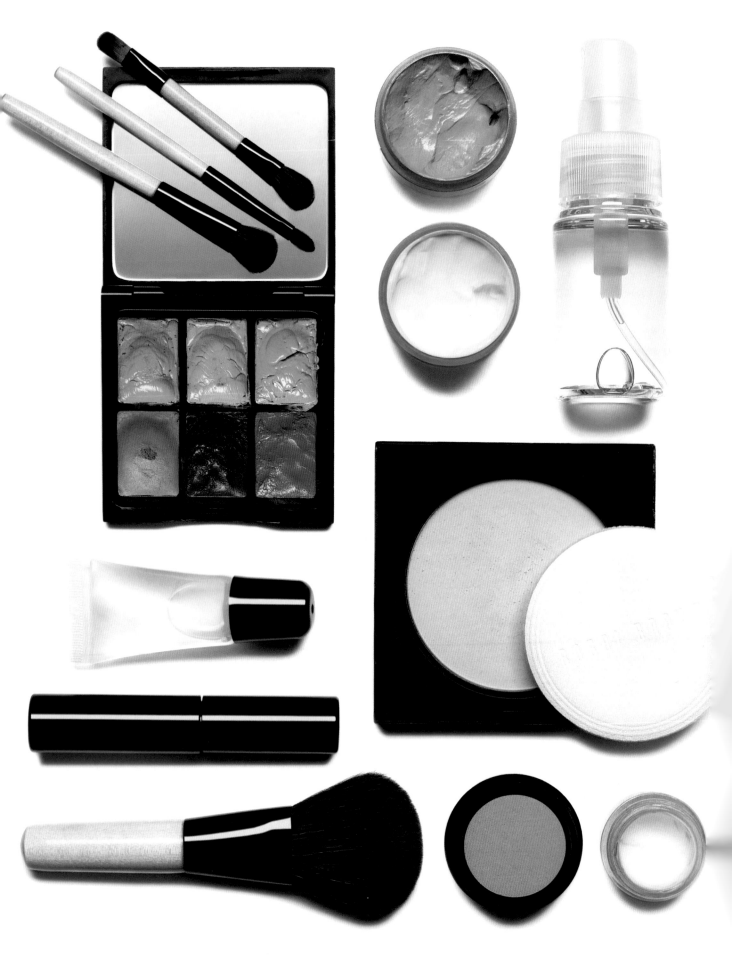

Chapter 2

EQUIPMENT

Being well organized is essential.

Whether you're a minimalist whose makeup kit rarely holds more than a lipstick and powder or a working makeup artist who routinely totes around a complete collection of cosmetics, it takes a plan.

MAKEUP KITS

Home Makeup

Organize your makeup either in your bathroom drawer, on top of the counter, or in a box. Keep basics and items used only occasionally separate. At least twice a year make sure your colors and formulas are working. Basics include:

Concealers and correctors

Foundation or tinted moisturizer

Powder (two colors)

Eye shadow (three to four basic colors)

Eyeliner (powder and gel)

Mascara

Blush (powder or cream)

Lipstick, gloss, lip pencil

Everyday Bag

Pack the following essentials in a small bag:

One or two palettes that contain your foundation, concealer, blush, and lip color

A compact of pressed powder with a mirror

A basic eye palette— the smaller the better

Mini mascara

Lip gloss

Mini brushes

Small sample sizes of face cream

Evening Bag

Tiny purses don't lend themselves to toting around lots of products, so you need to be selective. Pack the following items:

Lipstick or gloss

Lip pencil

A powder compact

Customizable face palette (containing concealer, foundation, blush)

Mini perfume

Breath mints

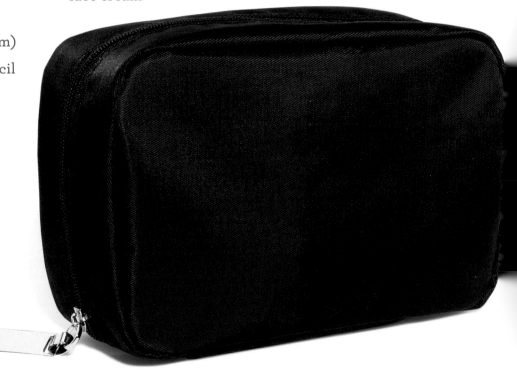

In Your Desk Drawer

It's worth investing in duplicates of your makeup to keep in your office to freshen up before a big meeting or for reapplying if you need to go straight out after work. These basics include the following items:

Concealer

Foundation

Pressed powder
(with mirror)

Blush

Lip balm, lip color,
and/or gloss

Black eyeliner and white or silver eye shadow to create an evening eye

Mini brushes

Travel toothbrush and toothpaste set

In Your Gym Bag

After a workout, you will want to clean your face and start your makeup from scratch. So be sure to bring the following items to the gym:

Face-cleansing cloths

Moisturizer

Customized face palette, or at least a tinted moisturizer, lip color or gloss, and mascara

For Travel

Keep your travel kit packed at all times so you never have to worry about arriving somewhere only to realize you've left something important in your bathroom cabinet. Invest in several small plastic bottles, label them, and fill them with your essentials. Purchase mini brushes, mascara, and a small eye palette. Include the following items:

Travel-size shampoo and conditioner

Body and facial moisturizers

Makeup palettes with all your basics

Mini mascara

Face powder, bronzer
(great for the travel weary)

Self-tanner

Lipstick or gloss

A brush roll of travel-size brushes

Tweezers

Hairbrush and hair spray

Perfume in a mini or compact version

Perfumed body creams are also great

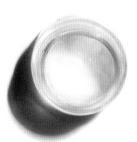

Tip

Collect deluxe samples from makeup counters — they are perfect for travel.

ESSENTIAL TOOLS

Brushes make all the difference in makeup application. Everyone from the most skilled makeup artist to the woman who wears only the basics can benefit from using the right tools. Consider investing in at least a few key brushes. High-quality blush, eye shadow, eyebrow, and eyeliner brushes are basic. Good brushes are not hard to find. Look at those made by makeup artists' lines as well as less expensive versions available at beauty and art supply stores. To find out which brushes you need and which ones are good quality, familiarize yourself with a variety of styles, shapes, and bristle types.

Assessing Brush Quality

Before purchasing brushes, you have to know what you are looking for and which brushes are worthwhile investments. Assess the quality of a brush by testing the way the bristles feel against the skin and by running your fingers through the bristles to make sure that they don't shed. It's important to test how a brush feels when you hold it in your hand. It needs to feel comfortable and easy to maneuver.

Tips

Brush Size
The brushes that come with most makeup compacts are too small and narrow for proper blush application. Toss them and use a brush designed specifically for that purpose instead.

Natural Bristles
Natural bristles (such as squirrel, goat, pony, or sable) are very soft and offer a more blended, natural application. They're best for working with powder-based products—blush, powder, and eye shadow.

Synthetic Bristles
Synthetic bristles are the best choice for brushes that will be used with creamy products, such as concealer, gel liners, and lip colors. They are generally stiffer than natural hair, so they give you greater control and a more precise application.

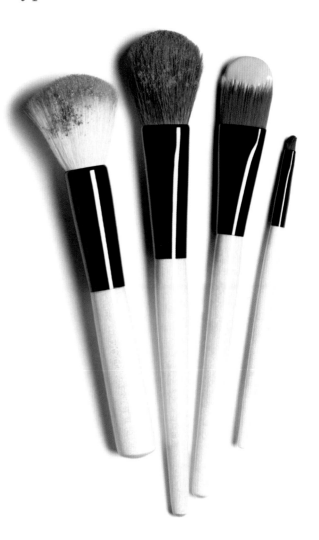

Tool Guide

This alphabetized glossary describes the different types of brushes as well as other tools you might want to keep in your kit. It will help you decide what brushes work best for a specific need or technique.

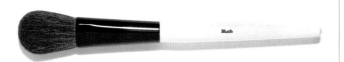

BLUSH BRUSH

This needs to be wide enough to cover the apple of the cheek. The bristles should be soft, natural hair with beveled and curved edges.

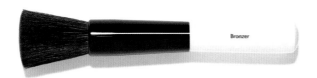

BRONZER BRUSH

This is thicker and fuller than a blush brush and has a flat profile. It is designed for sweeping and pressing bronzer over cheeks, forehead, nose, and chin to provide natural-looking warmth to the skin.

BROW BRUSH

A brush with stiff, short bristles cut on an angle. Designed for applying shadow to the brows. Look for a synthetic/natural blend of bristles, as the 100 percent synthetic brushes are too stiff and don't deposit color as effectively.

BROW GROOMING BRUSH

This is for brushing brows into place. It has stiff bristles cut straight across, like a toothbrush.

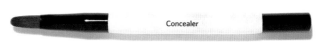

CONCEALER BRUSH

This should have firm but soft bristles that aren't too hard or scratchy, since the brush will be used on the delicate skin under the eyes. Look for a brush with glossy synthetic hairs, as these slip along the skin. The ends of the bristles should be tapered to help you place concealer in hard-to-reach spots, such as the inner corners of the eyes, and apply stick foundation to cover any redness around the nose.

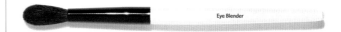

EYE BLENDER BRUSH

A soft, fluffy, natural-hair brush with long bristles designed to blend eye shadow and eliminate lines of demarcation on the lids after applying multiple shades. It is also great for applying powder to set corrector, concealer, or foundation around the eyes or over blemish cover.

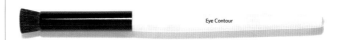

EYE CONTOUR BRUSH

A round, flat-head, natural-hair brush. Short, dense bristles apply a greater amount of shadow in the crease to contour the eye.

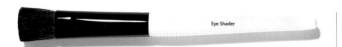

EYE SHADER BRUSH

A wide, flat-head brush that can gently sweep eye shadow color over the entire lid, from the lash line to the brow bone.

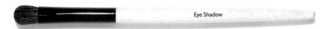

EYE SHADOW BRUSH

Wide enough to cover about half the eyelid. This brush has natural, soft, rounded bristles with beveled edges that deposit a sweep of shadow across the lower lid without leaving any harsh lines.

EYE SMUDGE BRUSH

A small-head brush with a slightly rounded point. This brush has soft, flexible bristles that help smudge liner to create a smoky look.

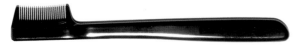

EYELASH COMB

This has straight, stiff (often plastic), fine teeth and is designed to separate lashes immediately after applying mascara (while the lashes are still wet). Mascara wands work just as well and are more convenient.

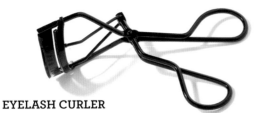

EYELASH CURLER

Look for a basic metal version with rubber pads. An eyelash curler shapes lashes into a natural-looking curl. Replace pads regularly. To avoid breakage, always curl the lashes before applying mascara.

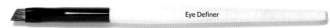

EYELINER BRUSH (ANGLED)/EYE DEFINER BRUSH

This small brush has very short, dense bristles cut on an angle. It is designed to use with shadow to strengthen thin brows or as an alternative to an eyeliner brush.

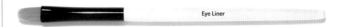

EYELINER BRUSH (FLAT)

With flat, dense, synthetic bristles that are slightly rounded at tip, this brush can be used wet or dry to apply a precise line at the lash line.

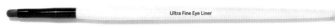

EYELINER BRUSH (ULTRA FINE)

The bristles on this small brush are synthetic, dense, and curve to a point. Perfect for the precise application of liquid or gel eyeliner.

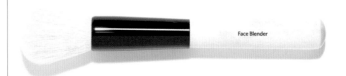

FACE BLENDER BRUSH

A natural or synthetic brush used to deposit shimmer, bronzer, powder, or blush.

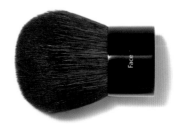

FACE BRUSH

A natural or synthetic fluffy, curved brush that can be used to apply bronzer, blush, or powder.

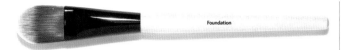

FOUNDATION BRUSH

Synthetic bristles in this full, flat-edged brush deposit just the right amount of foundation onto the skin.

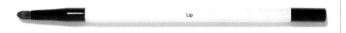

LIP BRUSH

Firm, long bristles come to a slightly pointed tip. This brush allows for the precise placement of lip color. Bristles can be either synthetic or natural.

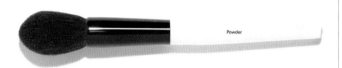

POWDER BRUSH

A natural-hair, large, fluffy brush with soft bristles that bevel to a slight point (for navigating around the nose and under the eyes). Designed for use with both loose and pressed powders.

Tip

Using Your Fingers

Nothing beats the warmth of the fingers to blend makeup into the skin. Lipstick can be blotted onto the lips to create a stain effect. Face cream, balm, or oil rubbed between both palms and then gently pressed onto cheeks adds moisture and a youthful glow to the face. I use my hands to warm concealers, blend foundation, and mix lip shades together. I also use my hands to work makeup into the face so that the makeup feels like a part of the skin and not like a mask.

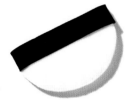

POWDER PUFF

A velour puff that's about the size of your palm. Designed to press powder onto the face to lock foundation in place. Can be hand washed or tossed in the dishwasher (at least once a week).

SPONGES

Disposable sponges are invaluable. Wedge-shaped ones are great for applying foundation around the nose and other hard-to-reach places, as well as for blending. Don't bother washing them—toss dirty ones, and take a new one. Higher-quality sponges can be washed and reused many times.

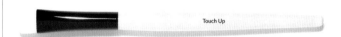

TOUCH UP BRUSH

Short, firm, natural-bristled brush used with foundation for spot touch-ups and for hard-to-reach areas around the nose and mouth. This brush can also be used to touch up concealer and apply eye shadow.

TWEEZERS

It's well worth investing in a good pair. Look at the Tweezerman or Rubis brands. Tweezers that are angled at the tip are easier to control than those that come to a sharp point. Always cover tweezers' tips with the included rubber cap when they are not in use.

SHOPPING FOR SUPPLIES

Whether you are starting your first professional makeup kit, replacing a few personal items, or looking for something new, shopping is a time to experiment, test cosmetics, and research trends. One of the best and easiest ways to stay current is to test the latest products on the cosmetics floor of any large department store. The makeup artist at the counter will show you new items and techniques. You can try the cosmetics and get information, all without any cost. Magazines and the Internet are great for research and information, but when you are ready for a purchase, it is important to touch and feel the products so you know the quality you are getting.

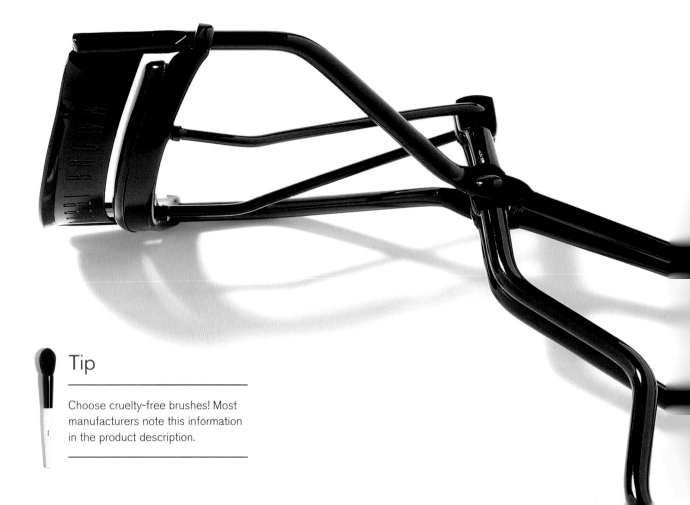

Tip

Choose cruelty-free brushes! Most manufacturers note this information in the product description.

It is a good idea to develop some shopping strategies to avoid frustration, intimidation, or impulse-buying. First, determine your budget. Makeup can be expensive. Estimate the cost of your supply needs, and add a realistic amount for trying new products. Making an inventory list of all the supplies in your makeup kit is very helpful. Use this as a shopping list, and just circle the needed items. If you want to replace something specific, you can take the container with you to the store. In a notebook, keep a page for jotting down any new products you might want to test. This is also a place to record product ingredients for comparison shopping. For the best service, shop when the stores are least crowded, generally in the mornings, early in the week. Let the makeup artist at the counter show you a new look or technique. Listen and ask questions. Be clear about your likes and dislikes. Ask for samples or trial-size containers of any products you like. Purchase a product only if you love the way the makeup looks and know that you will use it.

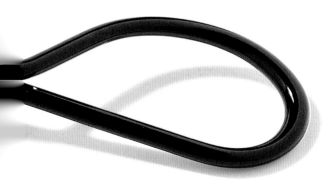

Sources

You will want to find several places to purchase makeup supplies that suit your needs and preferences. For testing and experimentation, store visits are very useful. Once you are familiar with a product line, it is faster and easier to do your shopping online. Most of the retailers and designers now have Web sites for quick and convenient shopping.

Department Stores

High-end brands are typically sold through dedicated counter areas in department stores. Most of the counter personnel are trained in makeup application and are able to provide information and advice. You can test the makeup before purchasing so you know exactly what you're getting. Some sales staff are paid on commission, so you may be pressured to make a purchase.

Drugstores and Pharmacies

These stores are convenient and carry a wide variety of mass-market products. Purchase basic supplies such as nail polish, cotton balls, makeup sponges, and cotton swabs at these retailers. Very few of the products can be tested before buying, so purchases might not meet your expectations.

Beauty Supply Shops

Makeup artists depend on these industry meccas for professional-quality products at budget-friendly prices. You will receive personalized attention and won't be rushed or pressured to make a purchase, because the sales clerks are not paid on commission. These stores will usually ship anywhere in the country.

Beauty Superstores

One-stop shops, such as Sephora and Ulta, offer a wide range of mass-market, prestige, and niche products. The staff is knowledgeable and willing to answer questions.

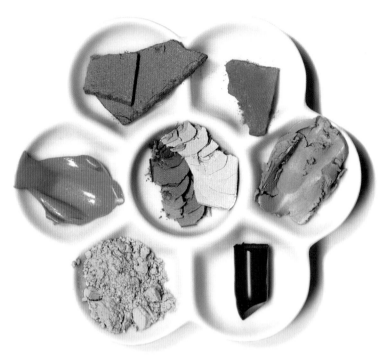

Purchasing Dos & Don'ts

Do buy multipurpose makeup, such as lip-cheek combinations.

Do shop in daylight for foundation.

Don't equate "dermatologist tested" with better quality. The claim does not guarantee that the doctor approved of the product—just that it was tested.

Do save your receipts. Many stores will refund your money within a specified period of time if you are not satisfied with a product. If any cream-based makeup smells or has an odd texture, take it back. It is probably old.

Don't toss leftovers unless the makeup is more than eighteen months old. When that lipstick or cream blush gets near the end, scoop the remainder into small, covered, compartmentalized boxes (palettes) that are available at art and beauty supply stores. Label the back of the palette with the color name for reference when you need to restock.

Specialty Stores

These freestanding stores offer a wide selection of products, often "indie" brands. This is a good place to find trend-driven shades, foundations, and concealers.

Catalogs

Shopping from catalogs specific to a brand is a convenient way to stock up on favorite shades of cosmetics. Once you are familiar with a product, this is a fast and easy way to order replacements, get a quick overview of new products, and see the latest fashion colors.

Discontinued?!?

Has your signature fragrance or favorite lipstick disappeared from the market? This happens for any number of reasons. It is possible that the product was not selling well, or it has been reformulated to meet new standards. Discontinued beauty products are available if you know where to look. Use the Internet to do your research. Visit the company's Web site first. There will generally be information available on discontinued products. Estée Lauder, for example, publishes item closings in advance on their Web site so that consumers can stock up. Specialty Web sites, outlets, and online auctions often carry these cosmetics and fragrances. Do be aware of expiration dates, however. Cosmetics have a limited shelf life and should not be used after the expiration dates posted by the manufacturer.

Finally, if you just can't locate your old favorite, make a plea. Either e-mail or write a personal letter asking the company to bring it back. Companies listen closely to their customers, and it is not unusual for specific colors or products to be resurrected thanks to consumer demand. At the very least, you will get a response from the company, usually providing reasons for the closing and often samples of similar products for you to try.

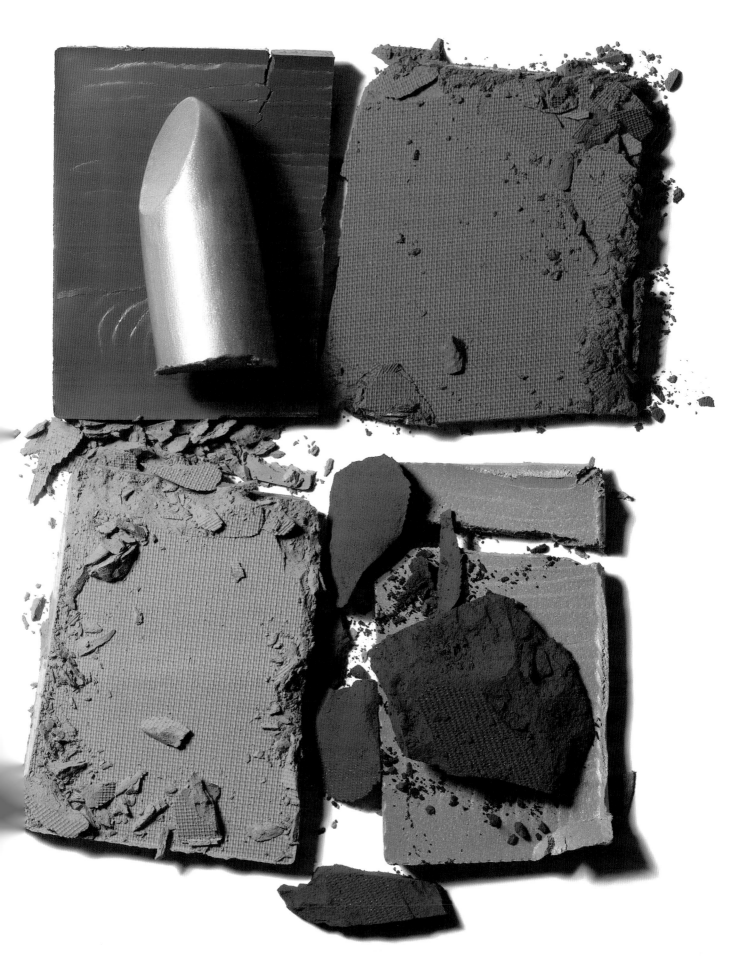

CARE & MAINTENANCE OF TOOLS & MAKEUP

Your makeup is only as good as the tools you use to apply it. Therefore, your tools must always be in their best working condition. That means clean brushes, puffs, and sponges; sharpened tweezers; makeup containers that are in perfect shape; and makeup that's not too old to use safely.

Brush Care

A good set of brushes will last several years if it is well cared for. This involves storing the brushes properly (either in a neat brush roll that has individual slots for each brush or upright in a pencil cup) and keeping them clean. To clean brushes, take a drop of brush cleaner or very gentle soap in your palm, wet the brush, and swirl the bristles around on your palm until they are covered in soap. (I love using baby shampoo.) Rinse thoroughly until all soap residue is gone. Do not immerse the brush head in water, because the hair is glued to the base, and even the most expensive brushes will come apart. Squeeze out excess moisture with a clean towel, reshape the brush head, and let it dry with the bristles hanging off the edge of a counter so the bristles dry into the perfect shape. Brushes can become mildewed if they rest on a towel while drying.

Clean all your brushes every month or two. For a quick cleaning in between washings, use a spray brush cleaner. Spritz it onto the bristles, and swipe them back and forth on a tissue until all product residues are removed from the brush.

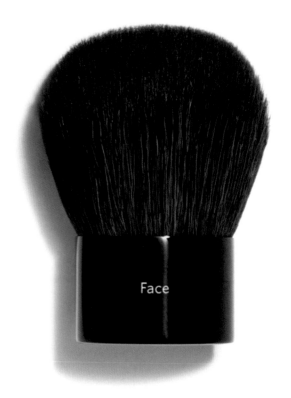

Face

Tip

Clean the sides of messy compacts with a cotton swab to keep them looking fresh.

Sponge Care

High-quality sponges can be washed many times before they need to be discarded. Alternatively, you can buy disposable synthetic sponge wedges at the drugstore that work well and are inexpensive. You can wash and reuse them only a few times before you throw them out.

Powder Puff Care

While drugstores sell disposable powder puffs, it's worth investing in a better-quality one. Hand wash the puff using the same liquid soap you use for your brushes, or toss it into your next load of laundry or on the top rack of the dishwasher.

Tweezer Care

When tweezers get dull—which happens with repeated use—they are no longer as effective at grabbing on to and removing small hairs. You can take them to a knife shop for sharpening. Some of the better brands, such as Tweezerman, come with a lifetime guarantee that includes free sharpening whenever necessary.

Eyelash Curler Care

The rubber pads that line the inside of an eyelash curler are there to protect the lashes, so when the pads start to wear out or break apart, they must be replaced. Many eyelash curlers come with a set of replacement pads. Keep a set on hand.

Makeup Care

Examine the contents of your makeup bag, drawer, or cabinet. Take out anything that's in a broken container or missing a cap. You can pour liquid foundation into a fresh bottle, scoop out creams and lipsticks and transfer them to small containers or palettes, and place capless pencils in zip-top plastic bags. Broken powder blushes and pressed powder compacts are irreparable and should be tossed. Weekly maintenance is far easier than semiannual overhauls.

You also need to get rid of any makeup that's past its expiration date:

Liquid and cream foundation	2 years
Concealer	2 years
Powder	2 years
Mascara	6 months
Lipstick	12 to 18 months
Lip and eye pencils	12 to 18 months
Eye shadow	2 years
Powder blush	2 years
Cream blush	2 years
Moisturizer	2 years
Eye cream	6 months
Sunscreen	2 years
Face cream	2 years

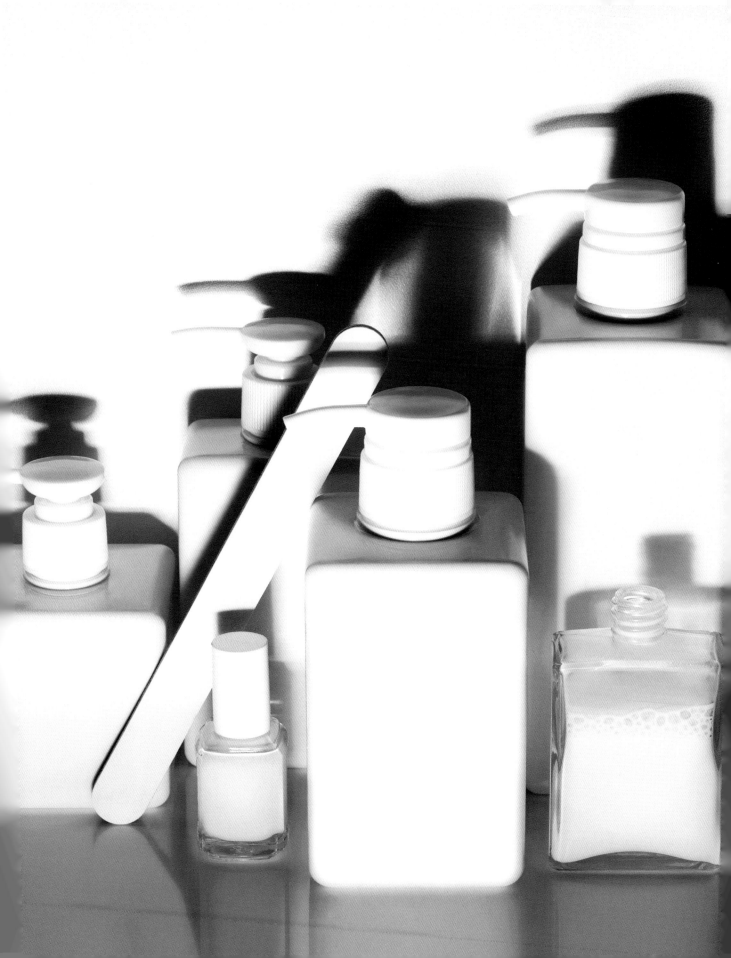

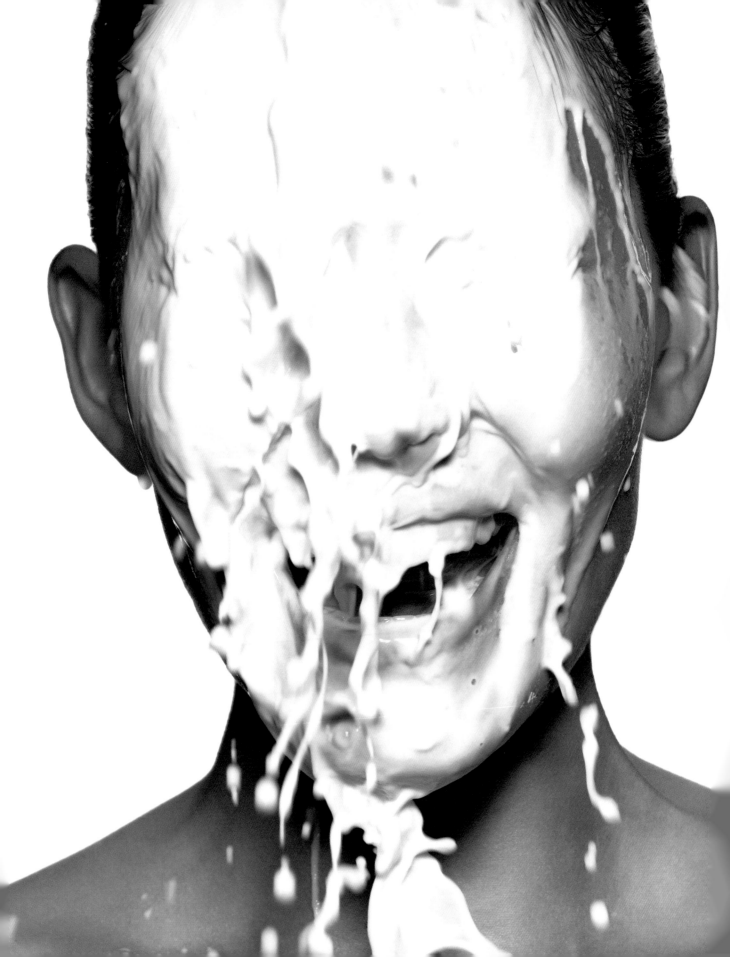

Chapter 3

SKIN

Beauty starts with smooth, healthy, glowing skin.

Anyone can learn to become a skincare expert by:

Understanding how **lifestyle** impacts the condition of the skin,

Knowing **how skin works,**

Learning the basics of skincare, including

How to **analyze** skin conditions,

How to **identify** skin types,

How to properly **care for skin,**

Knowing skincare **ingredients** and how they work
in order to select and use the appropriate products.

LIFESTYLE

Beautiful skin begins with a healthy lifestyle. While heredity may determine how your skin looks, behaves, and ages, you can improve it by taking good care of yourself. Skincare basics include eating the right foods, drinking plenty of water, exercising, getting enough sleep, protecting your skin from the sun, not smoking, and limiting your intake of both caffeine and alcohol.

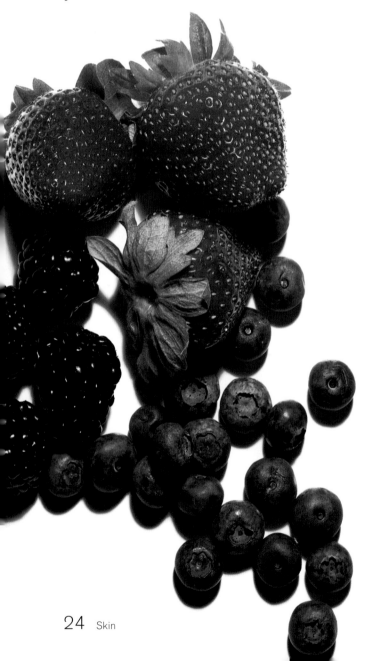

Nutrition

The health of your skin begins with good nutrition. New, living cells continually replace the dead cells on the surface of the skin. The growth of new cells is dependent on vitamins, minerals, and hydration.

Eat at least five servings of fresh fruits and vegetables each day. Remember to look for the "ACE" vitamins: A to help prevent aging, C to promote clarity, and E to protect against the environment. Vitamins A and C are most important for healthy skin and are plentiful in fruits and vegetables. Vitamin A is found in carrots, spinach, watercress, broccoli, sweet potatoes, and melons. Peppers, strawberries, oranges, grapefruit, and leafy greens all contain vitamin C. Also include whole-grain foods, nuts, dairy, fish, and beans in your diet. They are all foods rich in zinc, which promotes healing and reduces inflammation in the body.

Biotin is another nutrient needed for healthy skin, hair, and nails. It is sometimes identified as vitamin H and is part of the vitamin B complex. Foods such as peanut butter, whole grains, eggs, and liver contain biotin and can help prevent dermatitis and hair loss.

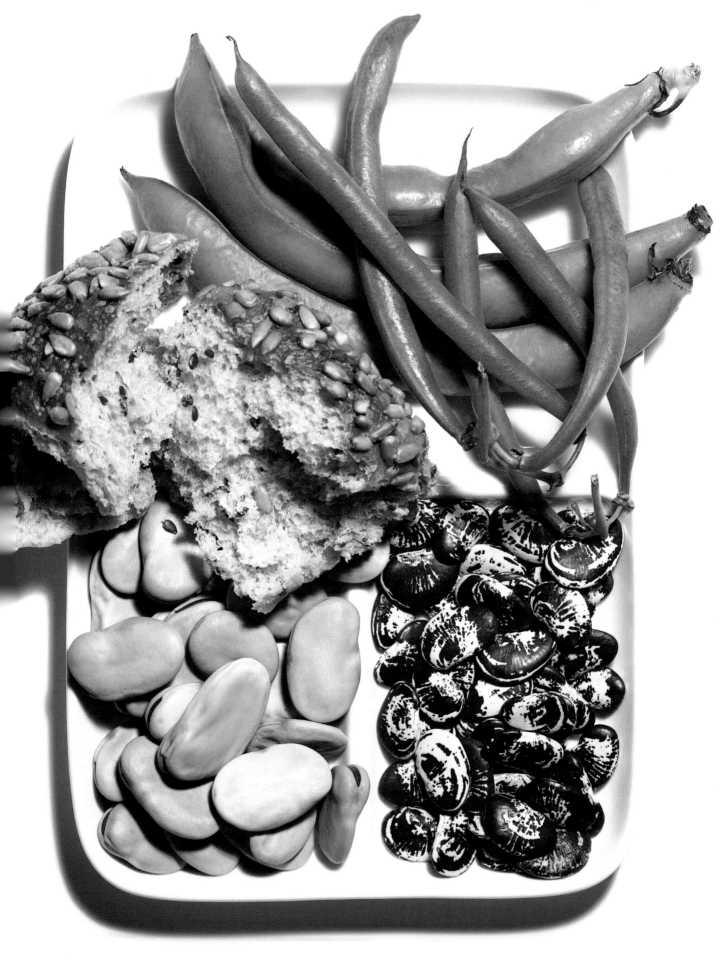

There are many advantages to taking your vitamins in food rather than in pill form. When you eat, you are never getting single, isolated nutrients. For instance, a bowl of leafy greens provides an abundance of several important vitamins, such as B, K, and E, as well as fiber and antioxidants. The fresh fruits, vegetables, and whole grains that provide fiber also naturally deliver vitamins and minerals and are low in calories. It is virtually impossible to consume dangerous levels of any vitamins or minerals through diet alone.

Your diet has a direct impact on not only your overall health and how you feel but also on how you look. Certain nutrients in particular are important for maintaining healthy skin, hair, and nails. Think of them as your beauty vitamins.

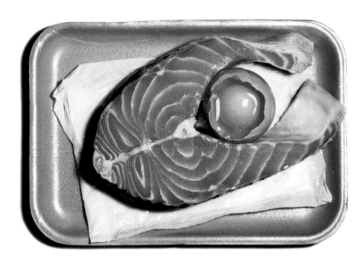

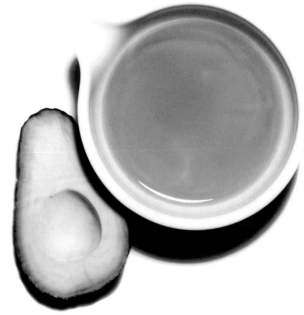

VITAMIN A

Antioxidant essential for the **growth and renewal of new skin cells. Topically applied, may boost collagen production and promote skin cell turnover.**

Egg yolks, dairy

VITAMIN B

Increases fatty acids in the skin, **promoting exfoliation and firmness.**

Yeast, eggs, liver, vegetables

VITAMIN C

Building block of collagen, the protein that gives skin its **structure, tone, and elasticity.**

Citrus fruits, broccoli, peppers, berries, tomatoes

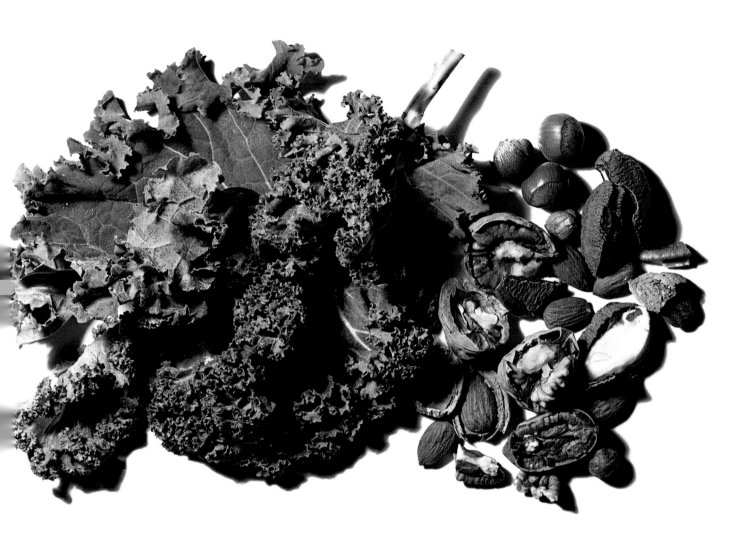

VITAMIN D

Essential for the **development of skin cells.**

Egg yolks, salmon, fortified milk, and other dairy products

VITAMIN E

Antioxidant that helps build and **maintain healthy skin tissue.**

Wheat germ, leafy greens, nuts, whole grains

FAT

Fat is also an important nutrient for the skin and the health of the whole body. **It is necessary for supple skin and soft, shiny hair.**

Incorporate unsaturated fats, such as the monounsaturated fats found in olive oil and avocado, with omega-3 fats, found in fatty fish and some seeds, into your daily diet.

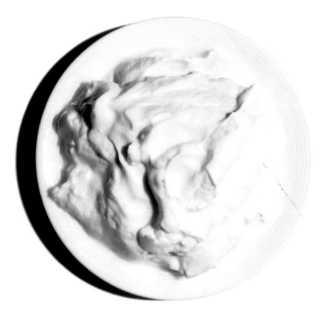

Keep these healthy foods on hand
for satisfying between-meal snacking:

Almonds

Plain, low-fat yogurt

String cheese

Chocolate protein powder

Protein bars

**Low-fat ricotta cheese
with a dash of vanilla**

Hard-boiled eggs

**Water with a bit of unsweetened
cranberry extract or lemon juice**

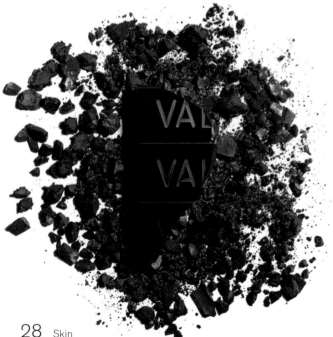

Our bodies are 80 percent water. Without sufficient hydration, the skin cells become dry and flaky. To keep the body, including the skin, hydrated, eat foods with a high water content, such as fruits, vegetables, and clear soups, and drink at least eight glasses of water a day. It is important to limit your intake of coffee and other drinks containing caffeine, as they are diuretics that remove water from the body and block the absorption of vitamins and minerals.

Exercise

Exercise is a skincare essential. Raising the heart rate through vigorous exercise increases blood flow, brings more oxygen to the skin, and cleanses impurities from the body through sweat. Just twenty to thirty minutes of exercise a day is enough to help boost your immune system, reduce stress, lower blood pressure, strengthen your heart, build stronger bones, increase your energy level, and improve your mood. Ideally, you want to do a mix of aerobic exercise and strength training. Aerobic exercise helps get the blood flowing, so take a walk, run, or swim regularly. With regular exercise, you build lean muscle mass and raise your metabolism. Since the metabolism slows with age, exercise is fundamental to weight management.

Sleep

Sleep is the time when the body's cells have a chance to repair and regenerate. Sleep deprivation stresses all of the body's systems, including the skin, and can result in headaches, irritability, lack of energy, or the inability to focus. The skin becomes less elastic and prone to outbreaks of acne or rashes.

Tip

Smile, be positive, breathe, and take a vacation once in a while.

Sun

Excess sun exposure is skin's number-one enemy. It causes premature aging, including wrinkles, loss of elasticity, and hyperpigmentation. Worse, over-exposure often causes deadly forms of skin cancer. Wear a broad-spectrum sunscreen with a sun protection factor (SPF) of at least 15 in the winter and 30 in the summer.

Smoking

Smoking also causes the skin to age prematurely. Nicotine impairs the blood vessels that provide skin with both oxygen and nutrients and rid the skin of impurities. It eventually robs the skin of oxygen, causing it to look dull and gray. With low levels of oxygen, the skin loses elasticity, which leads to sagging and wrinkling.

Alcohol

Skin problems can be caused by excessive alcohol intake. Alcohol can cause allergic reactions, such as hives and rashes. Some people have allergic reactions to salicylates, which occur in such foods as berries, bananas, beans, grapes, and wine. If a rash appears after you eat these foods, it is likely that beer and wine will also cause outbreaks.

Stress

Stress often shows up on the skin. Stress-related hormonal fluctuations can cause adult acne and other skin problems. While healthy eating and exercise habits help to combat the symptoms of anxiety and stress, finding mechanisms to deal with the underlying causes of stress is important.

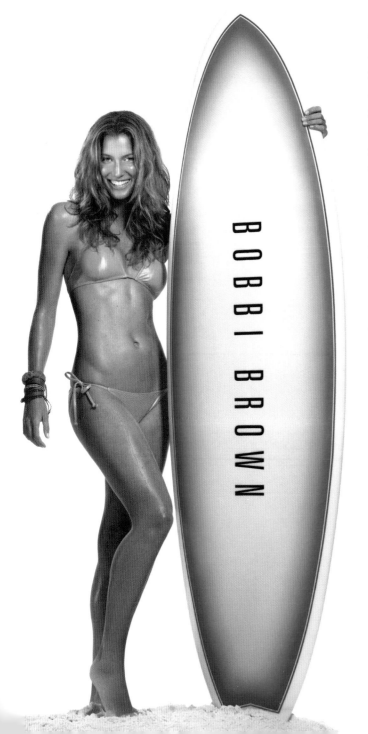

Tips

Drinking eight to ten glasses of water a day will help flush out toxins and keep all skin types clear.

Drink one glass of water each time you have a beverage that contains alcohol or caffeine.

SKINCARE BASICS

Few people have naturally perfect skin. With some knowledge, experience, good diet, and exercise, it is possible to greatly improve the appearance of the skin. The condition of the skin changes from day to day and season to season. Hormonal fluctuations, stress, pregnancy, medication, travel, and seasonal changes are only a few of the factors that can cause skin to act up. If you learn to recognize the various skin conditions, you will be able to choose the right cleansing options and moisturizers.

How the Skin Works

The skin is composed of three layers: a deep layer called the hypodermis, a middle layer called the dermis, and a surface layer called the epidermis. The epidermis gives immediate, visual clues to the condition and health of the skin, while the dermis determines how the skin responds and changes with age. The hypodermis, the deepest layer, contains a layer of fat, blood vessels, and nerves.

Skin's middle layer, the dermis, is composed mostly of collagen and elastin, which are proteins that give skin structure, strength, and flexibility. As we age, collagen and elastin production diminishes. The results show up on the face as a loss of firmness, rougher texture, more obvious wrinkles, and sagging.

Hair follicles, nerves, blood vessels, and sebaceous glands are also part of the dermis. Sebaceous glands produce sebum. This oily substance moves through the hair shaft to the top layer of the skin, where it covers the epidermis and provides a protective barrier against moisture loss. Too much sebum results in oily skin.

The outermost layer of skin, the epidermis, is several layers deep. Basal cells are created in the lowest layer and then migrate through a hardened layer to the stratum corneum, from which they fall off the body. The skin continually sloughs off the dead cells and grows new living cells. It takes about a month for a live basal cell to move to the top layer of the epidermis. As the cell moves toward the surface of the skin, it loses moisture and oxygen content.

On the surface of the epidermis is a layer of oil transported from the dermis by the hair follicles that forms a natural barrier, helping the skin to retain water. Harsh and scented cleansing products, exposure to chemical and biological pollution in the environment, and poor diet can remove this protective oil-based layer from the skin. This layer can be replenished with moisturizer.

Moisturizers work in several ways. First, they fill in the spaces between the relatively dry, or cornified, cells of the epidermis, making the skin feel and appear smoother. They also create a barrier on the skin, helping the skin retain water. The oil content in moisturizers works with the protective lipid coating of the skin to partially protect the skin from the air. Care must be taken in the selection and use of moisturizing products, as they make a huge difference in how the skin works. Hydration is the key to smooth, even skin, and moisturization is the external way to achieve it.

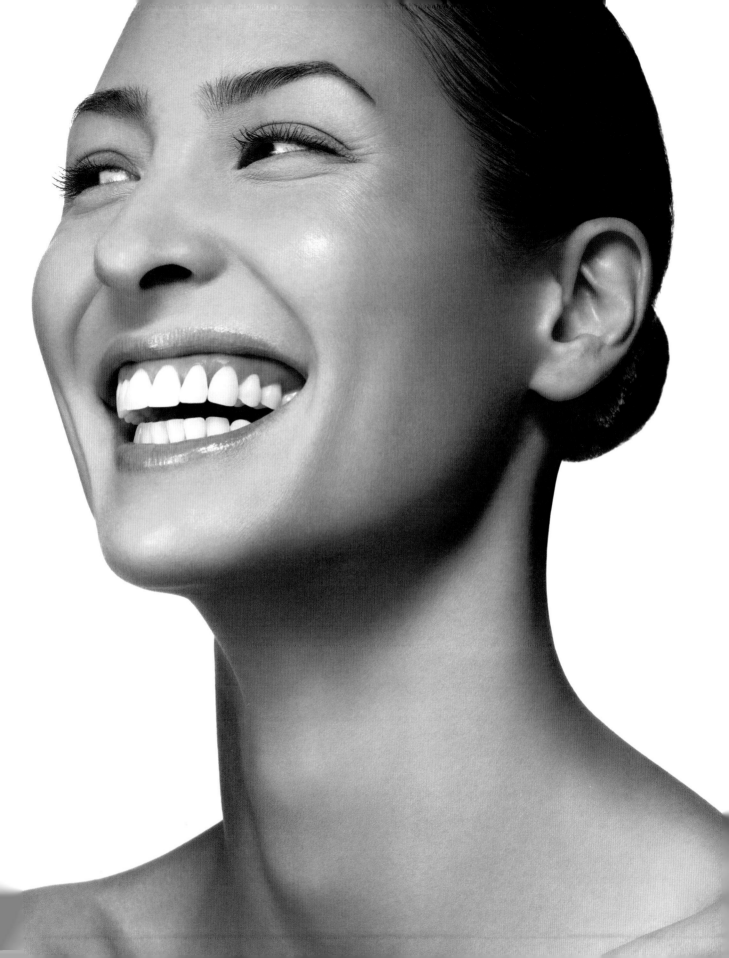

ANALYSIS OF THE SKIN

The following descriptions will help you recognize skin conditions and make decisions about skincare products.

Normal

Analysis

Comfortable-feeling

Smooth, even texture with small pores

Cheeks are the driest area, but not excessively so

May experience some shine and larger pores on the forehead, nose, or chin

Water and oil content in this skin is balanced

Care

Normal skin needs routine cleansing with a foaming cleanser, exfoliation twice a week, moisturization with lightweight lotions, and the use of a sunscreen to keep it healthy. A diet rich in vitamins A, C, and E helps keep skin smooth and soft. Sufficient fluid intake is important to maintain hydration and rid the body of toxins.

Dry/Extra Dry

Analysis

Feels tight after washing

May look dry or flaky

Feels rough and uneven; dehydrated

May be sensitive

Pores are small—almost invisible

Shows fine lines faster than other skin types

Care

Dry skin requires special care. A lifestyle that includes a healthy diet with foods high in water content, such as fruits and vegetables, and at least eight glasses of water a day keeps this skin type hydrated. Caffeine and alcohol cause dehydration, so limit intake to two cups or glasses a day. Using richer cleansers, limiting sun exposure, and using a good moisturizer can protect your skin's natural oils. Layering different textures of moisturizer can do wonders to hydrate the skin. Begin with lightweight face oil, and then layer a richer cream over that. Night creams with alpha hydroxy acids (AHA) help remove the dry, dead skin while moisturizing the new. Air-conditioning and heating create dry environments. Correct this in your home by using humidifiers.

Self-Test: Skin Analysis

Look at your own clean, unmoisturized skin in the mirror. Is the overall texture flaky (dry), shiny (oily), or smooth (normal)?

How does your skin feel after you wash it with your current cleansing regimen? Tightness through the forehead is an indication of dry skin.

How does your skin normally look by midday? Is there oil breakthrough or dryness even though you have moisturized?

What lifestyle factors are influencing your skin's current condition: stress? hormonal fluctuations? sun exposure? diet?

Does your skin have noticeable sun damage? How are you protecting yourself against the sun?

An accurate skin analysis will help you determine the most effective cleansing, hydration, and makeup products for your skin type and condition. However, when problem skin shows no improvement or worsens, see a dermatologist.

Oily Skin

Analysis

Oily skin is shiny, especially through the T-zone (the forehead, nose, and chin); it is a condition caused by overactive sebaceous, or oil-producing, glands.

May have large, visible pores

Frequent breakouts

Few signs of aging, such as fine lines

Care

Management of oily skin and the prevention of breakouts requires a healthy diet and a regular skincare routine. Cleanse the face at least twice a day to prevent dirt accumulation and to keep pores open. Use an alcohol-free astringent to remove excess oil. Use oil-free moisturizers to keep the skin from overdrying.

Combination Skin

Analysis

Oily through the T-zone

Dry cheeks or spot dehydration

Larger pores on the forehead, nose, and chin

Care

Care for this skin type requires regular cleansing, toning, and moisturizing of the oily areas and the use of a milder cleanser and denser moisturizer for the dry areas. Moisturizing products containing AHA will benefit this skin type.

Sensitive Skin

Analysis

Can range from dry to oily

Easily irritated by cosmetics, moisturizers, and cleansers

Sensitive and prone to redness

Itchy or blotchy

Care

Sensitive skin requires mild, nonperfumed cleansing products. Use an alcohol-free toner formulated for sensitive skin. Also, use cleansers and moisturizers specifically formulated for this type of skin.

Misleading Skin Conditions

Don't be fooled. The skin's condition can be quickly impacted by changes in environment, health, diet, and even current product choices for cleansing, toning, moisturizing, or makeup. There are many skin conditions that can hide your actual skin type. Redness, dryness, or flaking can be caused by a medical condition or medication. Skincare products can be overused, causing oily skin to become dry or flaky. Dry skin that is overmoisturized can appear greasy. Redness and irritation can be caused by low-grade allergies to cleansing, moisturizing, or makeup products, necessitating a change to gentler products.

CLEANSING & TONING THE FACE

Cleansers

The purpose of cleansing is to remove bacteria, makeup, and the dirt, sweat, and oil that build up on the skin each day. At *least* once a day, the skin needs to be cleaned with a formula that does not strip the skin of all its natural oils.

Makeup Remover Options

EYE MAKEUP REMOVERS remove eye makeup quickly and easily without harsh tugging or wiping. Look for oil-free, water-based formulas gentle enough for all skin types.

LONG-WEAR MAKEUP REMOVERS quickly and gently remove long-wearing and waterproof makeup. Look for products safe for contact lens wearers. These can generally be used for removal of lipstick and mascara or eyeliners.

CREAM CLEANSERS also work. See below.

Cleanser Options

Familiarity with these options will allow you to make the right choice based on your skin condition and type. Look for ingredients like wheat germ oil, which cleans without stripping, and glycerin, which attracts moisture to the skin's surface.

SOAP will deeply clean the skin and leave it feeling thoroughly cleansed and refreshed. Look for glycerin or cold cream soaps formulated specifically for the face. Glycerin creates a moisture cushion on the skin and a soft feel. Soap is best for oily skin types. Do not use body or bath soap, especially antibacterial soap. It will strip the skin and leave it feeling tight and dry.

GEL CLEANSERS typically foam or lather during use. These cleansers are formulated to dissolve oil buildup and fight blemish-causing bacteria without stripping the skin. They are best for oily or combination skin types that are prone to breakouts.

CREAM CLEANSERS are lightweight, water-based formulas that clean without leaving residue. These products contain oils and emollients along with cleansing ingredients and are recommended for normal to dry skin types.

OIL CLEANSERS work best on the driest of skins.

BALM CLEANSERS condition and moisturize the skin while cleansing. They leave a moisturizing cushion on the skin and are suitable for all skin types except oily.

EXFOLIATING CLEANSERS sometimes contain alpha hydroxy acids, such as glycolic or salicylic acid, and can be used several times a week to encourage cell turnover and dead skin removal. These products are gentle enough for all skin types. Some exfoliating cleansers contain beads or grains that loosen dead surface skin cells. These manual exfoliants should be used twice a week in place of the daily cleanser.

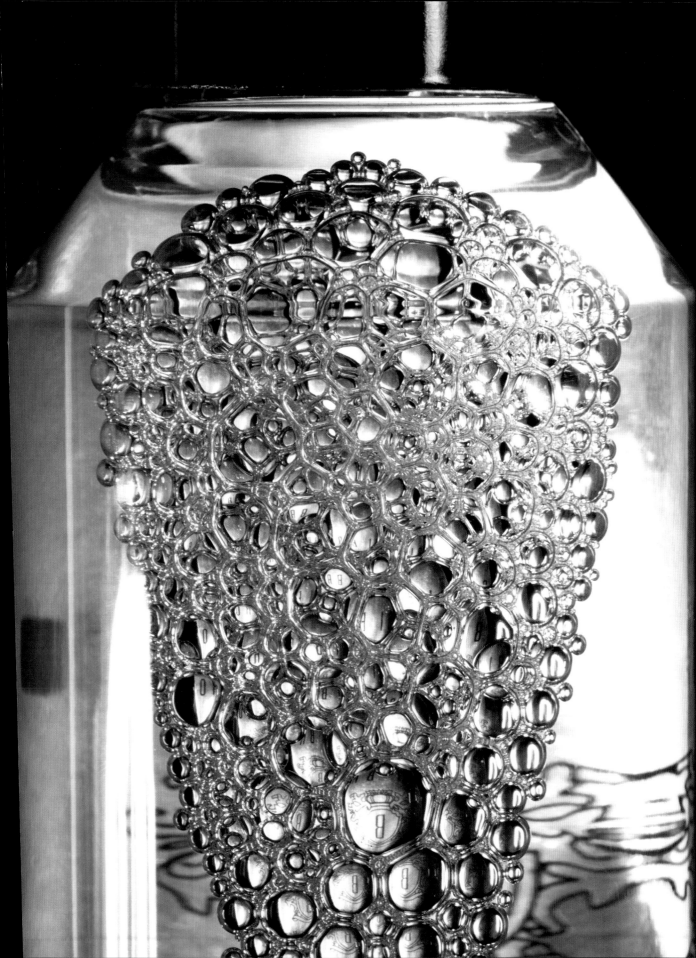

TREATMENT MASKS provide intensive supplements to the regular cleansing regimen. Oily and blemish-prone skin will benefit from the application of a clay mask, which helps to draw out impurities, reduce blackheads, and dry up excess oil. Dry skin, or any skin type that's been exposed to strong sun or wind, can be rejuvenated with a creamy hydrating mask. Masks containing cucumber, chamomile, aloe, or calendula are naturally soothing and good for irritated skin.

STEAMING THE SKIN helps remove impurities, stimulates circulation, and opens the pores. Herbs, such as lavender or thyme, added to a steam treatment stimulate the skin. Steaming can be helpful for all skin types.

MASSAGE stimulates circulation and helps to relax the facial muscles, giving the face a smooth and lifted look.

Toners

Toners stimulate circulation in the skin, remove any remaining dead skin cells or greasiness, and give the skin a smooth texture. Toners can be helpful for those who have very oily skin or who wear lots of makeup. Use a toner after cleaning the skin or as an interim cleaner to remove dirt and oil. During the summer, toners can be especially useful, as the skin is more oily and tends to attract more dirt and bacteria. Toners also help to restore the skin's natural pH balance.

While no cosmetic product can change the size of your pores, toners and astringents can make them appear smaller. These products work by very slightly irritating the skin, causing it to swell, making pores less noticeable.

To apply toner, pat the skin with a cotton ball soaked in the product of choice. You can also spray toner onto the face. Of course, cold water can just be splashed on the face instead.

Toner Options

Alcohol and water are the major ingredients in many skin fresheners, astringents, and toners. Other ingredients can include witch hazel, glycerin, rose water, vinegar, alum, boric acid, menthol, camphor, and other herbs. The major difference in the products is the amount of alcohol they contain. Alcohol strips the naturally occurring oils skin needs to be healthy, so look for a product without alcohol, especially if you have dry skin.

COLD TREATMENT with a splash of cold water is the best toner and can be used by those with any skin type. It closes the pores and improves the skin's texture.

SKIN FRESHENERS are very mild and contain water, such humectants as glycerin or rose water, and very little alcohol (less than 10 percent). Humectants help prevent the evaporation of moisture from the skin. These products are very gentle and are especially good for sensitive, dry, and normal skin.

SKIN TONICS are stronger, containing water, humectants, and up to 20 percent alcohol. Tonics are for normal, combination, or oily skin.

ASTRINGENTS contain water, humectants, up to 60 percent alcohol, and antiseptics. These are drying and only suitable for very oily skin or for application to specific problem areas. Witch hazel is an astringent.

Removing Makeup
& Cleansing the Skin

Secure hair off the face with a headband
or elastic.

**When wearing makeup, it is often necessary to
cleanse using a multistep process.** Start with a
makeup remover or tissue-off cream to dissolve
much of the makeup, avoiding the eye area.

The skin around the eyes is especially delicate
and can be easily irritated. There are makeup
removers specifically formulated for this area.
Take a cotton pad dampened with the product,
and rest or press it gently around the closed eye.
Wipe lightly. Do not tug or pull on the eye or
surrounding skin.

Apply cleanser to the entire face. With a
cleanser appropriate to your skin type, massage
the product into your skin with an upward circular
motion. Include the neck, under the ear lobes, and
the chin.

**Rinse the entire face, including the eye area,
with warm**—not hot—water.

Dry the face with the softest natural-fiber towels
you can find. Pat the face dry. Rubbing or hard
wiping creates small abrasions on the skin surface,
causing irritation, redness, and even swelling.

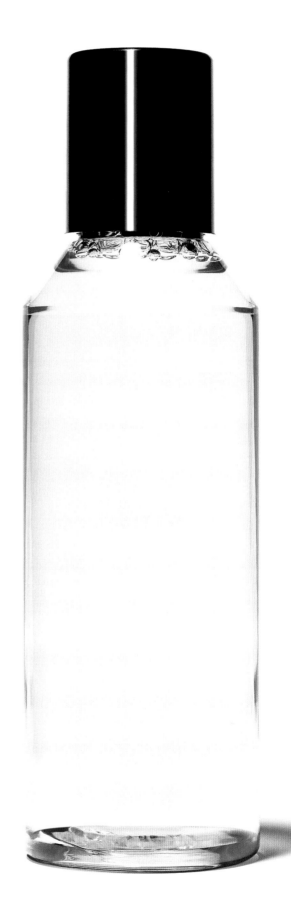

MOISTURIZERS & SUN PROTECTION

Hydration

The most important skincare step is ensuring hydration. Skin's tone and flexibility depends on the presence of water in the underlying tissues—water drawn from humidity in the air and moisture added to the skin's surface. Oil is the skin's natural protectant, preventing moisture from leaving the skin. Oil in the skin functions as a defensive barrier. It smoothes the texture and helps to maintain skin-cell health. When oil glands overproduce, the skin appears greasy, and when the glands underproduce, the skin becomes dehydrated and flaky. Adding moisture to the skin helps maintain skin firmness, smoothness, softness, and luminosity.

Facial Moisturizers

Moisturizer is the true fountain of youth. Moisturizers form a barrier between the skin and the environment that holds water in the epidermis. They hydrate and plump up the skin so that it looks smooth and bright. The right moisturizer will enhance the look, feel, and health of the skin and can even help temporarily eliminate fine lines and wrinkles. Moisturizers can also protect the skin from pollution, debris, and weather. The right skincare products help makeup go on smoothly, properly adhere to the skin, and last longer.

There are two types of facial moisturizers. Oil-in-water emulsions usually contain humectants, such as glycerin, which attract water. Added water from the environment is wonderful for the skin. The second category of moisturizer is the water-in-oil emulsion. These creams and lotions work by forming a water-trapping barrier on the skin surface. Look for the ingredient sodium hyaluronate, which locks in moisture and prevents it from leaving the skin. Humectants are often added to these products as well.

The major difference between moisturizing products is the ratio of water to oil. Even products labeled oil-free sometimes have small amounts of oil in them. You can sometimes find the ratio of water to oil on the label of a moisturizer.

PETROLEUM-BASED MOISTURIZERS are very effective at locking in moisture. They can, however, block pores and feel sticky.

VEGETABLE OILS are sometimes used as the base for moisturizers but in general are not as effective as mineral oils or animal fats.

INGREDIENTS SUCH AS VITAMIN E, COLLAGEN, PROTEINS, HORMONES, PLACENTAL EXTRACTS, AND AMINO ACIDS are sometimes added to moisturizing products.

VITAMIN A DERIVATIVES are added to anti-aging products.

CHEMICALLY ENHANCED products contain agents such as urea, glycolic acid, or lactic acid. They are formulated to improve the moisture-retaining ability of the moisturizer and are often recommended for dry skin.

FRAGRANCES are added to products to provide a pleasant aroma and to mask the odor of other ingredients.

All skin types benefit from the use of some type of moisturizer.

DRY SKIN needs a heavier, oil-based moisturizer that will absorb completely into the skin, leaving it feeling soft and supple. Oils are more effective than creams at preventing water evaporation. Look for the ingredients urea or propylene glycol, chemicals that keep skin moist.

NORMAL SKIN has a healthy moisture balance. Water-based moisturizers containing lightweight oils, such as acetyl alcohol, or silicone-derived ingredients, will help maintain healthy, normal skin.

OILY AND COMBINATION SKIN types benefit most from an oil-free, water-based moisturizer. Oil-free products are made from synthetic chemicals and contain little to no oils or animal fat. If you have oily skin, use all moisturizers sparingly. Look for products labeled "noncomedogenic," which means they are formulated to prevent clogged pores. Test moisturizers to find one that leaves a matte finish on the skin. This will minimize shine and the appearance of large pores.

SENSITIVE SKIN needs a moisturizer that does not contain fragrances or dyes and is designed for this skin type.

EXTRA DRY AND MATURE SKIN requires more moisture. Nourishing oils, dense creams, and balms are formulated specifically for both these skin types. These products help to temporarily plump up the skin, making it appear smoother and reducing the appearance of fine lines. Look for petrolatum-based moisturizers that also contain ingredients such as lactic acid or alpha hydroxy acids, which help to prevent dry skin.

Specially formulated moisturizers are needed for the area under and around the eye. The skin surrounding the eyes has smaller pores, is thinner than the rest of the facial skin, and is more sensi-

Tips for Moisturizing

Use a fast-absorbing eye cream under concealer to help skin look smooth, not crepey. The skin around the eyes is more delicate than the rest of the face. For puffiness and wrinkles under the eye, try using a richer formula containing shea butter or beeswax at night.

If your skin is very dry and dehydrated, use a super-rich moisturizing balm with ingredients like petrolatum, glycerin, or shea butter for better texture and for smoother application of foundation. Warm the balm in your palms before applying it to your face.

Layer different textures of moisturizers to achieve maximum results. For instance, use an absorbing cream with balms or oils.

If you have oily skin, try using an oil-control lotion on the forehead and nose to tone down shine. Oil-free formulas hydrate while helping to control overactive oil glands. Foundation applied over the lotion will hold better, too.

For dry, chapped, or cracked lips, apply a balm formulated specifically for lips.

Try patting a moisturizing balm onto your cheeks after completing your makeup. It will give a glow to your face and help the foundation look natural.

To create your own sheer, tinted moisturizer, mix face lotion with foundation.

These tests will help you to determine the ratio of oil to water in a moisturizing product.

Apply moisturizer to your skin. If the skin under the moisturizer is warm, there is a greater percentage of oil in the product. If the area is cool, there is a greater percentage of water. The science behind this is that evaporation cools, and water evaporates. Oil does not evaporate and therefore traps heat in the body.

Put a small amount of moisturizer on a tissue, and hold it over a lightbulb. Products with higher oil content will melt. The wider the area of melted oil, the greater the percentage of oil in the moisturizer.

tive. It is important to keep this area as hydrated as possible. Products on the market target specific problems. Before you go shopping for an eye cream, decide whether you want an eye cream that hydrates and prepares for concealer, or an overnight cream that is rich and emollient. Anti-wrinkle or anti-aging creams contain caffeine, retinol, alpha hydroxy acids, or vitamin C. Anti-darkening creams contain vitamin K or hydroquinone. Also decide if you want two different creams, one for night and the other for day. To avoid possible irritation of the eye, look for an eye cream that does not contain fragrance and has a pH close to that of tears (about 7.5).

Lips are often the first area of the face to wrinkle. Dry and chapped lips are a clear sign that you need to drink more water. While hydrating the body is the first step toward beautiful lips, there are many products that help keep them plump and smooth.

For personal use, have on hand two facial moisturizers, one lighter than the other. On those days when the skin needs more moisture, apply the lighter product first, and then layer the heavier moisturizer over that. Also find a moisturizing product formulated specifically for the under-eye area, lip balm, body moisturizer, and sunscreen. As your skin changes in response to lifestyle, season, or climate, you can treat it with the right hydrating product. Makeup artists carry a full range of moisturizers in their kits.

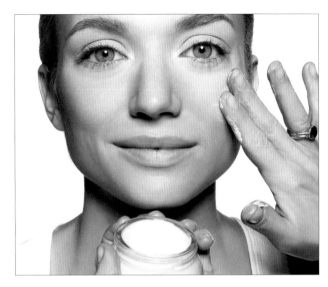

Moisturizer Application

Once the face is thoroughly cleansed and toned, and while it is still slightly damp, apply moisturizer using a clean sponge or your fingers. (Note: dense balms will work only on dry skin.) If you are using your hands to apply any makeup products, always wash them thoroughly so you don't transfer oils and bacteria to your face. Bacteria on the hands or makeup tools often cause breakouts.

Use about a nickel-size amount of moisturizer.

Warm the balm or moisturizer between your palms.

With firm, upward strokes, gently press the product into the skin until it is completely absorbed.

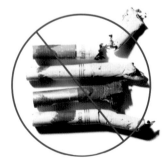

Smoking is always a horrible idea.

It severely damages your skin and lungs and is a common cause of cancer. It makes you smell and robs color from your skin and lips. Smoke breaks down the skin's defenses, depriving it of the oxygen it needs for healthy cell renewal. Repeated exposure to cigarette smoke causes the skin to lose its luster and tone and to wrinkle. Smokers often develop permanent wrinkles around the lips. Smoking is the one lifestyle choice for which balance and moderation are not options.

Sun Protection

Lines, dark spots, and uneven skin texture are *not* the inevitable effects of aging but are often the result of too much sun exposure. Overexposure to sunlight can also cause cancer. Too much sun is the skin's worst enemy. The only way to prevent premature aging and skin damage due to overexposure is to stay out of the midday sun when possible, wear protective clothing and hats, and always use the proper sunscreen.

Three types of radiation reach us from the sun. Visible and infrared light rays provide light and warmth. Ultraviolet rays are harmful. The sun's ultraviolet (UV) light falls into three wavelength bands: UVA, UVB, and UVC.

UVA RAYS have the longest wavelength and remain high in intensity all day. They penetrate through the epidermis and deep into the dermis, damaging newer cells. UVA rays are very dangerous and can cause cancers and sensitivity reactions.

UVB RAYS have a midrange wavelength, and like UVA rays penetrate the epidermis and continue into the dermis. These rays break down the organization of skin cells, causing wrinkles and broken blood vessels. They are highest in intensity from 10 a.m. to 2 p.m. and near the equator. Glass protects skin from UVB rays.

UVC RAYS have the shortest wavelength and are usually absorbed by the ozone layer. They are absorbed by the epidermis and can be very dangerous in

Tips for Protecting Your Skin from the Damaging Effects of the Sun

Whenever possible, stay out of the sun for long periods of time, especially between 10 a.m. and 2 p.m., when rays are strongest.

Protect exposed skin all year round. Wear sunscreen with an SPF (sun protection factor) of 15 to 30, depending on the season and length of exposure. Long-sleeved shirts and wide-brimmed hats provide some protection. Remember, the sun penetrates through loosely woven and wet clothing very easily, so wear sunscreen even when covered.

Avoid tanning beds. There is no such thing as safe tanning.

Wear sunglasses that wrap around the eyes and have 100 percent UV-blocking lenses. Most sunscreens are too harsh to use on the sensitive area around the eyes.

Select a sunscreen that protects against both UVA and UVB rays, sometimes labeled as broad-spectrum sunscreen. Many popular sunscreens will not adequately protect your skin from these harmful rays.

Apply liberally—about one teaspoon of sunscreen to your face and at least one ounce (about a shot glass) to your body each day. The face and hands are high-risk areas for cancer, so apply liberally to those areas.

If you have sensitive skin, use a cream-based product, and avoid sunscreens with tretinoin (Retin-A, Stieva-A, Retisol-A, Rejuva-A, Renova, Vitamin A acid), which dries the skin. Look for a fragrance-free, hypoallergenic sunscreen if you have any allergies to skin products.

Waterproof and water-resistant sunscreens are good if you are involved in swimming or sports. Waterproof products work for ninety minutes; protection with water-resistant sunscreens lasts thirty minutes. They need to be applied/reapplied twenty minutes before entering the water so that the product can bond with the skin.

Those who work out of doors might need frequent application of a sunscreen with a high SPF.

UVA rays are reflected from all light surfaces, including water, sand, snow, ice, and even concrete.

Children younger than six months old should not wear sunscreen but instead be covered and kept out of the sun.

large amounts. As the ozone layer thins, attention will need to be paid to these UVC rays.

Exposure to the sun produces the formation of molecules in the skin called free radicals. These molecules attack healthy skin cells, damaging and interfering with the production of new collagen. With the destruction of collagen fibers and hyaluronic acid molecules—both of which are responsible for preserving the volume and resiliency of the skin—skin loses its firmness, resulting in wrinkles. The sun can also damage the eyes and affect the immune system. UV rays can damage white blood cells and Langerhans cells, both essential to the skin's ability to fight viruses and other diseases.

For more information and to learn of new developments in sunscreen protection, these Web sites, listed recently in a *New York Times* article, might prove helpful.

Environmental Working Group
(lists products with UVA protection)
www.cosmeticsdatabase.com

The Skin Cancer Foundation
www.skincancer.org

American Cancer Society
www.cancer.org

American Academy of Dermatology
www.aad.org

British Columbia Centre for Disease Control
www.bccdc.org

Sunscreen Application

Apply sunscreen at least once a day, and use an adequate amount of the product.

Clean the skin before application.

Apply to cool, dry skin twenty to thirty minutes before exposure. Cool, dry skin allows sunscreen to bind effectively. When sunscreen is applied to warm skin, the open pores can become irritated, and rashes can develop.

Two applications help cover any missed spots.

Apply moisturizer and makeup over sunscreen.

Reapply during the day, depending on your rate of perspiration and the amount of sun exposure you get.

Tip

Use the equivalent of a shot glass of sunscreen—that's two tablespoons—to cover skin from head to toe.

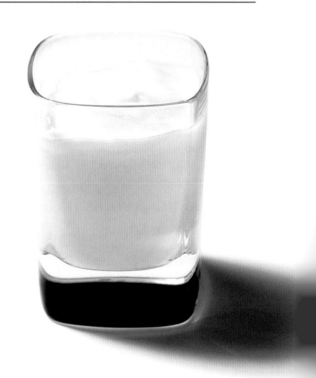

Skincare Glossary

There are many terms and ingredients associated with skincare products. What follows is only a basic list. While there are no miracles when it comes to the skin, a clear understanding of how ingredients function will help you select the right skincare products.

ALPHA HYDROXY ACIDS (AHAS) are naturally occurring acids found in fruits and milk, used topically to reduce the appearance of fine lines. AHAs help speed up the skin's natural exfoliation process, helping it shed dead skin cells. They can improve the texture of skin, unclog pores, and help prevent breakouts. Glycolic acid is one of the commonly used AHAs. Do not use products containing salicylic acid (a beta hydroxy acid), which is too harsh for general exfoliation, as they are intended for use only on problem skin areas.

ANTI-AGING: The best anti-aging formula is a healthy lifestyle. Nothing will stop the clock. Poor diet, excessive drinking, smoking, lack of exercise, and sunburn all accelerate the effects of aging on the skin.

ANTIOXIDANTS help protect the skin from damage caused by free radicals, molecules with an unpaired electron. They cause oxidation that can damage cellular material. Vitamins A, C, and E, beta-carotene, green tea, and grape seed extract are all highly effective antioxidants.

BALMS are super-rich moisturizers that target dry patches of skin on face, hands, feet, and body. Look for ingredients such as avocado extract or shea butter. For a subtle glow, I warm some in my hands and pat on the cheeks after applying makeup.

BASE is a term that generally refers to a product applied under foundation to smooth and protect the skin. Bases often contain a mix of vitamins, antioxidants, and anti-aging ingredients. Previous generations referred to foundation color as base.

BRIGHTENER: Makeup products sometimes contain light-diffusing particles and/or ingredients that inhibit oxidation. Both of these are referred to as brighteners.

COLLAGEN is a fibrous protein found in skin. When collagen levels in the skin are high, the skin appears firm. Levels of collagen decline as we age. As the support provided by the collagen is reduced, wrinkles begin to form. Injections temporarily replace lost collagen. The topical application of peptides may have a similar effect.

EMOLLIENTS (squalane, avocado oil, wheat germ oil, glycerin, lanolin, petroleum, shea butter, and others) hold moisture in the skin and make the skin soft and supple.

EXFOLIATORS are designed to help slough off dead skin cells. Look for scrubs designed for the face.

FIXERS are sprays that set makeup. Makeup is also typically set with powders.

GREEN TEA EXTRACT (*Camellia sinensis*) is a powerful antioxidant found in many anti-aging products that may slow down photo aging.

HUMECTANTS (glycerin, algae extract, sodium hyaluronate, urea, lactic acid, panthenol and others) absorb water from the air and help the skin retain moisture.

HYALURONIC ACID (sodium hyaluronate) is a fluid that surrounds the joints and is found in skin tissue. Aging slows the production of this acid, so it is often supplemented as an anti-aging treatment. It is used as filler for wrinkles (injection) and can be applied topically or taken in pill form. It is often added to moisturizer and works to hydrate skin.

OXIDANTS are unstable molecules caused by pollution, smoke, ultraviolet light, toxins, and other environmental factors. Also known as free radicals, they attack and damage the skin, leading to premature aging.

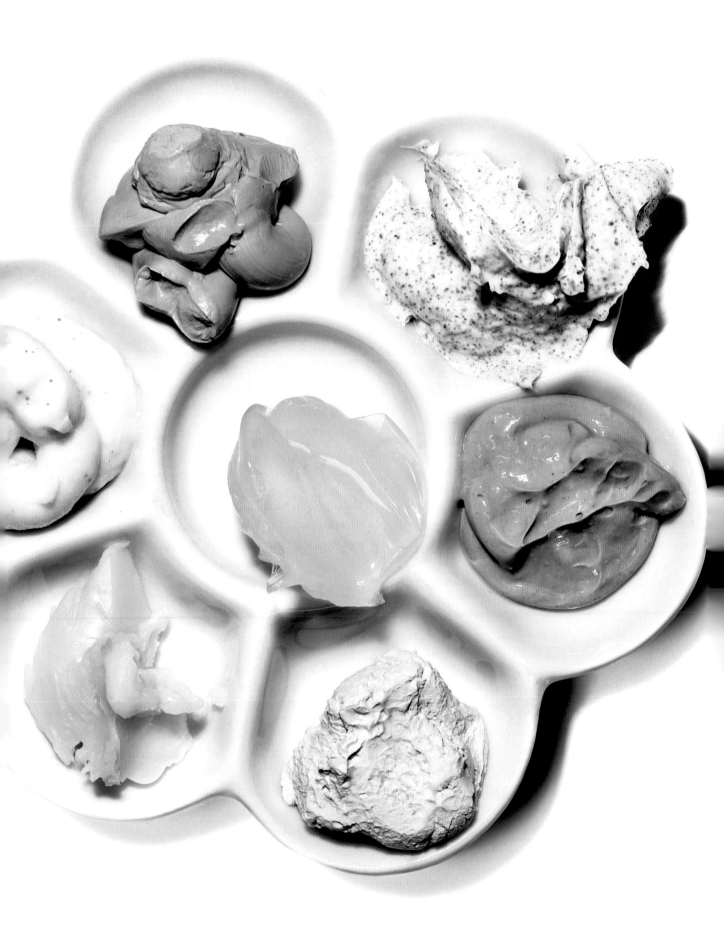

PEPTIDES are two or more amino acids bonded together, forming a linear molecule. The molecules can transfer biologically active agents (green tea, vitamin E, copper) to cells, renewing them. Algae peptides are used in some firming formulations. Copper peptides have been used for years to aid in wound healing. Labels might indicate that a product contains pentapeptides (five peptides) or polypeptides (many peptides).

PHOTO AGING is sun damage.

RETINOIDS (Retin-A, retinal, Renova) are powerful vitamin A derivatives used to fight acne and help build collagen to reverse visible signs of aging. The drug is effective in reducing fine lines around the eyes and mouth, not deep wrinkles. Inflammation and peeling are common side effects from use, which can last from two weeks to months. Because the drug makes skin more sensitive to the sun, use of a sunscreen is essential. Pregnant women and those planning a pregnancy should avoid this drug, since it is not known how much Retin-A is absorbed through the skin, and high doses of vitamin A can cause birth defects. Natural sources of retinoids include yams, tomatoes, fish-liver oils, melon, squash, and leafy green vegetables.

SERUMS are concentrated, corrective skin treatments that are packed with highly effective active ingredients that address specific skin concerns like dullness and uneven skin tone. Ingredients commonly found in serums include vitamin C, green tea extract, and white birch extract. For best results, serums should be applied after cleansing, before moisturizer.

SPF (sun protection factor) measures the degree of protection a product provides against the sun's UVB rays. The formula used divides the minutes it takes to burn wearing a thick application of the product by the minutes the same person takes to burn without any sunscreen. There is no current rating system for UVA protection.

SQUALENE (natural, unsaturated) is derived from shark-liver oil. It is very emollient and has some germicidal benefits.

TYROSINASE INHIBITORS (kojic acid, hydroquinone) all prevent browning or age spots on the skin. Licorice (*glycyrrhiza glabrd*) has been used for centuries to lighten and brighten skin.

VITAMIN B3 (niacinamide) is a water soluble vitamin found in yeast, eggs, liver, and vegetables that helps increase the amount of fatty acids in the skin, promoting exfoliation and firmness.

VITAMIN C (ascorbic acid) is an antioxidant that can reduce the appearance of hyperpigmentation and create a more even skin tone. It protects the skin from atmospheric pollution and from ultraviolet light. Vitamin C also helps convert inactivated vitamin E back to the active, antioxidant form of vitamin E. Vitamin C is involved in the formation of elastin and plays a role in converting proline, an amino acid, into collagen. Vitamin C increases collagen manufacture, reducing the appearance of wrinkles. The production of melanin is an oxidative process that causes pigmentation. As an antioxidant, vitamin C counteracts the oxidative process. High doses of vitamin C reduce the pigmentation of scars and make them less noticeable. Vitamin C is found in fresh fruits and vegetables.

VITAMIN E (tocopherol) provides antioxidant protection. All the cells in the body contain fatty acids that need protection against oxidation, which causes disease and symptoms of aging. Vitamin E protects the fatty acids (oils) against oxidation and rancidity. Vitamin E has been shown to act as a mild sunscreen, with a sun protection factor (SPF) of 3.

VITAMIN K helps to reduce ruddiness and promotes faster healing of bruising, swelling, and skin irritation.

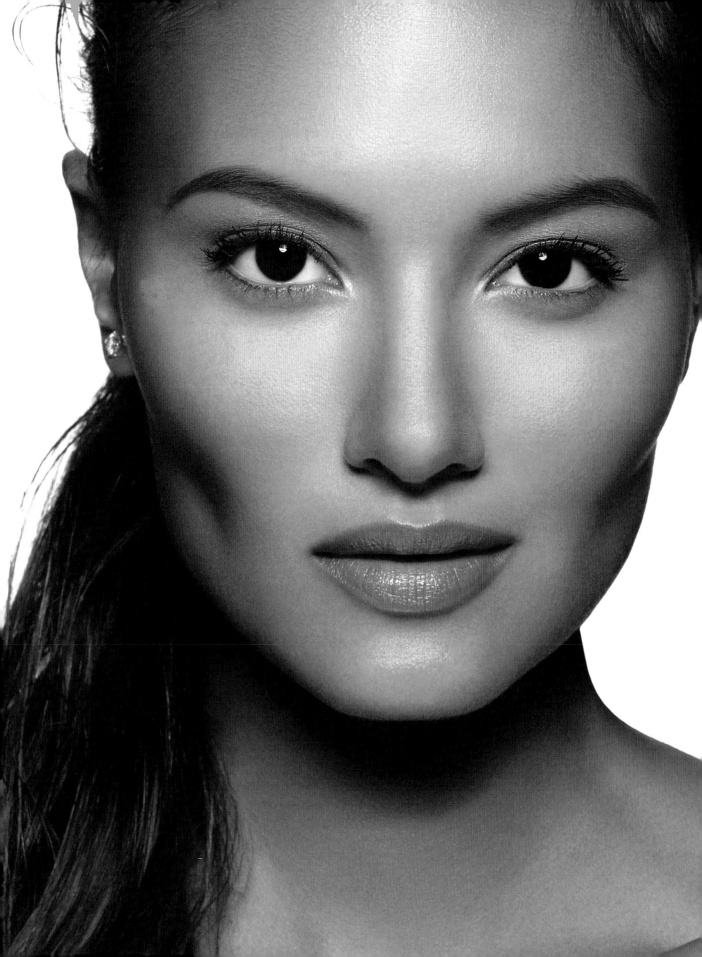

Chapter 4

FACE

The basics—**under-eye concealer, foundation, and powder**—are the secret to a great look. If the basics aren't right, the makeup won't be either.

PREPARING THE FACE FOR MAKEUP

Begin with these steps before applying any makeup.

Analyze the type and condition of the skin. This will determine the combination of skincare and makeup formulas to use. The condition of your skin changes each day, so make an assessment each morning.

Decide which products will improve the skin's current condition. That includes determining what weight moisturizer(s) are appropriate and whether an oil-controlling gel, a skin-soothing lotion, or a combination of skincare products is needed. Understanding how various ingredients work and the range of options available to you is important.

Choose the right foundation formula for the skin type and condition. Options include stick foundation, lightweight tinted moisturizer, denser tinted balm, fuller-coverage liquid foundation, powder, and oil-free formulas.

Select the correct foundation shade for the skin tone. It is important to select the foundation shade first.

Select an under-eye concealer one to two tones lighter than the foundation, and determine if a corrector is needed.

Select the perfect shades of powder to ensure that makeup stays fresh looking and lasts for hours. Choose a lighter powder to set concealer and that will double as an eye primer, and a deeper shade that works with the foundation tone. Test the color of the powder on the skin after applying foundation.

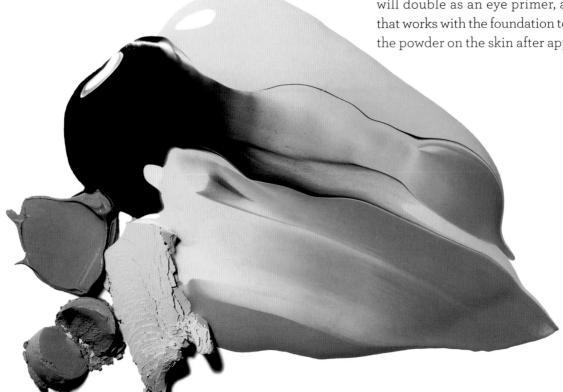

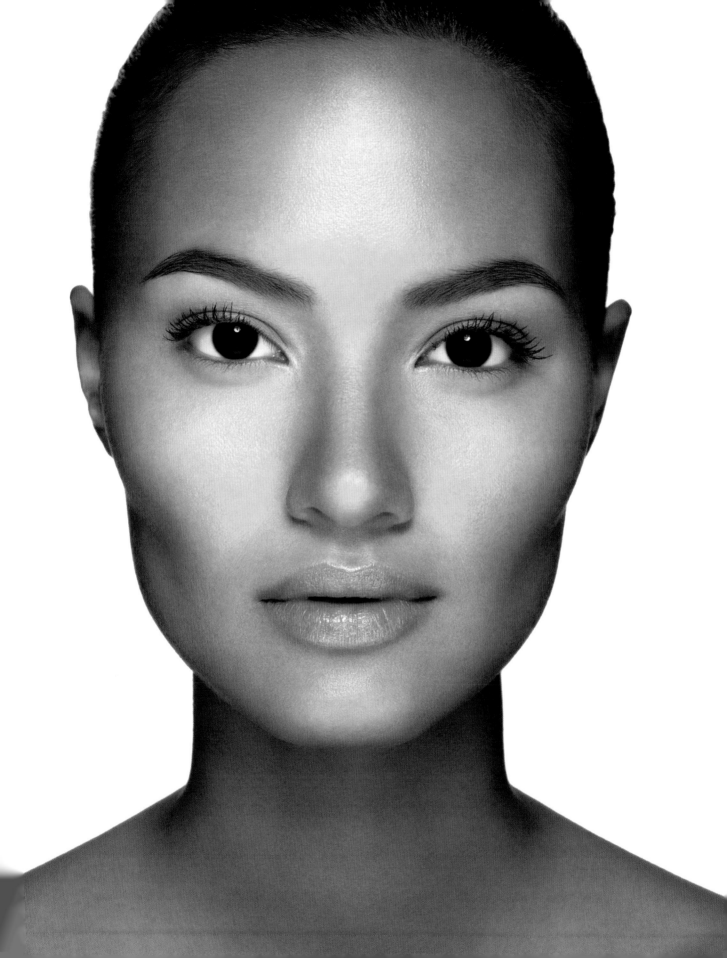

CONCEALERS & CORRECTORS

Correctors brighten the darkest areas under your eyes, allowing concealers to both lighten and blend. Concealers should blend into your skin, lightening dark circles and instantly making you look better.

Concealers are the secret of the universe.

While concealers are available that cover tattoos, spots, blemishes, scars, redness, and bruises, most people use a concealer to lighten dark circles under the eyes. Different concealers and correctors are formulated for each specific use. Pick a concealer and, when needed, a corrector designed for each of your problem areas. Under-eye concealers are not formulated for use on blemishes or areas of redness. They are creamier in consistency and lighter than the skin tone. Using under-eye concealer on areas of redness will only highlight the imperfections. Yellow-toned foundation that matches the skin tone is the best way to adequately cover blemishes, scars, and tattoos.

The application of under-eye concealer is the most important step in any makeup routine. Concealer is the one product that, when chosen and applied correctly, can instantly lift and brighten the face. Choose a color one to two shades lighter than the foundation. The skin under the eye is very thin, so the blue of the fine veins just under the surface tend to show through. A light yellow-toned concealer masks this blue discoloration and brightens the skin. For those with alabaster skin, a porcelain-toned concealer will work. Sometimes a stick foundation one or two shades lighter than the face can serve as an under-eye concealer for those who need very little coverage.

Correctors are available for extreme under-eye darkness. When a regular concealer cannot fully lighten the under-eye area, a peach or pink corrector is used to counter the purple or green tone. A regular yellow-toned concealer is usually lightly layered over the corrector to lighten the under-eye area. Occasionally, those with extremely deep purple or green coloration under the eye will not need the layer of regular concealer.

Tips

Some women need between two and four colors that can be mixed and blended to accommodate changes in skin tone under the eye, which can vary with the time of day, amount of rest, and hormones.

Sometimes a corrector is enough to solve the under-eye problem. Rules should be followed, but there should be flexibility for what works where. Sometimes something as bold as a bright pink or peach cream blush will work for very intense darkness.

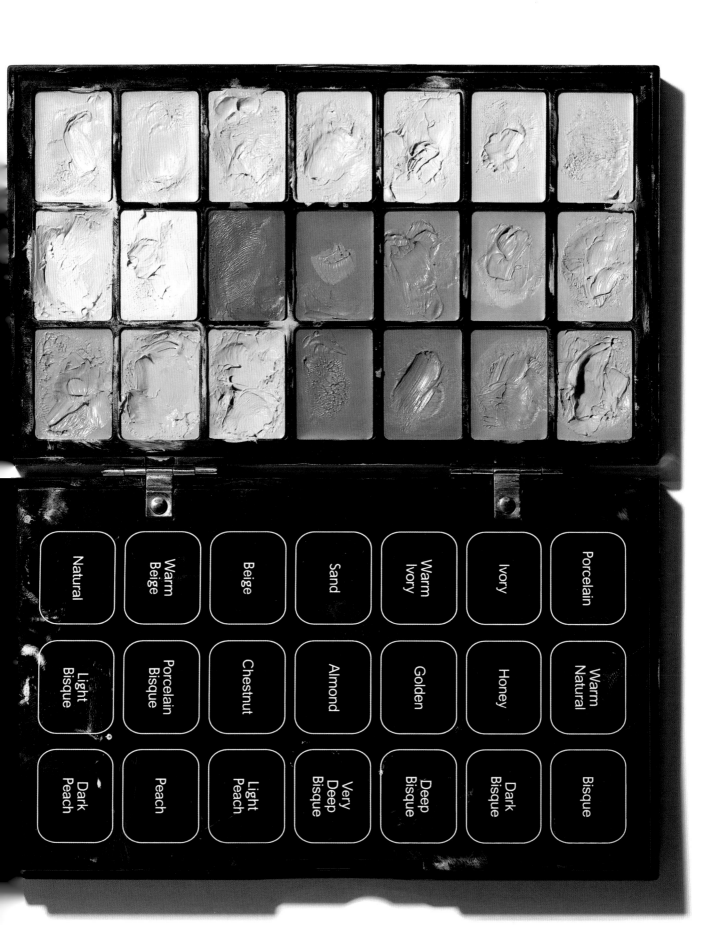

CHOOSING CORRECTOR COLOR

Correctors are for extreme under-eye darkness.
If your skin is pale, choose the lightest colors,
beginning with bisque or light pink. For deeper
skin tones, choose peach or darker peach.

Pink

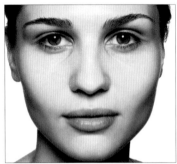

1

Begin with a
clean face.

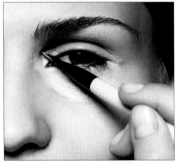

2

Apply corrector
beginning at the inner
corner of the eye and
continue underneath
close to the lashes, where
there is darkness.

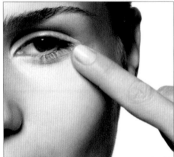

3

Gently blend by pressing
with your fingers.

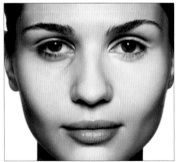

4

The corrector is
complete on the
right.

Peach

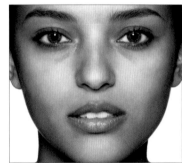

1

Begin with a
clean face.

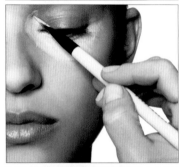

2

Apply corrector at the
innermost corner of
the eye and underneath
to cover the darkest
areas. Apply corrector
generously, making sure
there is enough to block
the darkness.

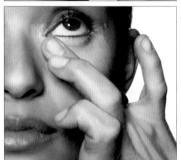

3

Gently blend and tap
with your fingers.

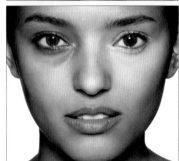

4

The corrector is
complete on the
right.

Darker Peach

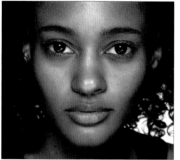

1

Begin with a clean face.

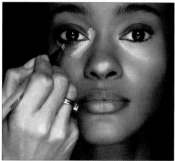

2

Begin at the innermost corner of each eye. This is the deepest, darkest area of the face, so apply the corrector densely.

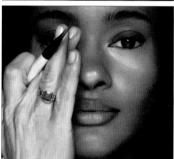

3

Blend with your finger and press the corrector into the skin. Never rub or drag your finger across the skin.

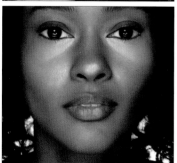

4

The corrector is complete.

CORRECTOR APPLICATION FOR ASIAN EYES

Even if you don't have a lot of darkness corrector still brightens the eyes.

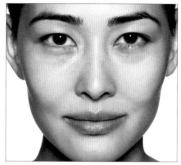

1

Begin with a clean face. Note the darkness is not severe.

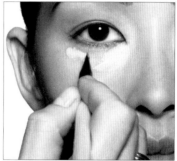

2

Cover the entire area with corrector.

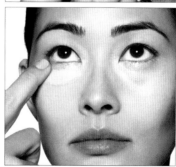

3

Gently blend with your fingers.

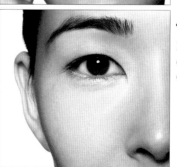

4

Note the difference even when the darkness is subtle.

CORRECTOR BRIGHTENS

Corrector can be pink or peach toned. Make sure it is applied up to the lashes and in the inner corner space between the eye and the bridge of the nose.

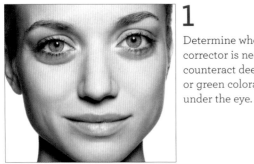

1

Determine whether corrector is needed to counteract deep purple or green coloration under the eye.

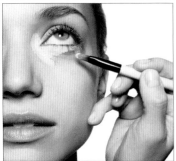

2

If corrector is needed, choose the color according to the directions on page 52.

Apply corrector using a small concealer brush and starting at the inner eye.

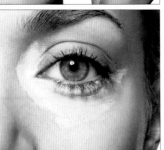

3

Apply corrector to all areas of darkness.

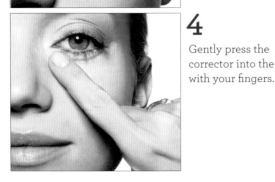

4

Gently press the corrector into the skin with your fingers.

Troubleshooting: Corrector or Concealer

If it creases
Using enough powder applied correctly is key. If you skimp, it will end up creasing.

If it's cakey
The ratio of eye cream to concealer is off.

If it's too light
Use an extremely light dusting of light bronzing powder to warm up the area.

If it's not bright enough or if it's too dark
Try to add a bit of fast-absorbing eye cream, then repeat corrector and concealer.

If the eye makeup transfers to the concealer
Use eye makeup remover, a cotton swab, or a sponge and remove all under-eye product. Start over with eye cream, and let it absorb before applying other eye makeup.

Clean brush between corrector and concealer steps.

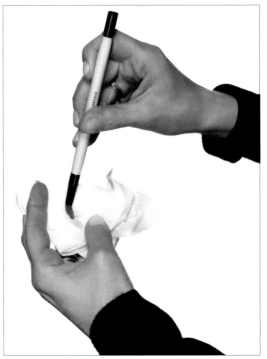

CONCEALER LIGHTENS

Concealer should be one or two shades lighter than your foundation and yellow in tone to blend as it lightens. Apply after corrector in most cases.

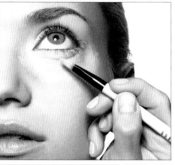

1
Apply concealer generously under the eyes starting at the recessed area at the innermost corner of each eye.

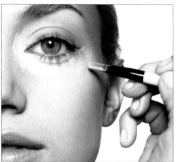

2
Cover the entire area below the lower lash line to cover any darkness or redness.

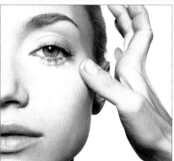

3
To blend the concealer, gently warm it between your fingers and then press it into the skin.

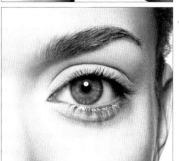

4
Set the concealer in place with a sheer loose powder.

POWDER SETS CONCEALER

Most women can use a yellow-toned, loose powder, but those with extremely fair skin may need a white-toned powder.

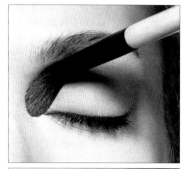

1
Using a brush that fits in the corner of the eye, dust the powder onto the skin.

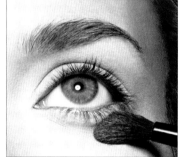

2
Brush the powder across the under-eye and sweep off any excess with the brush.

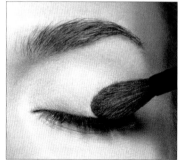

3
Sweep the powder across the eyelid.

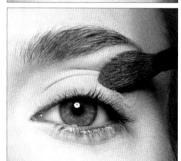

4
Apply the powder under the brow bone. Repeat two times if necessary.

FOUNDATION

Beauty starts with great skin. The right foundation will make you look like you're not wearing any foundation at all. You'll just have even-toned, great-looking skin.

The reason we wear foundation is to even out our skin tone and texture. When applied correctly, the result is skin that looks clear and smooth. But, what is most important is that the skin look better than it did without foundation.

Some women shy away from foundation because they associate it with thick pancake makeup that sometimes looks like a mask. But even the strongest makeup should have a natural-looking base.

Formula

Foundations are available in many different formulas. Choose one that is right for your skin and style and has a consistency you like to use. Use the following guidelines to choose your formula.

TINTED MOISTURIZER

For normal/normal-to-dry skin. Gives a sheer, lightweight coverage and is an alternative to foundation. Provides a totally natural look. Great for weekends.

TINTED FACE BALM

For extra-dry skin. Provides sheer coverage. Intensively hydrates and gives skin a dewy finish. Balm actually plumps the skin and reduces the appearance of fine lines.

STICK FOUNDATION

For all skin types except oily. Provides easy spot coverage and is also buildable for medium to full coverage. Best foundation for photography.

LIQUID FOUNDATION

For dry to extra-dry skin. Hydrates and smoothes, providing medium to full coverage.

MOISTURIZING COMPACT

For dry to extra-dry skin. Hydrating formulas provide medium to full coverage.

WHIPPED FOUNDATION

For combination skin and great for skin with texture. Balances the skin by hydrating dry areas and absorbing oil in the T-zone. Provides medium to full coverage.

OIL-FREE LIQUID FOUNDATION

For oily skin. For combination skin in the summer. Absorbs oil and smoothes while providing light to medium coverage.

OIL-FREE CREAM FOUNDATION

For normal-to-oily skin. Absorbs oil, providing medium to full coverage. A good choice to cover acne and large pores.

OIL-FREE POWDER COMPACT

For oily skin. Provides medium to full coverage. Because of the portable packaging, compact foundations are great for touch-ups.

MINERAL POWDERS

Suggested for very oily skin. (Be careful when choosing color. Oily skin can change color of powders, and they may appear dry and pasty.)

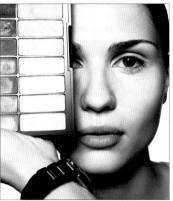 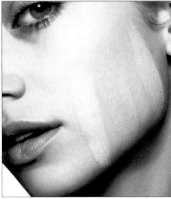 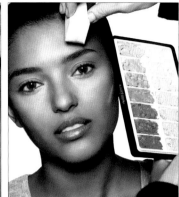

Finding the Perfect Shade

Once you have decided on the right formula of foundation, you need to find the right shade. The correct shade will disappear on the skin.

Make sure the foundation is yellow-based. Everyone has yellow undertones in their skin. Pink-based foundations look like a mask on most people. Only 1 percent need a pink tone: those who sunburn even in the shade. Foundation should not change the color of the face but simply even out the tone.

Test several shades of foundation on the side of your face, between the nose and the side of the cheek. Make a stripe of foundation in the preferred formula from cheek to jawline, gently blending into the skin. Also test a shade lighter and a shade darker for comparison. The correct shade will disappear.

Double-check the selected color on forehead. Sometimes women have darker skin on the forehead, and the foundation shade that matches here will work better for the whole face.

Always test foundation in natural light. Walk to a window or doorway to check the match. The swatch that disappears into the skin is the right shade. Do not test foundation on the hand or arm, as the face is rarely the same color as the rest of the body.

If your skin tone gets darker in the summer or on a vacation, you may need to adjust the foundation tone. Keep a deeper shade of foundation on hand to accommodate changes in skin tone. It can be blended with your regular foundation if you are between shades or used alone when skin is darkest.

Oily skin sometimes turns foundation darker. Check and adjust accordingly.

Stick foundation that is a shade or two lighter than the skin tone can be used for light under-eye coverage instead of concealer.

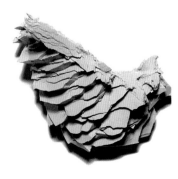

Tip

For those with combination skin, foundations are now available with both silica beads, which soak up oil, and lecithin, which hydrates skin. Moisturizers and oil-control lotions can be applied to parts of the face that need it to counterbalance the foundation choice.

Tools

The right tools help you apply foundation quickly and easily, with great-looking results. Sponges, also called makeup wedges, are used with foundation. Makeup can be applied directly to the sponge or face and gently blended into the skin. Some prefer to use a foundation brush. The synthetic bristles of this brush type can be used with all foundation formulas for a smooth and even application. Fingers are the best tool for warming and blending makeup into the skin.

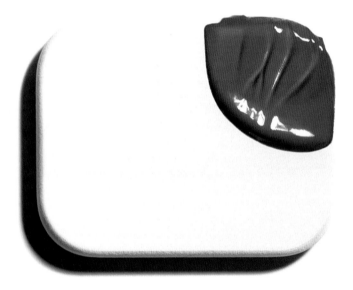

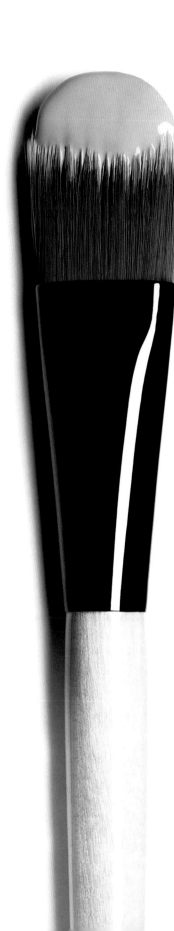

Tips

While sponges are a convenient and sanitary way to apply makeup, they can't replicate the direct control and warmth of using the fingers and hands. You can use the hands to warm a product before application. Foundation, concealer, lip color, and even pencils spread more easily on the skin if they are at body temperature. Use the fingers to apply makeup for complete control over placement of the product. Always thoroughly clean the hands and nails before applying makeup.

To see the true effect of the foundation, let it settle for a few minutes. Then blend or layer in more foundation in spots where it is needed.

FOUNDATION APPLICATION

To get the even-toned, great-looking skin you want, you need to choose the right color, texture, tools, and formulas. Always begin with a test to choose the color that's the closest match to your natural skin tone, and then follow the simple steps for proper application.

Troubleshooting: Foundation

Wrong color

Add a layer of darker foundation or darker powder bronzer or face powder to balance the face color. Select the tone properly. Sometimes the skin needs yellow, red, orange, or blue. The face color should match that of the body.

Color doesn't match neck

Instead of lightening the face, darken the neck with warm bronzer.

Face has a lot of redness

Use a sheer coat of foundation, making sure the skin tone can be seen through it. Use bronzer lightly on the face, neck, and chest to blend.

Orange-peel texture coming through

First try a light moisturizer on your palms to warm it up. Then press it into the skin. Layer with more foundation. If this doesn't work, take the foundation off. Greatly hydrate the skin. Wait two minutes and change the foundation formula to work with the skin.

Pasty-looking skin

The color is too light. Check the color following the tips below.

Yellow-looking skin

The color is too dark. Recheck the color on the forehead and cheek. Switch to another color and correct with bronzer. Some women need to use two shades on different parts of the face during different times of the year.

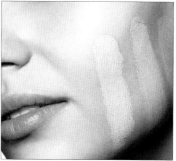

1 Swipe each shade to choose a color. Gently blend into skin. The correct color will look like your natural skin tone.

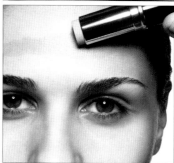

2 Check the color to be sure it matches the forehead.

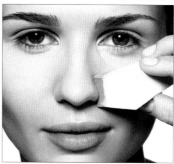

3 Begin applying a small amount of foundation around the nose.

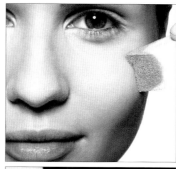

4 Blend the foundation upward into the hairline. Apply foundation all over or only to the parts that need it. Use your fingers to press the foundation into the skin to fully blend.

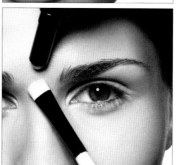

5 Use a blemish stick after the foundation to cover red spots or blemishes.

THE BEAUTY OF DIVERSITY

Through my work as a makeup artist I've had the good fortune to travel around the world and meet women of diverse backgrounds. Through these travels I've learned that women of all ethnicities—from Asian to Middle Eastern and Latina—want the same thing when it comes to their skin. They want their skin to look smooth, even, and flawless. Each ethnicity has its own unique (and beautiful) traits and I believe in using makeup that enhances, rather than masks, these traits.

Asian Skin

"Isn't yellow foundation going to make my skin look more yellow?" is a question that I often hear from my Asian customers when I recommend foundations with yellow undertones. I've experimented with countless foundations over the years and I've found that yellow-toned foundations always look the most natural—especially on Asian skins.

Many Asian women are prone to and concerned about sunspots, which are the result of sun damage. Aside from wearing sun protection every day, the best way to deal with sunspots is with corrective peach- and pink-toned concealers. Some women have skin with yellow undertones and yellow surface tones. For them, I suggest covering the sunspots with a medium-toned peach corrector. If the concealer is too light in tone it will look gray on the sunspot, so you may have to try a few different tones to find the right one. Other women have skin with yellow undertones and pink surface tones (often the result of skin irritation due to using bleaching agents). The best way to cover their sunspots is with a medium-toned pink bisque corrector. As I mentioned earlier, you'll know the concealer is too light if it turns ashy when it's applied on the sunspot. After applying the corrector, gently smooth on a yellow-toned foundation in a shade that matches your skin perfectly.

Black Skin

There are many variations in skin tone among black women, so consider the following advice as general guidelines rather than hard and fast rules. Black skin tends to be darker across the forehead and perimeter of the face, and lighter on the middle parts of the face, including the cheeks. The trick when applying foundation is to create a seamless look between the light/golden and dark/warmer parts of the face. Some women like enhancing the golden tones in their skin, and other women like playing up the warmer tones in their skin. It's a matter of personal preference and it's important—whether you are doing your own makeup or you

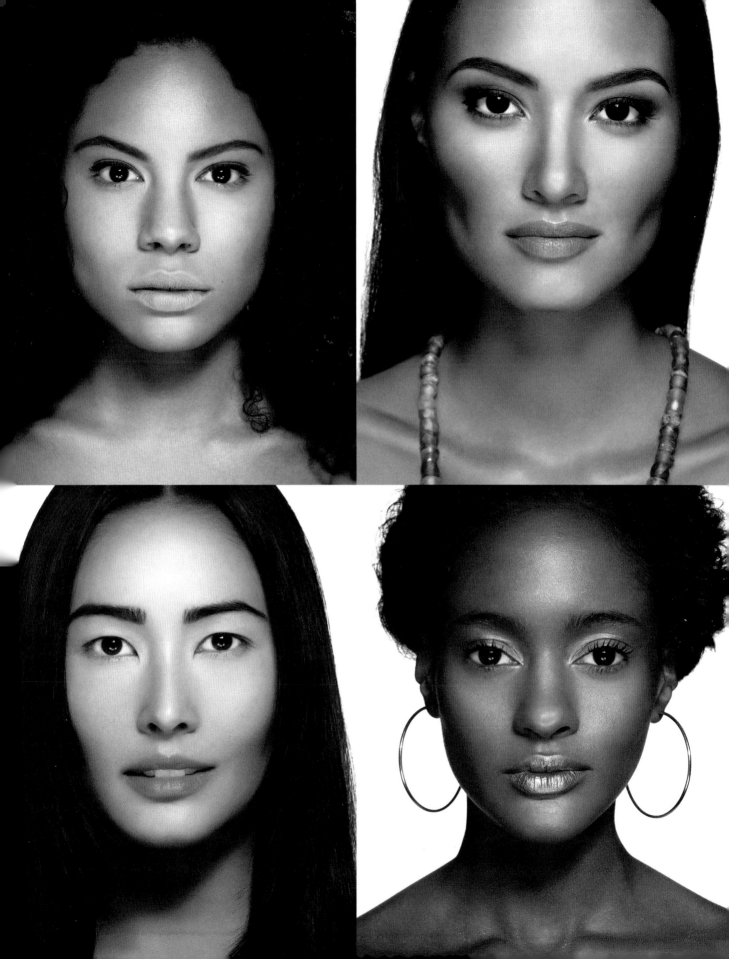

are a makeup artist working with a customer—to know which tones you're going to focus on.

If you want to go golden, choose a tinted moisturizer or sheer foundation that matches the skin on the center of your face. Apply the tinted moisturizer/sheer foundation just on this area, then use a coppery bronzer on the other parts of the face to diffuse the transition between the lighter and darker areas.

If you want to go warm, choose a tinted moisturizer or sheer foundation in a shade that falls between the lighter and darker parts of the face. Applying a dark shade of foundation all over the face will look unnatural so the idea here is to tone down the difference between the light and dark areas. Look for a yellow-based foundation that has a bit of orange, red, or blue to it, depending on how deep the color of the skin is. Lighter black skin looks most natural with yellow-based foundation that has a touch of golden orange. Very dark skin looks best with yellow-based foundation that has warm cinnamon tones. In all instances, if the foundation looks ashy or gray on the skin, it's not the right shade.

Latin Skin

Latin women generally have golden skin with olive undertones. Some women have pink surface tones (around the nose and mouth, and on the cheeks) due to skin irritation and sensitivity. Latin skin tans very easily, turning a golden cinnamon during summer months. Alternately, in the winter months, skin tends to take on a yellow-green cast.

Bronzer is a great year-round beauty staple for Latin skin because it can be used in the summer to add warmth to your foundation, and in the winter to counteract sallow coloring. Latinas range in coloring from fair to dark so one shade of bronzer does not fit all. If you are fair, choose a bronzer that has pinky-red tones to it. If you are darker, choose a brownish-red bronzer. When shopping for foundation, look for a yellow-based golden shade to complement the natural tones in your skin. Be careful not to go too golden with your foundation, however, because skin will start to look orange.

Middle Eastern Skin

Middle Eastern skin is very similar to Latin skin in that it is golden with olive undertones. Many women complain of extreme darkness under the eyes. The best way to cover their purplish-green and brownish-green under-eye circles is with corrective peach- and pink-toned concealers. If you have golden surface tones, use a peach-toned concealer one shade lighter than your foundation to cover your dark circles. If you have pink surface tones (due to sensitivity), start with a peach-toned concealer to cancel out the darkness, then layer on a pink-toned concealer to brighten the under-eye area and make it similar in tone to the rest of the face. In most instances this combination of concealers will offer enough coverage. If you still see under-eye darkness, you may have to layer on a third concealer—a yellow-toned one in a skin-tone-correct shade

Multiethnic Skin

Many beautiful mixed-race women need to be open and observant about what makeup looks natural. Basic rules apply, but sometimes these women need multiple products or bronzers as mix-ins to make foundation look great.

MULTICOLOR FOUNDATION & POWDER APPLICATION

Some dark skins need two colors of foundation and two powders to create the perfect foundation to even out skin tone.

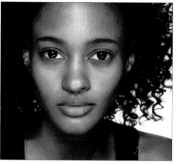

1 Check if forehead is darker than the rest of the face.

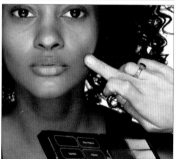

2 Check the side of the face as well as the forehead.

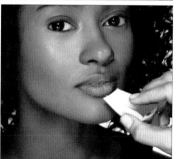

3 Apply lightest foundation color around the mouth.

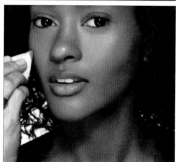

4 Use lighter color or mix light and dark foundation for cheeks.

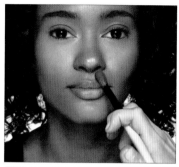

5 Apply warm-color face powder all over the face to set the foundation.

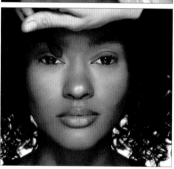

6 Apply yellow powder on lids.

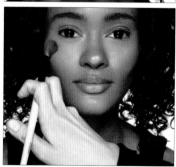

7 Apply yellow powder over concealer.

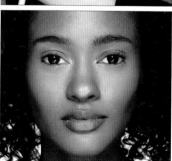

8 The end result is skin that is even and one tone.

SPECIAL SKIN CONDITIONS

Some faces need more than the basic application of foundation to look fresh and flawless. Others do best with the thinnest layer of expertly blended foundation. In special cases, you will need a skillful hand and specific application techniques. The best makeup artists recognize skin conditions, treat them appropriately, and use the perfect combination of product and technique to make the skin look its best. These product suggestions and techniques for various special skin conditions are basic guidelines. The trick is knowing when the makeup is working and when it needs to be changed. Experimentation is usually needed to achieve the desired results.

ROSACEA

A sheer, tinted moisturizer will diffuse redness. Too dense a product can make the face look masklike. Correct with a bronzer.

COMBINATION SKIN

Use moisturizer on areas of dry skin and an oil-absorbing lotion on the T-zone. Use an oil-free foundation all over the face during the summer, consider a more moisturizing formula for the winter. Either formulation can be used on specific areas of the face as needed.

EXTREMELY DRY SKIN

Use rich moisturizer followed by a creamy, moisturizing foundation. Don't use powder. Balm or oil can be applied lightly on top of foundation.

BLEMISHES

Using a concealer brush, apply oil-free cover stick or foundation to the blemish. Try to match the skin tone exactly. Concealers, which are a shade or two lighter than the face, should not be used on blemishes. Pat the area lightly. Do not rub. Blend into a small area directly around the blemish. Powder to lock the product(s) in place. Continue with foundation.

HYPERPIGMENTATION (IN GENERAL)

Apply a foundation tone or spot concealer a shade lighter than the skin to the affected area with a small brush. A bronzing gel can be blended into the skin starting at the cheek area, working around the face. This will help blend the more pigmented skin. Layer foundation that matches your skin tone over the concealer and/or gel for a flawless finish. Experiment, as concealer alone is often too light and will highlight the spot rather than cover it effectively. Set foundation with powder.

BIRTHMARKS AND PORT-WINE STAINS

Several layers of concealer are needed to cover areas with very dark pigmentation. First, apply a pale yellow–toned foundation or concealer that is three to five shades lighter than the skin tone. Then, apply one that is only slightly lighter than the overall skin tone. Finally, apply a full-coverage foundation that matches the skin tone. Set with powder. Again, experiment to find the right tone and formulations to effectively cover very dark spots.

SCARS AND TATTOOS

It may not be possible to cover scars and tattoos completely. If stick foundation or cover stick does not cover them, try using Covermark, a heavy-duty concealer designed for tattoos and scars. Apply foundation that matches skin tone to the whole face, and set with a powder that matches the skin tone.

UNEVEN SKIN

Skin is sometimes darker through the forehead or through the area of the lower mouth. Two different tones of foundation can be used to match each of the skin tones. Blend well to create an even transition between tones. Bronzer can be used over foundation to even out skin tone. A gel bronzer applied to moisturized skin prior to foundation evens the skin as well. Foundation can then be applied where needed.

FRECKLES

Rather than using a heavy foundation to conceal freckles, let them show through. Use a tinted moisturizer that evens out skin tone, and consider using a bronzer to finish.

ACNE

Start with the right skincare regimen, and use oil-free moisturizers. Apply blemish cover stick with a small, clean brush, or spot conceal with an opaque foundation only in those areas where needed. Use a tinted moisturizer or lightweight liquid foundation to even out the skin tone. The trick is to blend away the discoloration without applying heavy coverage.

WRINKLES

Hydration is the key to creating smooth-looking skin. Exfoliate regularly with a gentle scrub or an alpha hydroxy acid cream. Use water-infused hydrating ultrarich moisturizers and creamy makeup formulas. For lines around the lips, use a lip balm. Choose a creamy lipstick and matching pencil to prevent feathering.

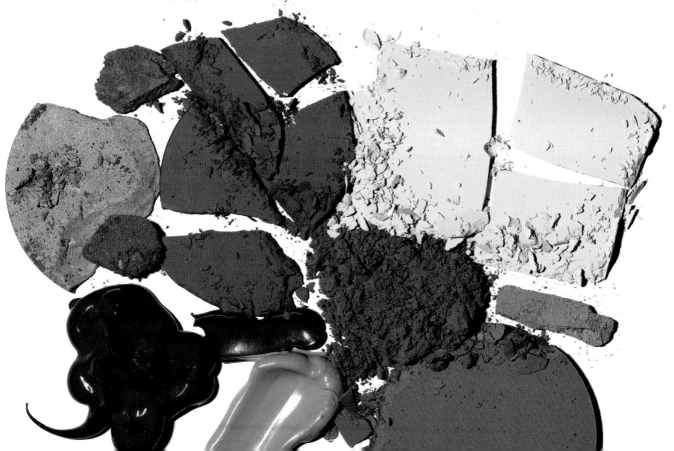

POWDER

A light dusting of powder sets concealer and foundation for hours, keeping the skin looking fresh.

Choosing the Right Powder

Color

Like foundation, powder works only when it is the right shade. For most people, the right powder has a yellow undertone. While the color of the powder will vary to match the foundation, it is the yellow-toned base that will give warmth to the skin. White powder is right only for those with alabaster skin. Translucent powder is not invisible or transparent and only makes skin look ashy.

Texture

Pressed powder is best for touch-ups. It dispenses a small amount and comes in a convenient compact. It is great for those who like a very natural look. Loose powder is denser and provides more coverage. Depending on the application technique, loose powder can be matte or sheer. Not everyone needs powder. Those with very dry skin might use powder only to set under-eye concealer.

Tools

The right tools will supply the perfect amount of powder. Using a powder puff will give powder a smooth, opaque finish. A powder brush will allow a sheer finish. A clean powder brush is also used to remove excess powder after an application with a powder puff. A small concealer brush can be used to apply powder to the corners of the face—under and around the eyes and around the mouth and nose.

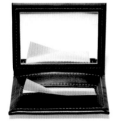

Tip

Oily skin can turn powder yellow or orange with time. Sometimes you have to choose a lighter color.

To avoid powder buildup on oily skin, use an oil-blotting paper before touching up.

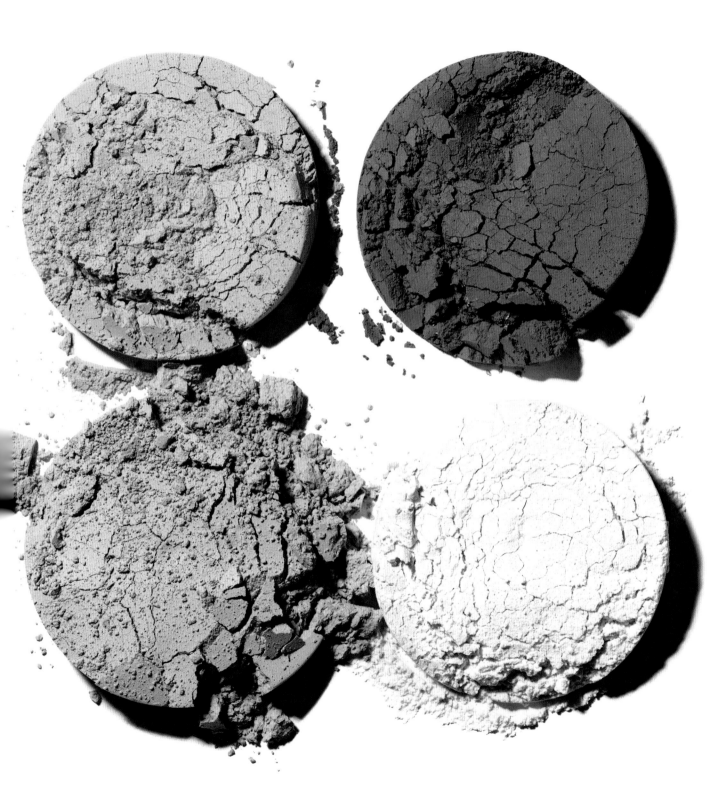

FACE POWDER APPLICATION

Some people with very dry skin can skip putting powder on the face. But everyone needs powder over concealer.

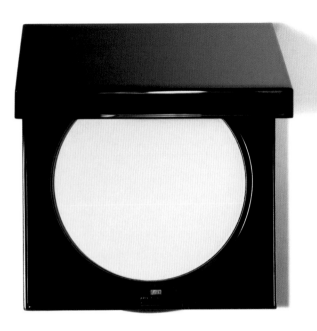

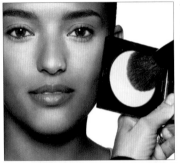

1
Choose the color according to the directions on page 66.

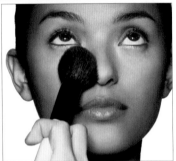

2
Apply powder with either a brush or a fluffy powder puff.

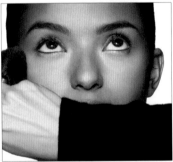

3
Dust the powder across the cheek and forehead.

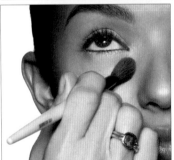

4
Switch brushes to apply powder on top of the concealer. This powder is often lighter in color than the face powder.

Troubleshooting: Powder

After an application of concealer, foundation, and powder step back and observe what you have done. Do the products blend seamlessly and invisibly into the skin? Do you see any darkness or redness? Do *not* continue with any other makeup until the skin looks the best it can. If you need to improve how the skin looks, stop and look. Can it be corrected with a bronzing product? Or should you begin again using a different product?

Ashy
Warm up the powder color and/or add bronzer.

Orange
Is the skin oily? Did it change? Switch to paler powder and wait to check the results.

Flaky
The skin is too dry.

Cakey
Make sure you have enough moisturizer on the skin. It's also possible to have too much. The foundation-to-moisturizer ratio may be giving the powder too much grab.

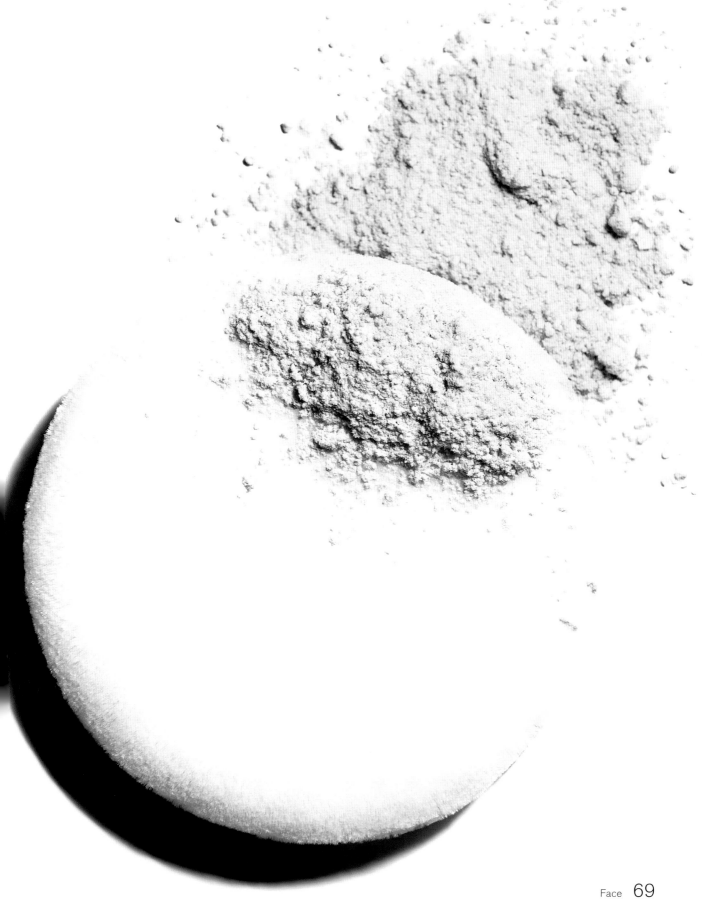

BRONZER & SELF-TANNER

Bronzers and self-tanners imitate the healthy look of the sun. They are also used as correctors to warm up the complexion. Applying bronzer is a great way to add a healthy glow all over the face and to even out color differences, especially through the neck. Bronzers work on all skin tones except porcelain because bronzer can make porcelain skin look dirty. Self-tanners can be used on the face and body to add color and hide flaws. When used on the face, apply self-tanner several hours before applying makeup, and don't forget your neck and ears (and remember to wash your palms with soap and water). Bronzer works as a blush for very dark skin. On all other skin tones, blush should be used over bronzer to add a pop of bright color.

Color: How to Choose

Bronzers work best when the skin looks natural. They can be brown-, red-, blue-, orange-, and sometimes yellow-based.

ALABASTER SKIN (Gwyneth Paltrow skin color)
Pinky shimmer or peach

LIGHT (Drew Barrymore)
Beigy brown with a bit of pink

MEDIUM (Sienna Miller)
Browny pink with only a bit of orange for warmth

MEDIUM-DARK (Jennifer Lopez)
Brownish orange

DARK (Vanessa Williams)
Brownish red

DEEPEST (Venus Williams)
Brownish blue

Formulas

Bronzers are available in flat or shimmering powder, gel stick, and cream formulas. Self-tanners are available in cream, gel, and spray, and are often mixed with moisturizer to get the best results.

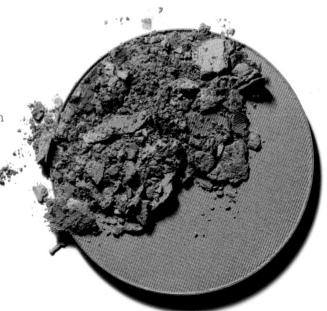

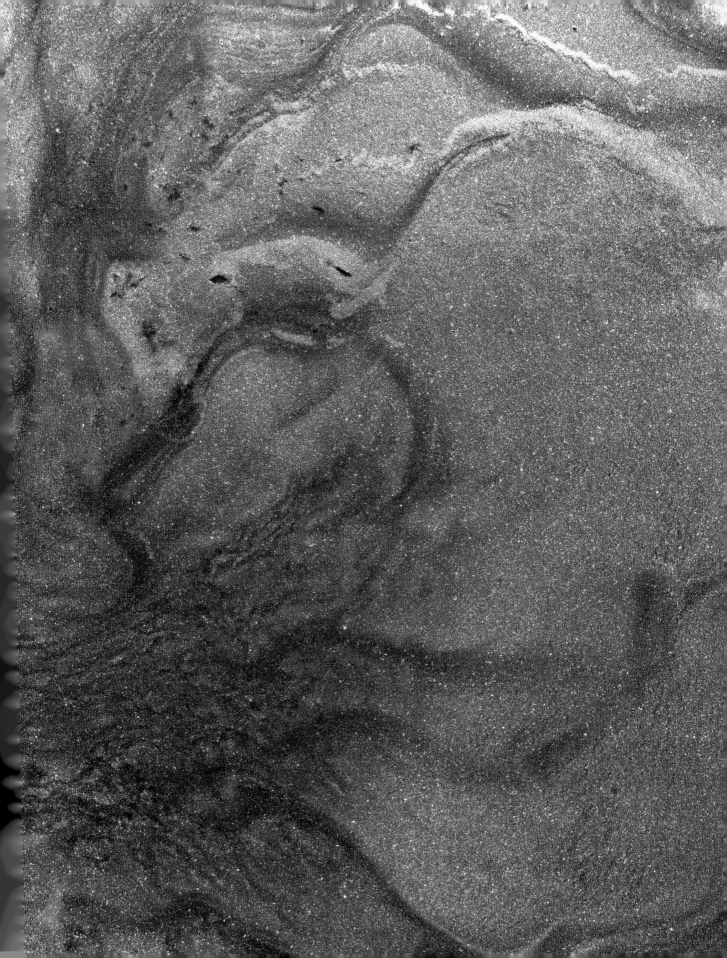

POWDER BRONZER APPLICATION

Powder bronzer is the easiest to apply. I use it to add a tint of color to the skin and to correct light foundation or red skin.

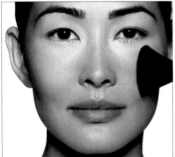

1

Using a large, flat brush, apply a small amount of bronzer for even distribution. Start on the apples of the cheeks.

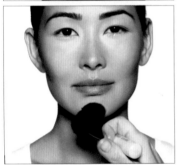

2

Next, dust over the nose and chin.

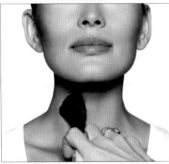

3

Brush bronzer onto the neck area.

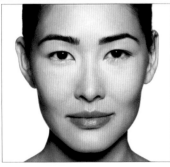

4

Turn the face to either side to make sure the color is well blended.

GEL BRONZER APPLICATION

This formula is sheer and can correct foundation if necessary, but it is a bit harder to blend than others. It works well on men.

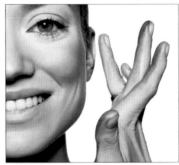

1

Choose the color to enhance your natural shade.

Begin at the apple of your cheeks.

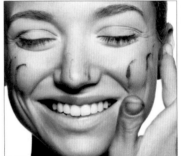

2

Gently apply bronzer to the cheeks, forehead, nose, and chin. Apply lightly. You can always add more.

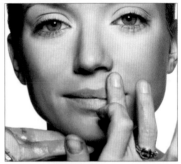

3

Apply bronzer lightly to the areas around the lips, forehead, neck, and ears.

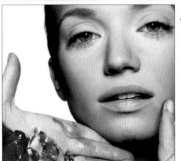

4

Blend with a clean hand. Add more bronzer if necessary.

Bronzers as Correctors

Some women have more color on their face and chest and less on their neck. Use bronzer to warm up the paler skin on the neck. For those with very red areas, sunspots, or rosacea, bronzers can be used to even out the skin tone.

Self-Tanner

Use self-tanners to add color to any area of the body including the face. It's an easy way to mask cellulite and veins on the legs. On the face, self-tanner can brighten up a tired complexion. It can be difficult to decide which product to use so it's important to test in a hidden spot before applying all over.

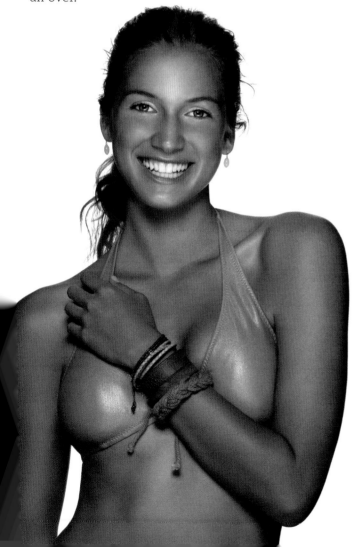

Self-Tanner Application

Prepare the skin. Always apply self-tanner to clean, smooth, makeup-free skin. It is best to exfoliate first if there are any rough patches. Knees, elbows, and heels are often areas with coarse, dry skin.

Apply a light, even layer. Wait for the color to develop, and then apply a light second coat for a deeper tan. It is easier to build color than to fix mistakes.

Do not forget to apply the product to the neck and ears for a natural-looking result.

Wash your hands immediately after using self-tanner. The product will stain palms and the skin between the fingers.

Wait ten minutes after applying self-tanner to the face before applying any other makeup or getting dressed.

Most self-tanners take an hour or more to develop into a "tan," so plan ahead.

Troubleshooting: Dark or Streaky Self-Tanning Results

Fade overly dark color by exfoliating the skin in the shower with a washcloth or loofah. Then, thoroughly clean the skin with cold cream or baby oil. Some self-tanners can be removed with lemon juice. Fix streaks by applying an additional light coat of self-tanner on the lightest parts of the skin.

BLUSH

Blush is used to create a healthy, pretty look. Blush can also be used to create the dramatic contouring sometimes seen in fashion shows and the theater.

Pick a skin-type-appropriate formula that you find easy to use. Different formulas can be used, depending on the desired finish or time of year. For the most natural look, match the blush color to that of the cheeks when flushed from exercise. You can also pinch the cheeks and look at the tone; match that color. By holding several shades of blush next to the cheek, you will see which add a lift and can eliminate those that are too dull or orange. The right shade will add a pretty brightness to the face without looking obvious.

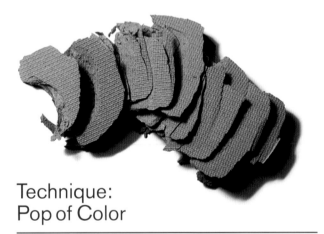

Technique: Pop of Color

Using two shades of blush, apply your natural color and then add a pop of a brighter color on top. The natural shade looks great at first, but often fades easily. The brighter shade alone is often great for evening, but too much of a contrast for every day. This layering technique offers natural brightness. When using a bronzer, skip natural color and layer the pop color on top. Using a natural shade on top of bronzer makes the cheeks look dirty.

Blush Formulas

POWDER is the easiest formula to use. It blends easily and works on all skin types.

GEL delivers sheer color, but blending is a bit more difficult. It works well for smooth skin.

CREAM goes on smoothly and leaves a dewy finish, which is great for dry skin.

CREAM/POWDER goes on as cream and dries to a long-lasting powder finish. It is best for normal skin.

CHUBBY PENCILS are very portable and easy to blend. They are best for normal to dry skin.

CHEEK TINTS are similar to gels. They go on sheer for a stained look and can be difficult to blend. Tints work only for smooth skin.

POT ROUGE provides blendable color for normal to dry skin types. These products are usually creamy in texture and packaged in pots. They provide a sheer stain on the cheeks and medium coverage on the lips.

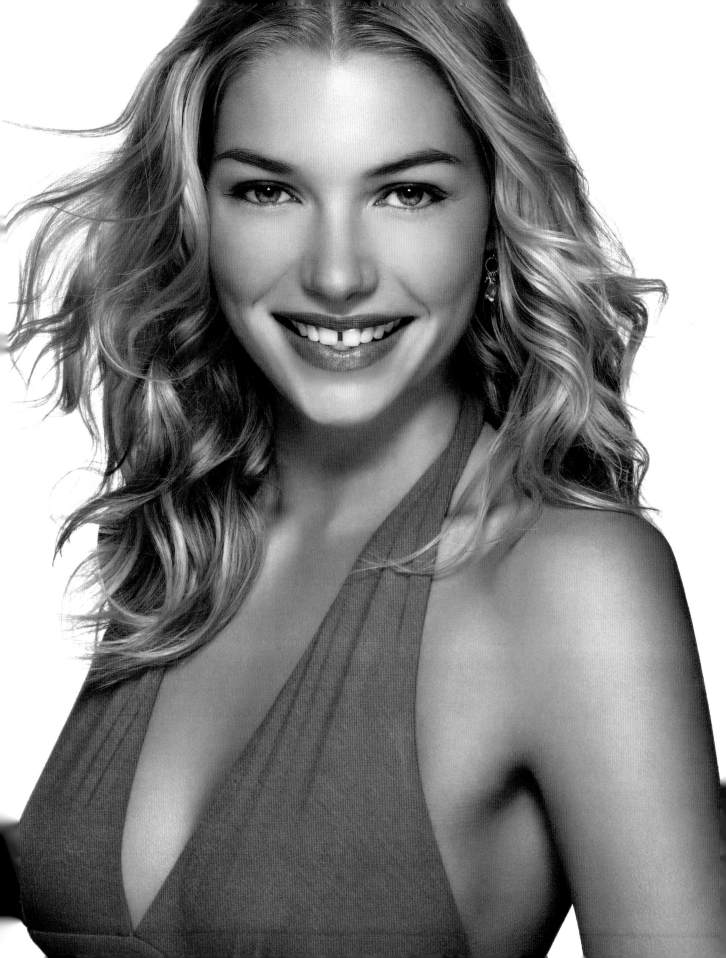

POWDER BLUSH APPLICATION

Powder is the easiest blush formula to use. Make sure your brush is totally clean, or it will affect your color choice.

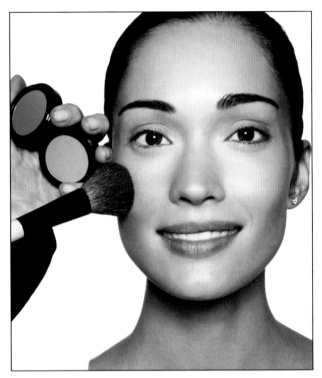

1 Smile and apply the product to the apple of the cheeks.

2 Blend toward the hairline, then down to soften the edges.

3 Blend thoroughly, keeping the most product on the highest part of the cheekbones.

4 Step back and consider the results. Turn your head to each side. Your face should look absolutely natural and balanced. A powder puff or fingers can be used to soften and correct a heavy application.

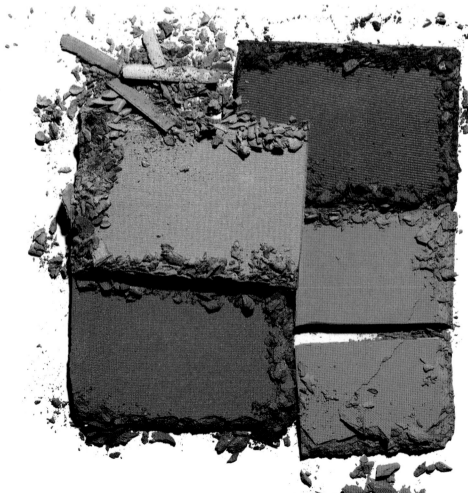

Tip

Never use blush on the eyelids as it is too red and will make the eyes look sore and tired.

CREAM & GEL BLUSH APPLICATION

Cream and gel formulas should be saved for smooth skin. Powder formula is better for textured or blemished skin.

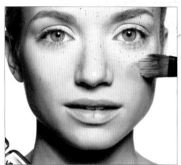

1

Apply over clean skin or foundation. The product can be applied with fingers, a foundation brush, or a sponge.

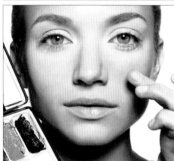

2

Use sparingly at first. You can always add more product if needed.

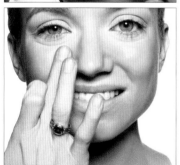

3

Smile, and apply the product to the apples of the cheeks and up toward the hairline, then down to soften the edges.

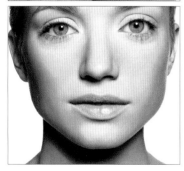

4

Blend thoroughly, keeping the most product on the highest part of the cheekbones.

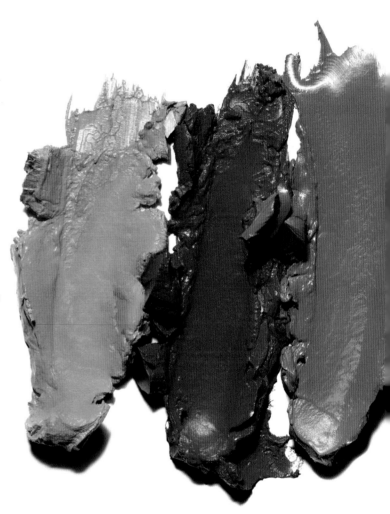

Troubleshooting: Blush

Blush streaks
Your foundation probably wasn't powdered, or you've used too much moisturizer under the foundation.

Looks flat
Layer cream rouge or balm on top of the color for a glow.

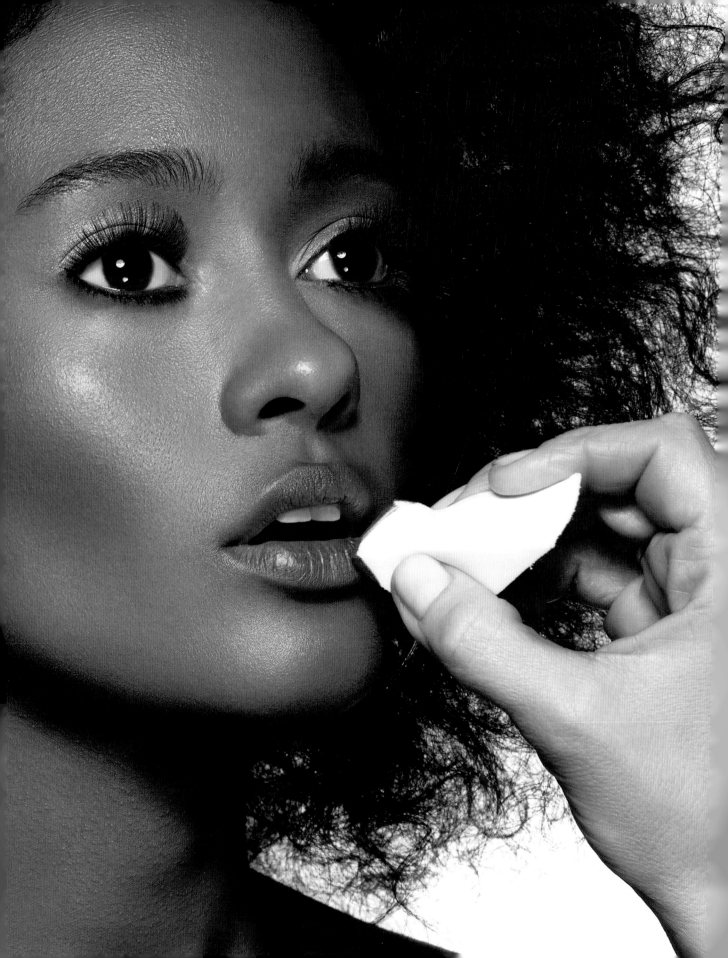

Chapter 5

LIPS

Applying lip color is one of the simplest of all makeup steps and is **a great way to instantly change a look.** Lip color applications range from simple, blotted-on stains to combinations of lip pencil, lipstick, and gloss. The right shade works with the skin tone and complements the natural color of the lips. You can choose from a wide range of product formulas, which include matte, sheer, shimmery, and creamy lipsticks and glosses.

COLOR & APPLICATION

Finding the Perfect Shade

To identify the best basic lip color, remove all makeup. The perfect neutral shade—pinky brown, nude, beige pink, rosy brown, pink, chocolate, or blackberry—will generally be close in tone to the natural lip color. The one that looks good on the naked face is the right neutral, everyday, mistake-proof color. It should not look ashy, orange, or pink but like an enhanced version of the natural lip color. Some women might need more color, and the shade that works best without makeup could be bright or dark rather than neutral. You know you have found the right shade when it enhances the skin tone, makes the eyes look brighter, and gives the face a lift.

Once you have identified the right neutral or everyday shade of lip color, you have the basis for selecting more dramatic colors. Most lip colors with the same undertone as the natural shade will look flattering.

Guide for Selecting Lip Color

NATURAL COLOR OF LIPS	LIPSTICK SHADE				
Pale Lips	beige	sandy pink	light coral	pale pink	bright red
Medium Lips	brown	rose	pink	orange	warm red
Dark Lips	brown	deep red	plum	deep chocolate	deep raisin/berries
Two-toned Lips	chocolate	blackberry	deep plum	deep raisin	deep red

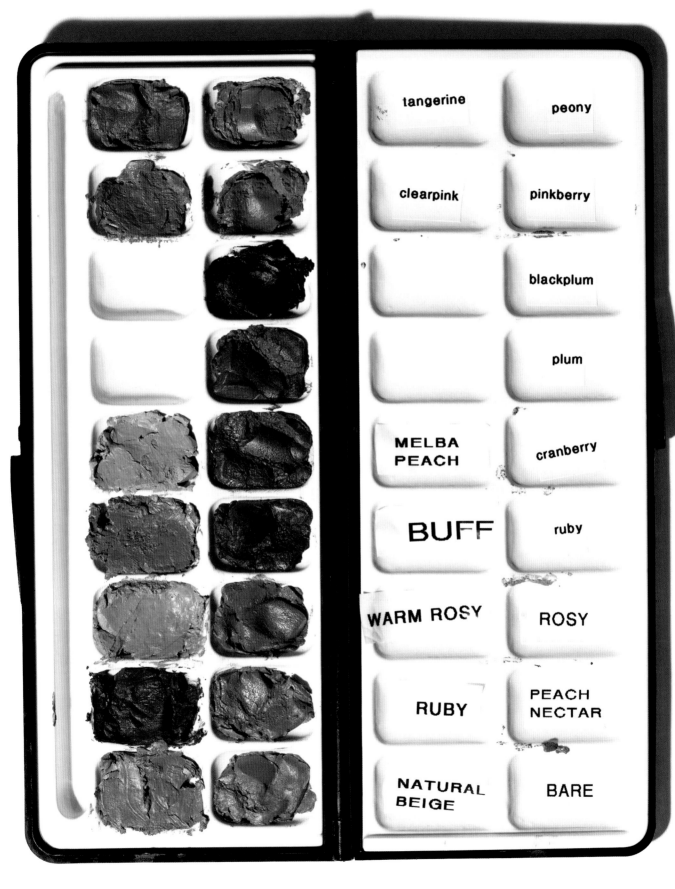

tangerine

peony

clearpink

pinkberry

blackplum

plum

MELBA PEACH

cranberry

BUFF

ruby

WARM ROSY

ROSY

RUBY

PEACH NECTAR

NATURAL BEIGE

BARE

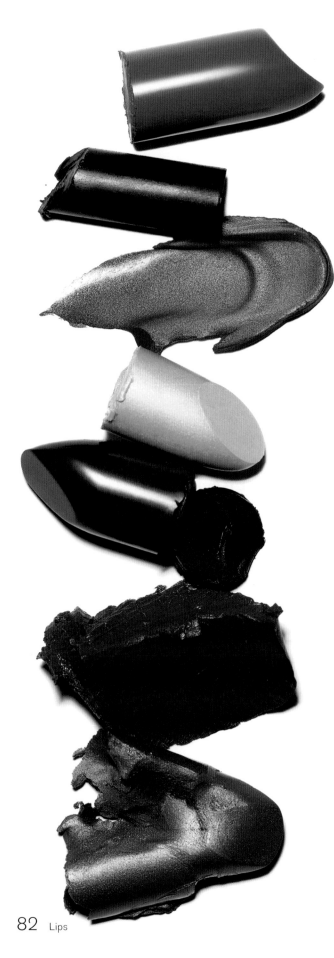

Formula

MATTE PRODUCTS are dense and last longest. They contain less moisture than other products, so they adhere to the lips and don't fade as quickly. They are not appropriate for very dry lips.

SEMIMATTE PRODUCTS are less dry than matte products and don't last as long. They work best on textured or dry lips and give off a soft sheen.

SHEER COLORS are see-through, forgiving, and easy to use.

STAINS provide long-lasting, highly pigmented color.

TINTS, like sheer glosses or balms, protect the lips with moisturizing formulas that usually contain sunscreen.

BALMS are tinted or clear formulas and help soften the lips.

GLOSS STICKS are hybrids, between sheer lipstick and gloss. They add a bit more pigment than lip gloss does but both are see-through and moist.

LIP GLOSSES provide hydration, sun protection, and sheen. This formula is great for making the lips look fuller and for layering on top of other lip colors.

CHUBBY LIP PENCILS will both define lips and provide a creamy matte texture. They are long lasting but can be a bit dry.

LIP LINERS define the lips and keep lipstick on longer when used on the entire lip area.

LIP COLOR APPLICATION

Mixing and blending are fun but it's always great to find a color that works directly out of the tube. Never buy a color that the makeup artist has to "fix" to work on you.

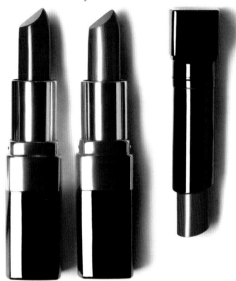

Troubleshooting: Lip Color

For pale lips use pastel shades, such as pale pink or light beige. Deep tones appear very dark on pale lips, so apply them with a light hand.

Very dark lips look best with blue-toned and deep, saturated lip color. Very pale shades of lipstick can appear gray or ashy on dark lips.

For uneven colored lips that are either dark with pink inside the lower lip or one darker and one lighter lip, you can choose to enhance or conceal the natural colors. Use a light shade that corresponds to the lighter lip color to enhance and bring out the paler lip, or use a deeper shade for a dramatic, full-coverage look. To even out tone, use a sheer, dark lipstick as a base on the lighter area, and then apply regular lipstick.

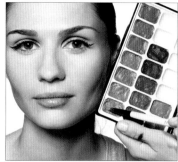

1

Choose the color and apply it using a lip brush or directly out of the tube.

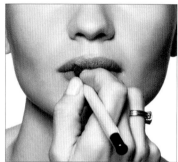

2

Beginning at one corner of the mouth, apply an even layer of color over the entire lip area.

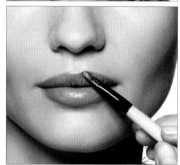

3

Keep the color within the natural lines of the lips. Use the brush to accurately line the lips.

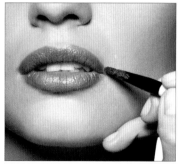

4

Continue the application to the other corner of the mouth. Always apply the color into the corners on both top and bottom lips.

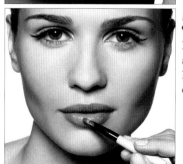

5

Fill in the bottom lip and any missed areas. Press your lips together to evenly distribute the color.

LIP PENCIL APPLICATION

It's so much easier to match the lip color than to use a dark color that has to be blended.

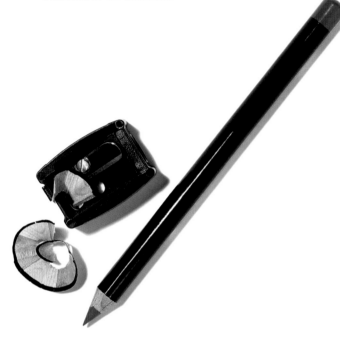

Tips for Long-Lasting Color

Some lip color products are long-lasting, but often those formulas are far too dry. Here are some techniques that provide extended wear to regular lipstick formulas.

Use a lip pencil that matches the natural color of the lips to line and completely fill in the lips. This base helps hold lip color in place. Layer lipstick on top.

Use pencil on top of lipstick to create a waxy barrier.

Blotting lipstick with your finger presses color into the lips and will create a stain that will last.

A bit of powder or blush patted on top of lipstick will keep it on longer.

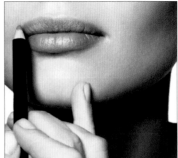

1
Begin by choosing color that matches the lips or lipstick. Begin lining the top lip.

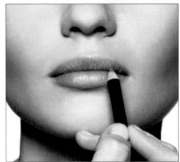

2
Extend the line across the top lip.

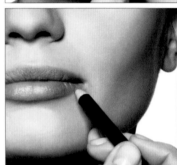

3
Define the line across the bottom lip.

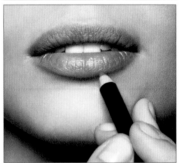

4
Line underneath the lower lip.

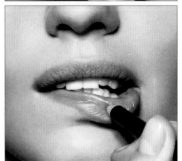

5
Fill in any missed areas and blend.

LIP GLOSS APPLICATION

Lip gloss gives a nice shine and can make the lips look a bit fuller. Don't overdo it by applying too much.

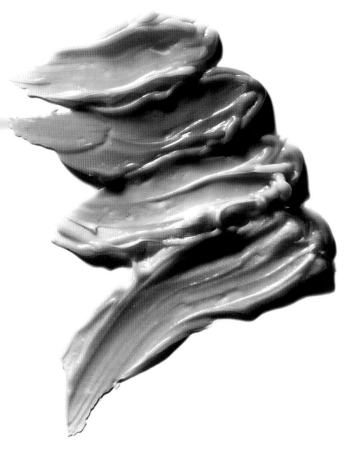

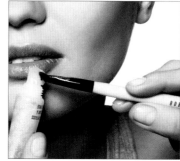

1

Apply gloss to a lip brush or directly to the lips.

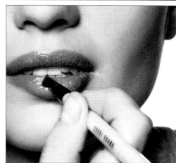

2

Using the brush or your finger, begin at the middle of the lips.

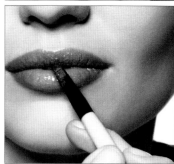

3

Apply gloss to both the top and bottom lips.

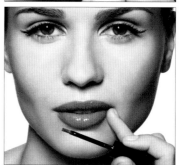

4

Wipe the edges of the lips when finished.

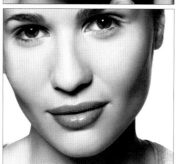

5

The lips look fuller and hydrated.

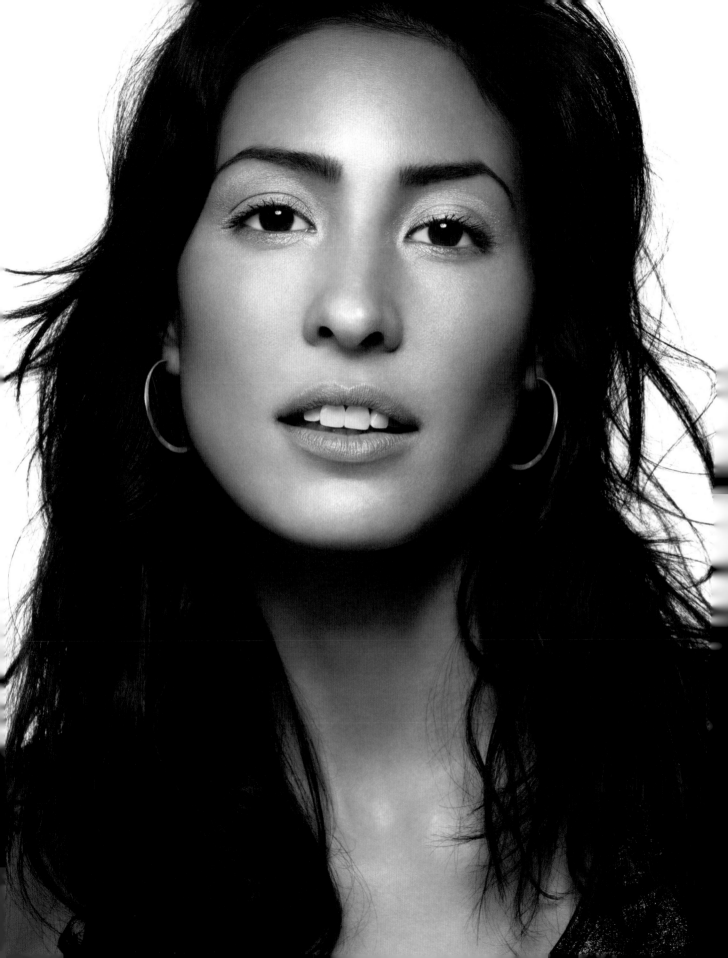

Chapter 6

EYES

The purpose of eye makeup—whether it's simple black mascara or dramatic contouring shadow—**is to make the eyes stand out.** When it's done right, eye makeup can give the appearance of **brighter, more beautiful eyes.** Here I cover the basics, like choosing flattering shades and lining the eyes, as well as advanced techniques, like creating a smoky eye and applying false lashes.

EYEBROW SHAPE & DEFINITION

You have seen what a difference a great frame can make to a painting. It is the eyebrows that form a frame for your eyes. Beautifully groomed eyebrows make a huge difference. It is possible to transform a face with just tweezers, shadow, a brow brush, and brow gel. A professional will help you find your ideal shape. Once the brows have been groomed, it is easy to do your own upkeep.

All brows benefit from added definition. Brow brushes and combs quickly tame and shape the brow hair. Brow shapers define, control, and shape the brows quickly and easily while adding just a bit of color.

Brow-Grooming Supplies

Brow brush

Brow pencil

Clear brow gel

Tinted brow gel

Brow shadow

Tweezers

Baby scissors for trimming extra-long or curly hair

Color Chart for Eyebrows

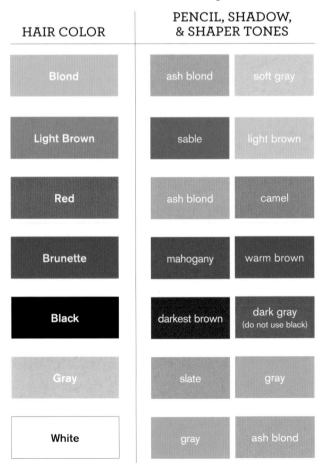

HAIR COLOR	PENCIL, SHADOW, & SHAPER TONES	
Blond	ash blond	soft gray
Light Brown	sable	light brown
Red	ash blond	camel
Brunette	mahogany	warm brown
Black	darkest brown	dark gray (do not use black)
Gray	slate	gray
White	gray	ash blond

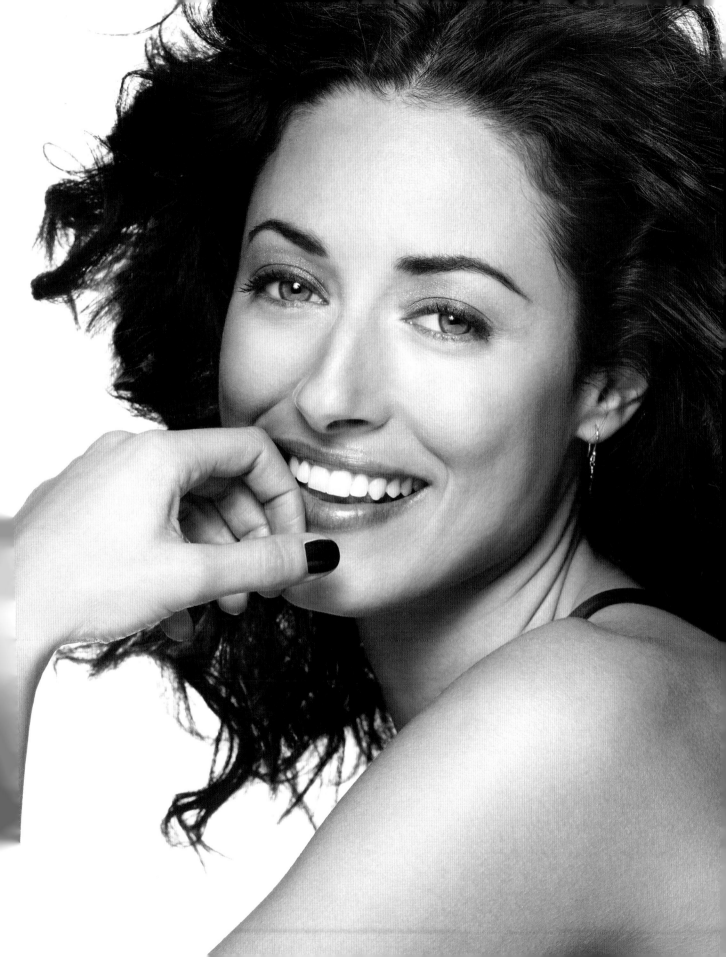

HOW TO SHAPE BROWS

The start of the brow should follow an imaginary line drawn from the outside of the nose to the inside corner of the eye.

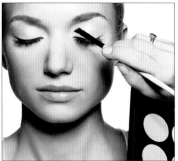

1

Choose the color that matches your eyebrows and hair.

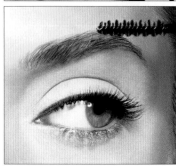

2

For a natural option, use eyebrow mascara to create the look of a natural brow.

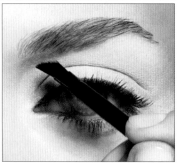

3

For more definition, use powder shadow. Start at the inner corner of the brow. Make sure you fill in all the gaps in the brow hair.

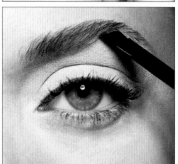

4

Bring the brush to the center, creating an arch, and then turn the brush and go down.

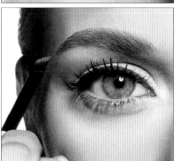

5

Make sure the brow is long enough.

Special Cases

Nonexistent brows

Brows damaged by overtweezing, age, or chemotherapy can be drawn in to look quite natural. Use a pencil the color of original brows, and softly draw in the shape. Layer a complementary color of powder shadow with a brow brush to fill in and soften.

Bare spots

Bare spots can be filled in with light strokes of pencil or with powder shadow. If neither works, try layering both.

Brows too far apart

Brows too far apart can be corrected by filling in missing brow areas with light pencil strokes. Balance the brows carefully. Layer powder shadow on top.

Tadpole brows

Tadpole brows can be reshaped with shadow. Fill them in to create a straight line.

ASIAN BROWS

Asian women often have sparse brows and need to fill in the brows to match a full head of hair.

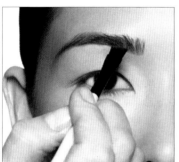

1
Begin at the inside of the brow.

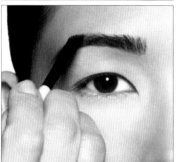

2
Fill in the brow using a shade that matches it. Use the powder to add density so it matches the hair on your head.

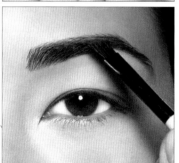

3
Lightly stroke along the length of the brow.

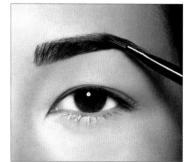

4
Continue all the way up the arch, turning the brush as it goes down.

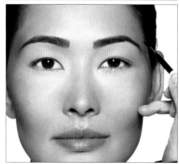

5
Make sure the brow is long enough.

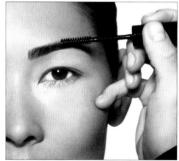

6
Use a clear eyebrow mascara to brush up an unruly brow.

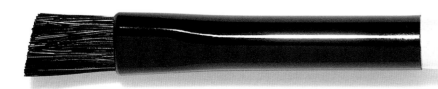

TWEEZING

It's best to get a professional shaping to begin. It's easier for upkeep. Tweezing after the shower is less painful than at other times.

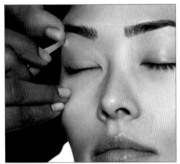

1
Begin by cleaning under the arch of the eyebrow. Remove a few hairs at a time, checking the results as you go.

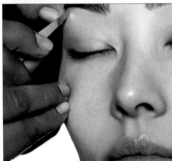

2
Slowly tweeze, moving inward toward the thickest part of the brow.

Tip

Some unruly brows will benefit from trimming long hairs with baby scissors.

Grooming Brows

To fill obvious holes or lengthen overplucked brows, use either pencil alone or a pencil-to-powder method. Using an eyebrow pencil in a shade that matches the brow color, fill with a light, feathery stroke, mimicking the look of hair. If using a powdered eye shadow, choose one that closely matches the hair and brow color. Using a stiff, flat, angled brow brush, pick up a small amount of color, and tap off the excess. Lightly stroke the shadow from the inner corner of the brow along the entire length to fill it in. Stroke color along the upper edge of the brow to accentuate the arch and give a "lift" to the eye area.

Apply shadow color only to the hair of the brows.

Finish with a coat of clear brow gel to set and tame any unruly brow hairs.

Look at your brows. Does the shape and intensity of color look natural and balance the face? A dusting of powder can soften the color if needed. Use a brow shaper to tame unruly brow hairs.

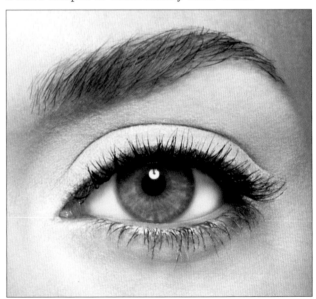

The Perfect Brow
The start of the brow should be aligned with the inner corner of the eye. The arch is three-quarters of the way across the brow from there.

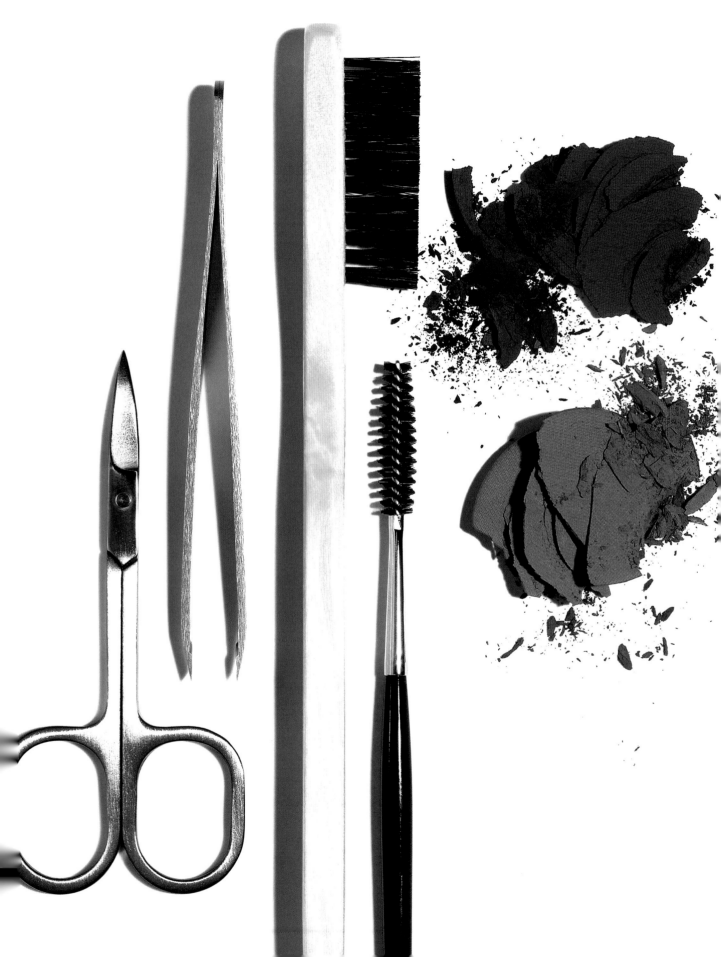

EYE SHADOW

Eye shadow helps accentuate the eye and makes eye color stand out. It is also used to correct eye shape.

Formula and Texture

Eye shadow is available in many formulas and textures: powder, cream, and pencil, matte, sheer, shimmery, glittery, creamy, glossy, etc.

The Basic Eye

Most of the time, a simple, natural look works best. For everyday application, pick shades of shadow that bring out the eye color rather than shadows that make a statement. The basic application is a simple, three-step process.

Crease Color or Contour

If you want to create depth or contour, choose a slightly deeper medium-toned shadow to sweep in the crease of the eye. Crease contour creates definition for puffy or deep-set eyes and can make a stronger eye statement for evening. Begin the shadow at the outside edge of the crease, and move inward with your brush. Softly layer the shadow, repeating and blending until you achieve the desired effect. Always use a blending brush or finger to create a smooth look.

Eye Shadow Color Chart

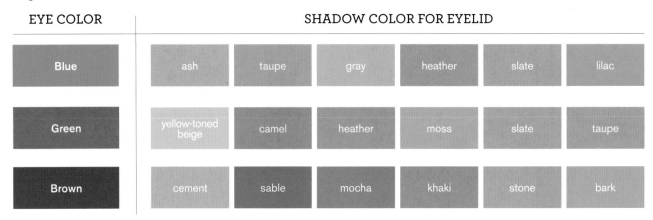

EYE COLOR	SHADOW COLOR FOR EYELID					
Blue	ash	taupe	gray	heather	slate	lilac
Green	yellow-toned beige	camel	heather	moss	slate	taupe
Brown	cement	sable	mocha	khaki	stone	bark

BASE EYE SHADOW APPLICATION

Use a light shadow color as a base on the lids; apply it with a full shadow brush that covers the entire lid from lash line to browbone. This step creates a clean slate for the other shadows. It also keeps moisture away from the lid and takes away any discoloration. For some women who prefer a clean eye look, this may be the only shadow that's needed.

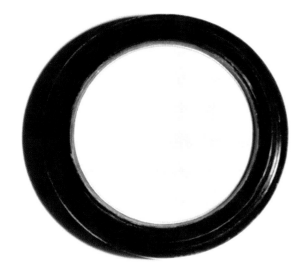

Tip

Avoid eye shadows with red and purple undertones if you have redness around the eyes, as these colors will make your eyes look tired. Stick with neutral, brown, or gray colors, but beware that some browns and grays have so much red in them that they should not be used.

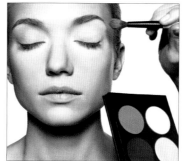

1 With a full shadow brush, apply a light shade (also known as your base color).

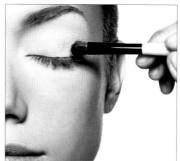

2 Apply color from the brow bone down to the lash line.

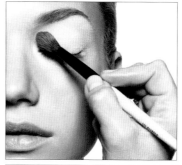

3 Don't forget to cover the inner corner of the eye.

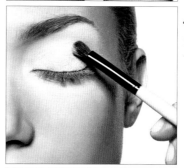

4 Brush all the way up to the brow.

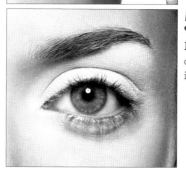

5 Make sure the eyelid is covered and the shadow is dense enough.

MEDIUM SHADOW & CONTOUR APPLICATION

This step starts with a color that doesn't need to be blended to deepen the lid. Next, a deeper color is layered as a contour.

Contouring for Eyes

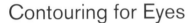

These tips can help change the look of your eyes, making them stand out or correcting a full, puffy eyelid.

Deep-set eyes need to be brought out with light and medium to deep medium shades of shadow. Colors that are too dark recede and will make the eyes look even more deep set.

Wide-set eyes will appear closer together with a sweep of shadow one to two shades darker than the foundation tone at the inner corner of the eye. When applying liner, thicken the line a bit at the inner corner, and do not extend it past the outer corner of the eye.

To make eyes look bigger, line your eyes all the way around.

To make eyes look more oval, top and bottom liner should meet at the outer corners. Then contour shadow from the lash line along the eyeliner outward and into the crease.

To make large eyes look smaller, use a soft shadow color as a liner at the lower lash line. The shadow should be several shades lighter than the top liner.

To make eyes look less puffy, apply contour shadow at the outer corners and blend it as you move in toward the nose.

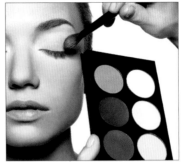

1
Choose a medium-tone shadow for the lid.

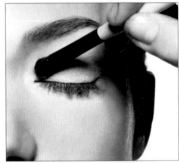

2
With a medium fluffy shadow brush, apply color to the lid.

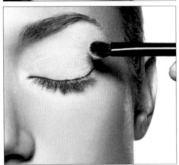

3
Continue applying from the lash line to the crease.

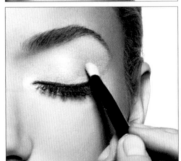

4
Layer a deeper medium shade on the outer corner and blend as you apply it. The correct shade will require little blending.

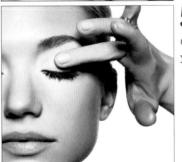

5
Continue blending with your fingers.

PLAYING WITH COLOR

Neutrals work for most applications but color is fun to play with.

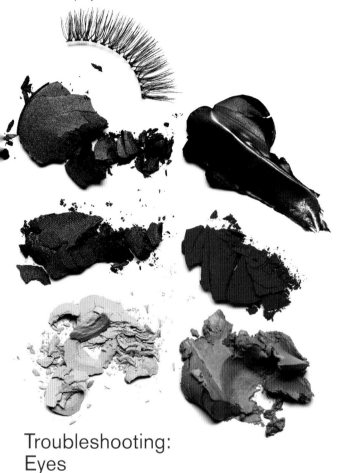

Troubleshooting: Eyes

Eye shadow flakes on the face.
First try a clean powder brush to sweep it off. If this doesn't work, use a nonoily makeup remover on a cotton swab or makeup sponge to gently clean the flakes off the skin. When creating a smoky eye, be sure to do the eyes first, clear the area of flakes, and then apply concealer and foundation.

You've made wings when trying to contour.
Using your finger or a cotton swab, wipe away, going up, and then blend toward the eye.

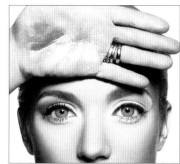

1 Choose a shade that you like.

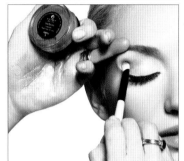

2 Cover the entire lid three-quarters of the way to the brow bone, blending as you go.

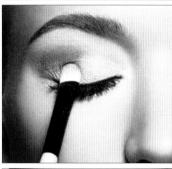

3 Layer with bold color.

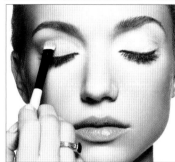

4 Blend the color with your fingers or a clean brush.

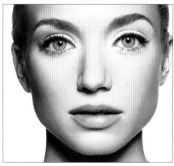

5 Experiment with different colors to find the shades you like most.

CREAM SHADOW APPLICATION

Choose a formula with or without powder in it. If it doesn't contain powder, be sure to apply it over powder.

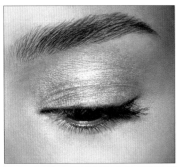

1
Apply cream shadow base or base powder color to hold the color on the eyelid.

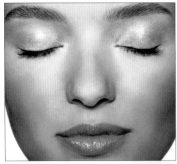

2
Apply cream shadow across the whole lid to three-quarters of the way up.

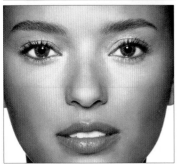

3
Make sure you apply shadow high enough on the lid and layer a second coat to be sure it's dense enough.

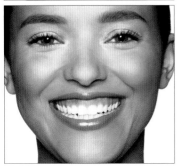

4
Check how the shadow looks. Add more as needed. You can use one or multiple colors.

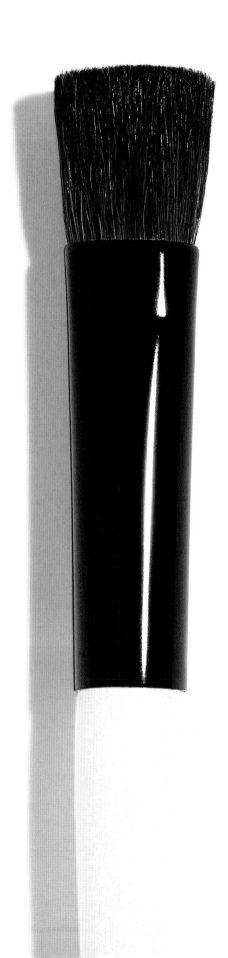

ASIAN EYE SHADOW APPLICATION

Always enhance the eye's natural shape and don't try to change it. It's never appropriate to use a dark color in the crease.

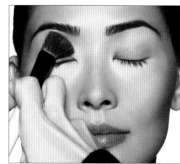

1

With a full shadow brush, apply a light shade (also known as your base color).

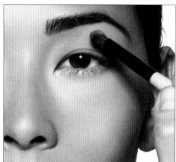

2

Choose medium-tone shadow for the lid and apply it three-quarters of the way up to the brow.

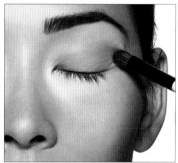

3

Sweep color all the way to the crease, blending as you go up.

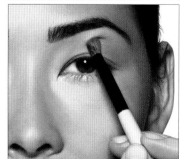

4

Apply a deeper color on top of the first color for density. Blend.

EYELINER

Eyeliner is the ultimate way to define and enhance the eyes. It frames the eyes, makes them appear larger, and really makes them stand out. Liner can also be used to improve the shape of the eyes. Its application needs to be generous enough to be visible when the eyes are open to make the most impact. Many women achieve a beautiful, defined look using liner only on the top lash line. For those who use liner on both top and bottom lash lines, it is important to keep the top thicker than the bottom. To avoid the appearance of tiredness and darkness under the eye, apply a relatively thin or smudged line as close as possible to the lower lash line.

Liner Formulas

There are several eyeliner formulations: powdered shadow, eye pencil, and liquid or gel liner. Each has its advantages and specific application techniques.

SHADOW LINERS are easy to apply, dry or damp, and can be long-lasting if applied correctly. Using shadow liner requires a good eyeliner brush—one that is thin, stiff, and flat, with either a straight or a slightly rounded tip.

EYELINER PENCILS are easy to apply but may smudge. Pencil liners have a creamy consistency that smears if they are not set with either eyeshadow or face powder.

LIQUID, CAKE, AND GEL LINERS are the most difficult to apply, but with practice, you can achieve incredible results. These liners are extremely long-wearing, very precise, and a good choice for creating dramatic looks.

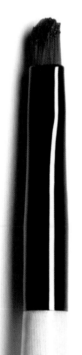

Special Techniques

Dark circles look darker when liner is applied on the lower lash line. Bring concealer up to the lash line, and use only mascara on the lower lashes.

Make eyes look more intense by double lining. Use a dark shadow with a dry eyeliner brush, then repeat with a liquid liner or wet brush using a slightly thinner line. The gradation in depth from the lash line will give a dense look to the lashes. The technique can also be reversed—gel can be softened with shadow.

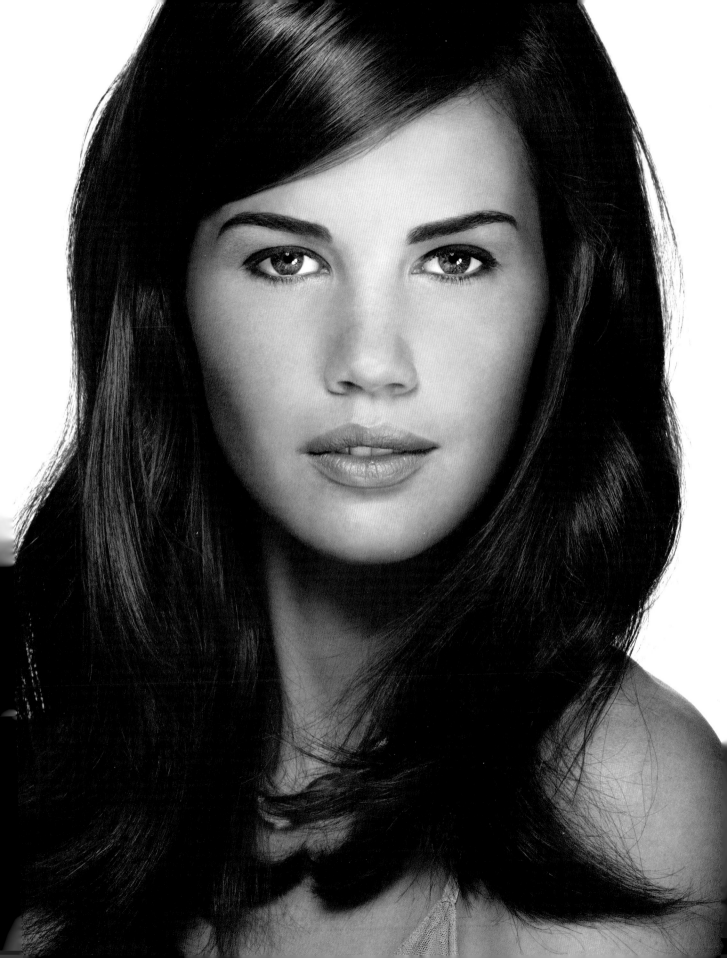

GEL, LIQUID & CAKE LINER APPLICATION

These formulas are the longest lasting. Mastering the techniques for using them will be worthwhile. Always line the whole lid across, with a thicker line at the outer corner, gradually thinning the line toward the inner corner.

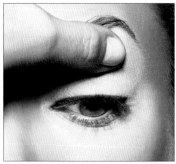

1
Begin lining in the middle of the lash line and move to the outside corner of the eye. Gently lift the lid to get close to the eye.

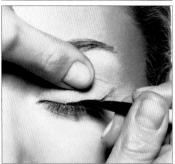

2
Apply the liner in smooth strokes.

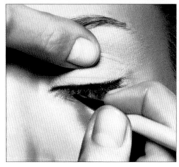

3
Next, apply the liner all the way to the inner corner of eye.

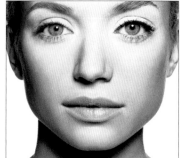

4
See the difference with one eye lined.

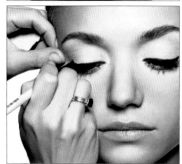

5
Repeat with the other eye.

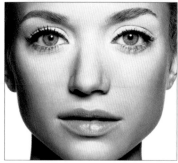

6
Note the difference when both eyes are lined.

Tip

Do not leave space between the eyeliner and the lash line. If, after application, there is a small space, fill it in with the same shade of powdered eye shadow.

PENCIL LINER APPLICATION

Pencils are easy to use but are not long lasting and can smear. Layering powder shadow on top will help with these drawbacks.

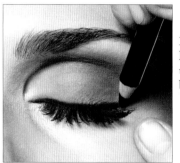

1

Draw the pencil across the lash line and blend gently using a clean finger or brush.

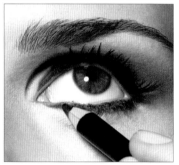

2

Using short feathery strokes can result in a more natural effect.

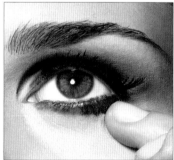

3

To soften, smudge the line using your finger or a brush.

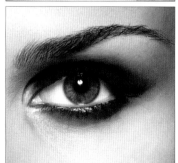

4

To give a pencil line staying power, use a liner brush to sweep a layer of powdered eye shadow in a corresponding shade over the pencil.

Eyeliner Dos & Don'ts

Don't apply liner to the inside rim of the eyelids, except for a theatrical effect or a fashion shoot. You risk infection and injury. And, rather than making the eyes stand out, lining inside the rim actually makes the eyes appear smaller.

Don't line just the bottom of the eye.

Do line all the way across the lids! You can line just the top and not the bottom, but don't line either lid halfway. Lining from the inner corner to the outer corner will help open up the eye.

Do apply liner as close as possible to the lash line, making sure there is no gap. This has the added benefit of making the lashes look fuller and lush.

Do apply liner thinnest at the inner corner of the eye, and thicken it as you move outward. This accentuates the eye's shape and gives the eyes a lift.

Do make the top and bottom lines of liner meet at the inside and outside corners to make the eyes appear larger. Not connecting the lines makes the eyelids appear too round and small.

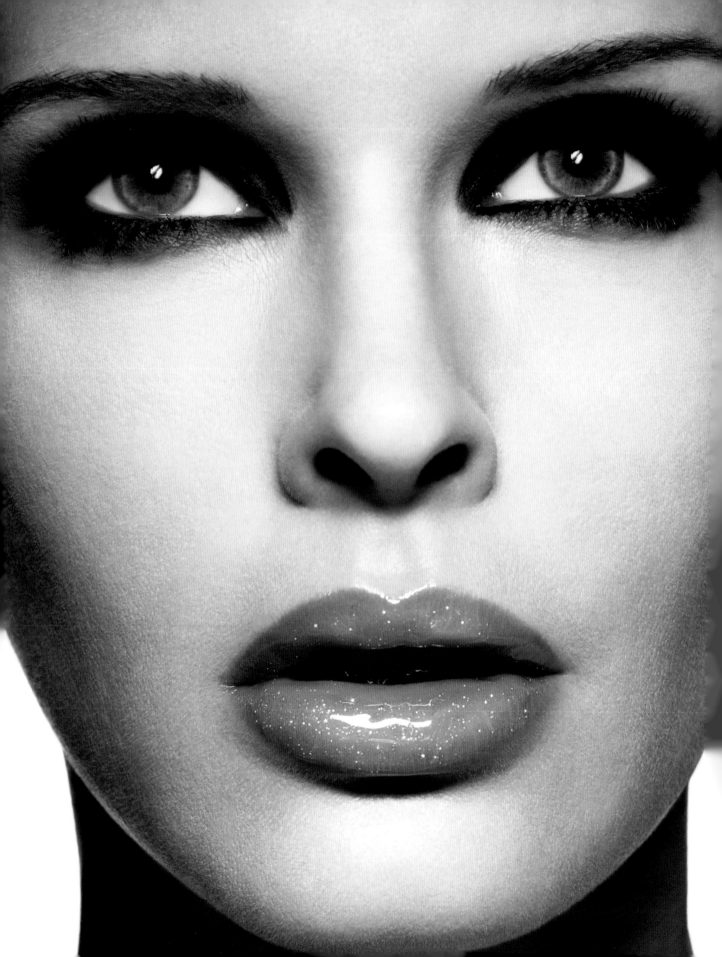

Special Effects

For evening or other special occasions, you may want to use bolder, more dramatic eye-makeup techniques.

Smoky Eyes

Prime the eye area with an all-over white base that will allow the darker colors to blend. Apply a slightly darker shadow on the lower lid, from the lash line up to the crease and use a deeper one in the same color family layered on top. The standard technique described above can be used to line the lower lashes, keeping the application lighter and balanced with the upper eye. Apply a double layer of liner, first using a dry brush and then a gel or pencil. Extend the liner line slightly beyond the outer corners of the eyes. Then reapply the liner a bit heavier and repeat two more times if desired. Always add multiple coats of mascara. Smudge and blend.

Glam Eyes

This look is great for New Year's Eve or the Oscars. Over a white base, layer cool colors, such as gray and slate. Build the depth of the color gradually, from the lash line to the crease. Finish with a strong liner application along the top lash line only, ending in an upward-sweeping point. Sweep a metallic or shimmery color over the lid layered from medium to dark. Finish with false lashes or three to four coats of black mascara.

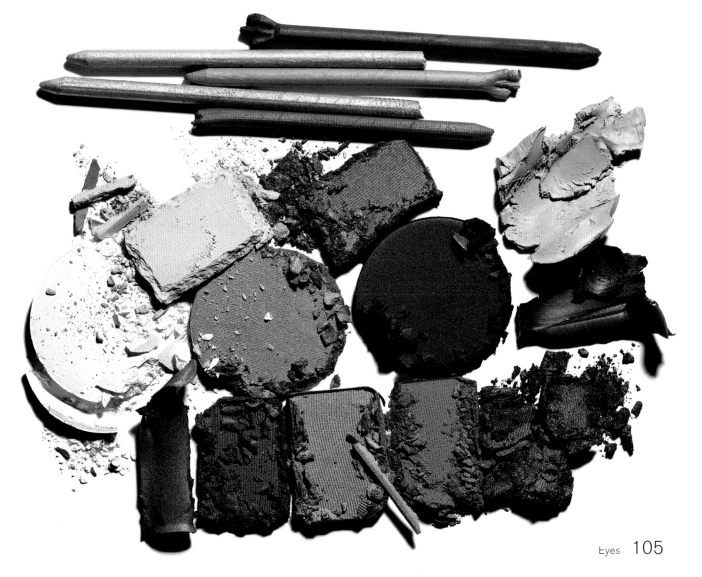

SMOKY EYE APPLICATION

A smoky eye is the most dramatic look for evening—it's pretty and sexy. Remember to keep layering the color and continue to check until you like the look.

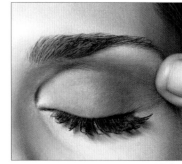

5
Use your finger to soften the shadow.

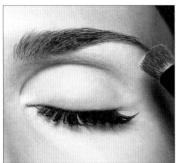

1
Start with white shadow on the entire lid.

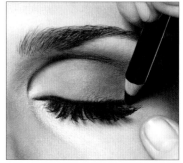

6
Start at the outside corner, using pencil or dark shadow or liner.

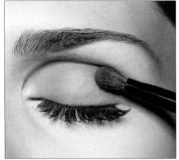

2
Choose a medium, smoky color for the lower lid. Apply it three-quarters of the way up.

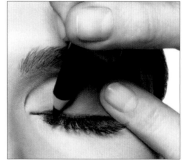

7
Apply in smooth strokes to the inner corner of the eyelid.

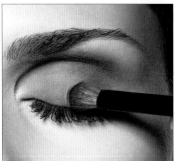

3
Continue to layer the color to make it darker. Add a deeper color on top and in the crease to intensify the look.

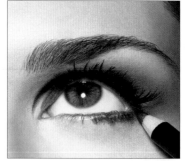

8
Line underneath the eye beginning at the outside corner, moving toward the inner corner.

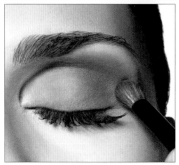

4
Concentrate on the crease. Continue to layer the shadow deeply enough to create a dramatic effect.

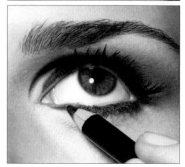

9
Line as close to the lashes as possible.

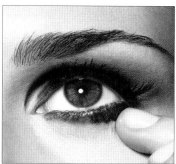

10

Soften the line using a clean finger or Q-tip.

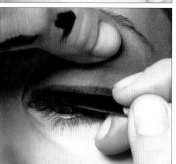

11

To give the pencil line staying power, use a liner brush to sweep a layer of eye shadow over the pencil.

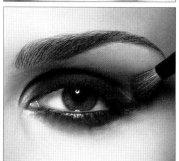

12

Smudge the line to create a smoky look, somewhere between liner and shadow. The liner can be thickened.

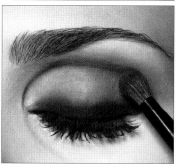

13

Reapply to add more definition. Continue layering and checking for the effect you desire.

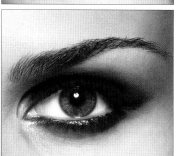

14

Final smoky eye.

For a more dramatic look, adjust your lip color.

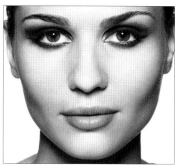

Smoky eyes with pale lip color.

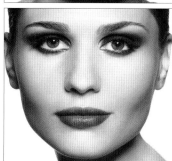

Smoky eyes with medium lip color.

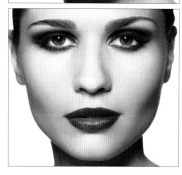

Dramatic look with smoky eyes and dark lipstick.

ASIAN LINER APPLICATION

For Asian women, lining the eyes is a very important step in making the eyes stand out.

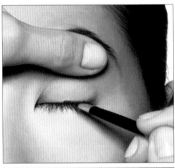

1
Gently pull the eyelid and start in the middle.

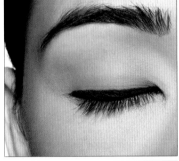

5
Repeat the steps on the other eye.

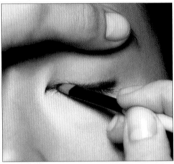

2
Go in close to the lashes.

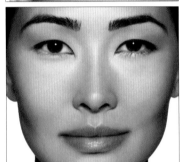

6
Lined eyes.

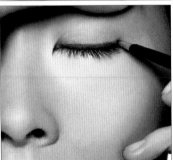

3
Extend the line all the way across.

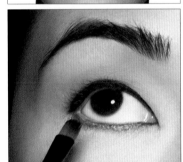

Optional:

If you choose to, line under the eye. Asian eyes look best with a very soft shadow line.

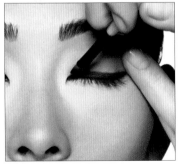

4
Reapply to make the line thicker.

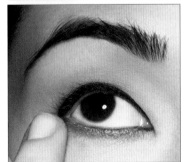

Blend the liner with your fingers.

ASIAN DRAMATIC LINER APPLICATION

It's important to check the result of the eyelining when the eyes are open. You need to make the lines thick enough to show.

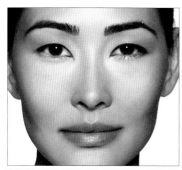

1

Simple eyeliner.

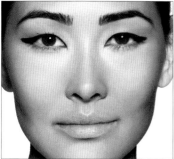

2

For more drama, make the line thicker.

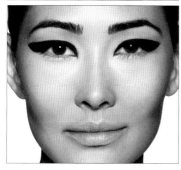

3

And thicker.

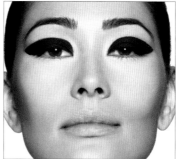

4

Or go way out.

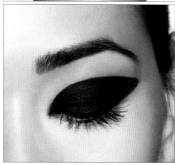

5

Make the line thicker along the lash line and see how far you want to go.

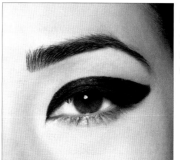

6

If you use strong eyeliner, skip the eye shadow in the crease.

Permanent Solution?

Just say no to tattooed liner. It never looks natural, and the color usually fades to an ashy gray or blue color over time. Deep brown eyeliner can freshen and help the line look natural again.

EYELASHES

Lashes open up and emphasize the eyes. Most lashes are transformed with a sweep of mascara and the use of an eyelash curler. Black mascara is always my first choice. For women with very fair coloring or those who have naturally blond lashes, mascara is a must. Product choices include mascara, curlers, and false lashes.

Formulas

THICKENING MASCARA is designed to make lashes appear fuller. To avoid clumping, wipe the wand before use; following application, the lashes can be separated with a lash comb, or separate them as you go.

LENGTHENING MASCARA is a thinner formula than the thickening product, so it lengthens lashes in a way that looks natural.

WATERPROOF MASCARA is great to use on those occasions when you anticipate tears or sweat, or in humid climates. The product can be removed only with an eye makeup remover specially formulated for waterproof products.

COLORED MASCARAS are fun for the very young and for making theatrical or fashion statements. Henna-colored mascara can work for those with light red hair.

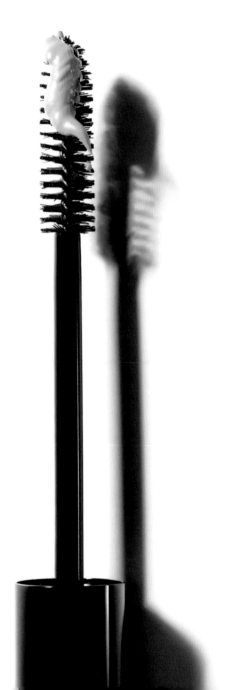

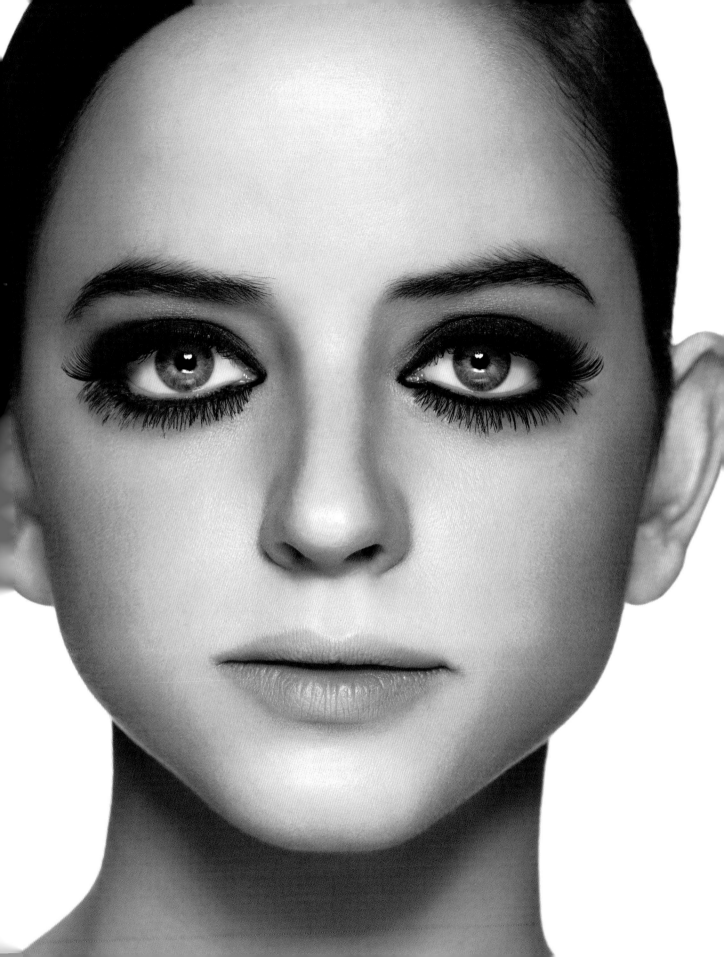

EYELASH CURLING

Start with clean lashes. Gently lift the lid, hold the curler in front, and move the arm up to curl lashes. Hold for five to ten seconds.

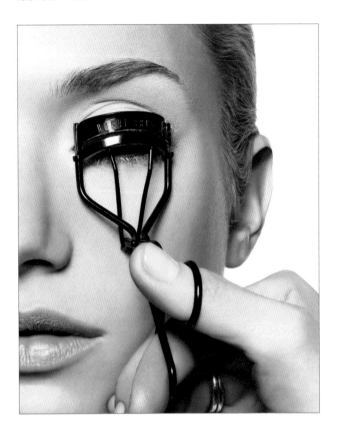

Tips

You can also curl lashes by gently pressing them up with your fingers as the mascara dries.

The blackest of black mascara makes eyes stand out the most.

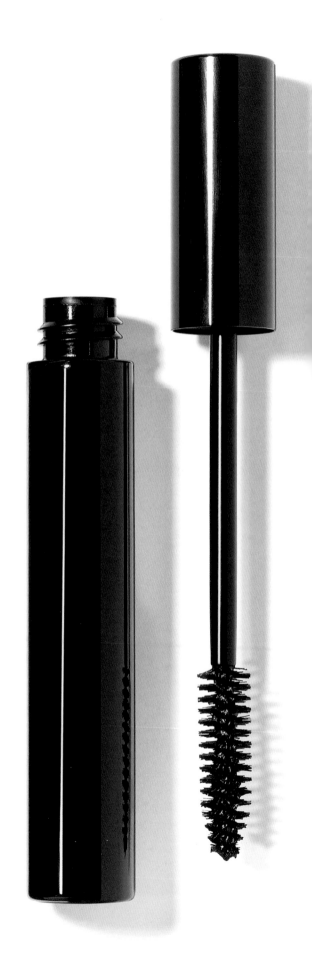

MASCARA APPLICATION

When applied properly, mascara will both define your eyes and make them stand out. Remember, you'll need two to three coats for impact.

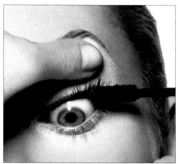

1

Wipe the tip of the wand. Gently lift the lid. Looking down, begin at the outside of the eye.

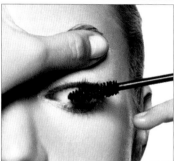

2

Move the wand in close to the nose.

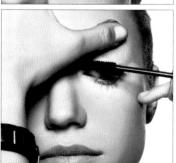

3

Be sure to apply mascara close to the base of the lashes.

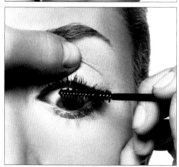

4

Separate the lashes as you go along.

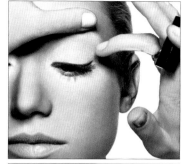

5

If you smudge the mascara, wipe it instantly before it dries.

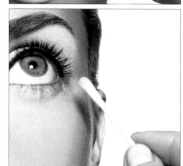

6

If mascara dries on your skin, use a Q-tip to clean it up with a bit of non-oily makeup remover.

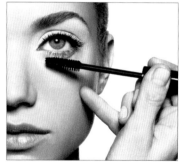

7

Wait a few seconds before beginning the lower lashes. Apply mascara lightly to the lower lashes.

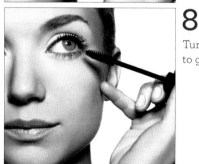

8

Turn the brush at an angle to get all the lashes.

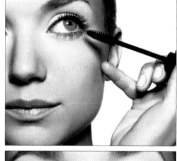
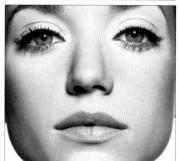

9

The finished product.

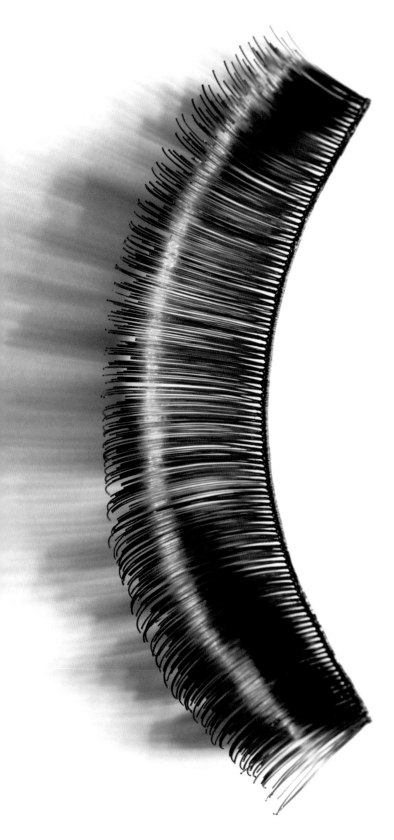

False Eyelashes

False eyelashes are used to create a more dramatic-looking eye and for special effects. Lashes can be applied individually, in a small section, or in a full band. Eyelash glue comes in white, clear, and black. I prefer black as it blends into the lash line.

Eye Makeup Removers

Eye makeup removers are available in liquid, lotion, and cream formulations. Find a product that thoroughly removes your eye makeup without causing any irritation or stinging. Generally, a non-oily product will remove makeup quickly and easily. However, when using waterproof makeup, oil-based removers are the most effective. Place a nickel-size amount of the product on a cotton ball, and gently press through the eye area to dissolve the makeup. If needed, repeat this process until the cotton ball comes away clean.

Troubleshooting: Eyelashes

There are many effective ways to create the illusion of lashes without false eyelashes.

Sparse eyelashes
For those with sparse lashes, try smudging dark shadow at the lash line with a liner brush and then applying two thin coats of mascara.

Pale lashes
Very light colored lashes sometimes don't look natural with black or very dark mascara. Try light brown or henna-colored mascara for a natural look.

No lashes
When lashes have been lost due to alopecia or chemotherapy, a double application of powder shadow in a smoky shade helps create the illusion of lashes. First, use a damp brush and powder shadow to line the lid close to the lash line, and then smudge the dry shadow from the lashes upward.

FALSE EYELASHES APPLICATION

This takes time, patience, and practice. Many women go to a professional to have them applied.

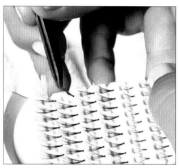

1
Use a lash tweezer to pick up a lash. Begin with small lashes.

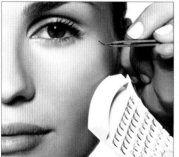

2
After dipping the lash in glue (use dark glue instead of clear) give it a few seconds to air dry partially.

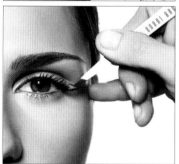

3
Start at the outside of the eye.

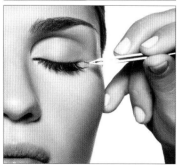

4
Close your eye to continue the application.

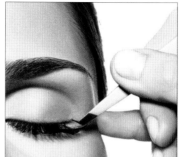

5
Gently build the lashes toward the center, using five to ten lashes.

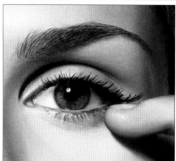

6
Use your finger to hold each lash until it dries.

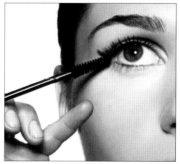

7
After the glue dries, apply mascara.

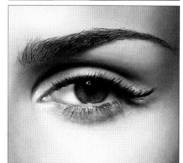

8
The finished product.

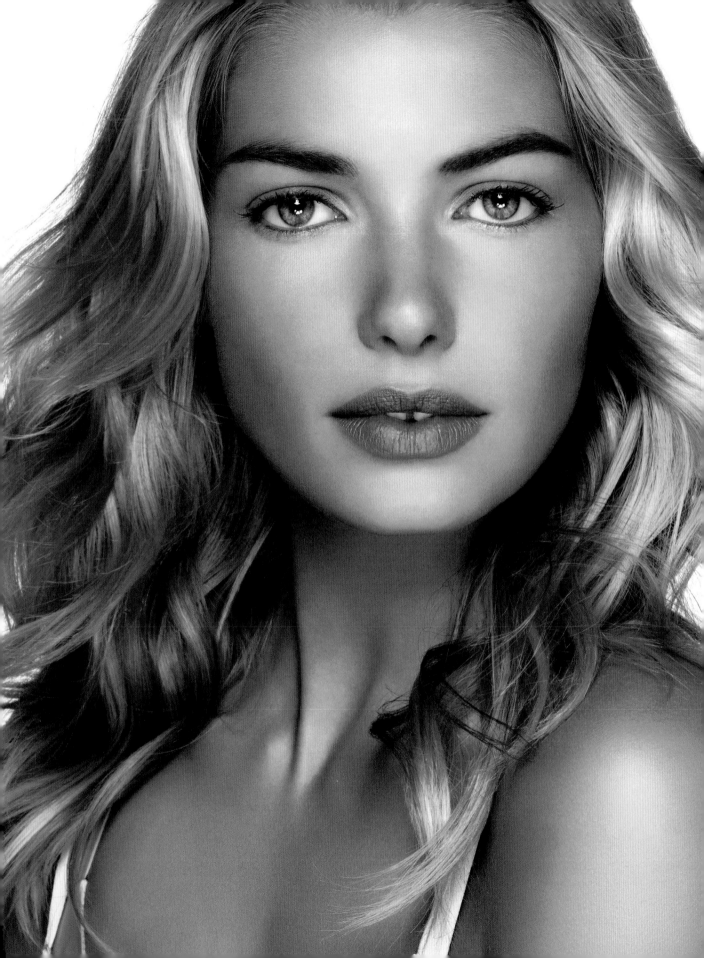

Chapter 7

TEN-STEP GUIDE TO PERFECT MAKEUP

Makeup is simple. When you know how to apply it and have an organized makeup drawer, it should take only five to ten minutes. **Practice is the key.**

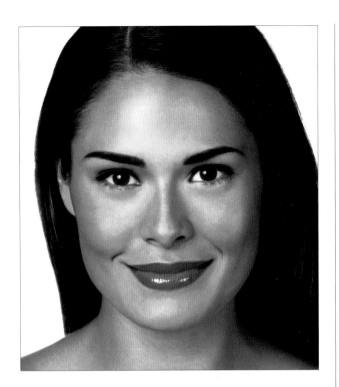

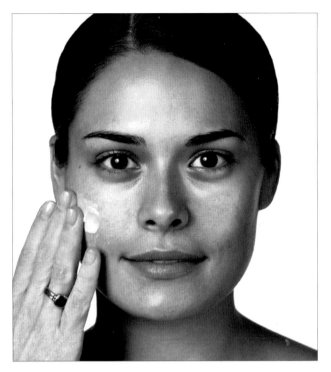

A basic, simple look requires ten steps. Make sure you apply makeup in the correct sequence.

Pre-Makeup

Moisturizer is the key to fresh-looking skin. It creates the perfect base for makeup. For normal skin, use a lightweight moisturizing lotion. For dry skin, use a rich hydrating cream or balm. For oily skin, use an oil-free formula that hydrates and helps control oil production.

Always begin with a lightweight eye cream to ensure that under-eye concealer goes on smoothly and evenly.

When skin looks dull, use an exfoliant to help slough off dead skin cells.

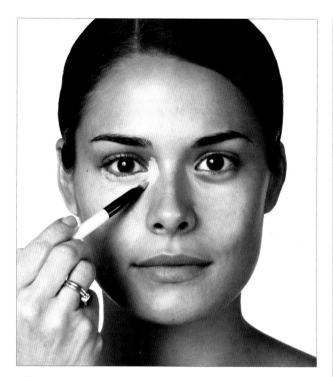

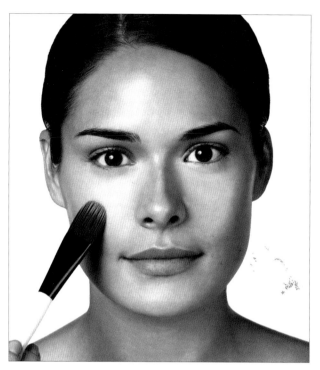

Step 1

Corrector/Concealer

First, neutralize darkness with a pink- or peach-toned corrector. Apply with a brush to the deepest or darkest area to prepare for concealer. (Sometimes you can stop here if the coverage is enough.)

Next, choose yellow-based shades of concealer and layer them over the corrector underneath the eye. Using a concealer brush, apply underneath the eye up to the lash line and on the innermost corner of the eye. Blend by patting with your fingers.

Last, apply pale yellow or white powder with a brush or puff to set the concealer in place. Also apply powder onto the eyelid to take away shine or darkness.

Under-eye concealer should be one to two shades lighter than your skin tone. If the concealer looks ashy, it is too light. If it looks very yellow, it is too dark.

Applying concealer on the spot next to the inner corner of the eye will open up your eyes and give you a fresh, bright-eyed look.

Step 2

Foundation

To find the perfect foundation shade, swatch a few shades on the side of the face and forehead, and check the colors in natural light. The shade that disappears is the right one.

Use a brush, sponge, or fingers to apply foundation where the skin needs to be evened out—around the nose and mouth where there is often redness. For full, all-over coverage, use a brush, sponge, or fingers to apply and blend foundation to the outer edge of the face.

To cover blemishes, spot-apply foundation stick or blemish cover stick in a shade that matches the skin tone exactly. Pat with your finger to blend. Repeat if necessary.

It's a good idea to have two shades of foundation—one for the winter months and a slightly darker one for the summer, when skin color tends to be darker. You can blend the two for spring and fall.

For a sheer, casual alternative to foundation, use tinted moisturizer to even out skin tone.

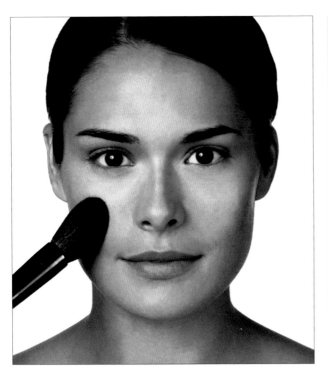

Step 3
Powder

For crease-free, long wear, apply loose powder in a pale yellow tone (or white, if you are very fair) over concealer using an eye blender brush or a mini powder puff.

Apply powder in the correct shade for your skin tone to the rest of the face using a powder puff or powder brush.

If skin feels dry, dust powder only around the nose and forehead.

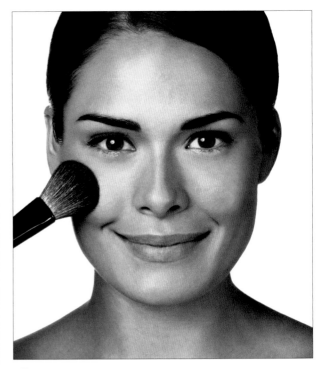

Step 4
Blush

Smile and apply a natural shade of blush on the apples of cheeks. Blend up toward the hairline, then downward to soften the color.

For long-lasting results, layer a pop of brighter blush on top.

For an extra glow, dust a shimmer powder on the cheekbones with a face blender brush, or use a creamy formula applied with your fingers.

Tap or blow off excess powder blush from your blush brush before applying. It is easier to build color in a few light layers than to remove excess color and start over.

Pot rouge or cream blush is a good option for dry skin.

To add a warm tint to skin, use a bronzer on areas where the sun normally hits the face—cheeks, forehead, nose, and chin.

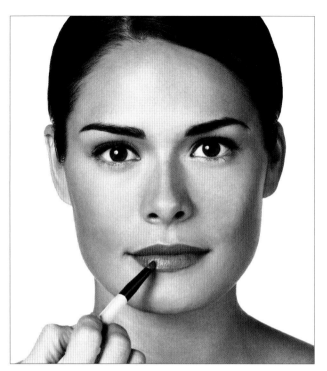

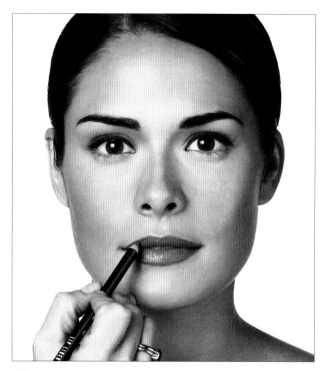

Step 5

Lipstick

Start with clean, smooth lips.

Neutral lipstick shades and sheer formulas can be applied directly from the tube. Use a lip brush to apply darker or brighter colors, which require precise application.

Use the natural color of your lips as a guide when choosing a lipstick shade. The most flattering shade will either match or be slightly darker than your lips.

If you have thin lips, choose light to medium lip color shades, as dark shades have a minimizing effect.

Step 6

Lip Liner

To achieve natural-looking definition and to keep color from feathering, line lips with a lip liner after applying lip color. Use a lip brush to soften and blend any hard edges.

To make your lipstick or gloss longer lasting, line and fill in lips with lip liner before applying color.

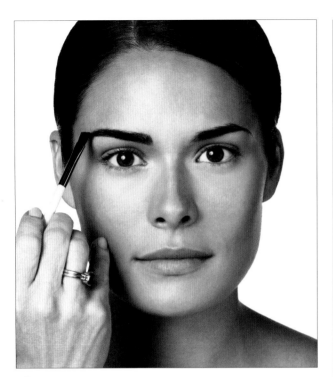

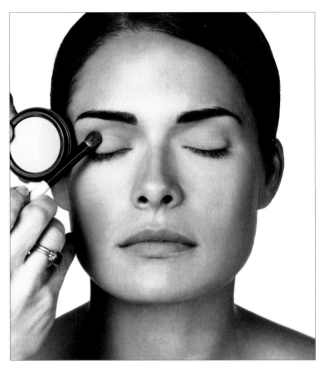

Step 7
Brows

Define brows using shadow or pencil in the color of your eyebrows and hair.

To apply shadow, begin at the inner corner of the brow, and follow its natural shape using light, feathery strokes.

Set unruly brows in place with a brow shaper.

Fill in sparse areas or holes in the brow with an eye pencil. For the most natural look, layer powder shadow on top.

Soften too-harsh brow color by pressing loose powder onto the brows with a powder puff.

Step 8
Eye Shadow

Sweep a light eye shadow color from the lash line to the brow bone.

Dust a medium eye shadow color on the lower lid, up to the crease.

Apply contour color if needed to fleshy part of lid as a correction and to add depth to eye.

Face powder on bare lids helps create a smoother-looking surface for eye makeup and keeps shadow from creasing.

For a longer-lasting look, use a long-wearing cream shadow.

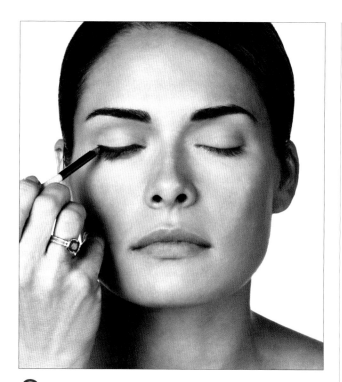

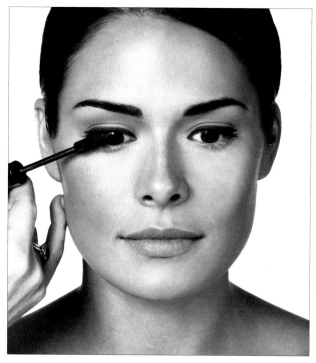

Step 9
Eyeliner

Line the upper lash line with a dark shadow color. Apply damp or dry.

After lining the upper lash line, look straight ahead to see if there are any gaps that need to be filled in. If you also line the lower lash line, make sure the top and bottom lines meet at the outer corner of the eye and that the lower line is softer.

Black eyeliner is the secret to gorgeous, sexy eyes. Layer black liner on top of your normal liner (just on the upper lash line).

Step 10
Mascara

Choose your mascara formula based on your needs and desired effect. Thickening mascara gives individual lashes a denser look and is ideal if you have a sparse lash line. For lashes that are enhanced but still natural looking, choose defining and lengthening mascaras. Waterproof mascara is a good choice if you want a long-lasting look or if your mascara tends to smudge.

When applying mascara, hold the mascara wand parallel to the floor and brush from the base of the lashes to the tips. Roll the wand as you go to separate the lashes and avoid clumps. Always apply two to three coats.

If you choose to curl the lashes, do so before applying mascara. Curling lashes after applying mascara can break the hairs.

True black mascara makes the most impact. Choose brown for a softer look.

FACE CHART

The purpose of a face chart is to have
a reference of a makeup lesson. Many
women tape them to their mirrors while
they try to recreate the look.

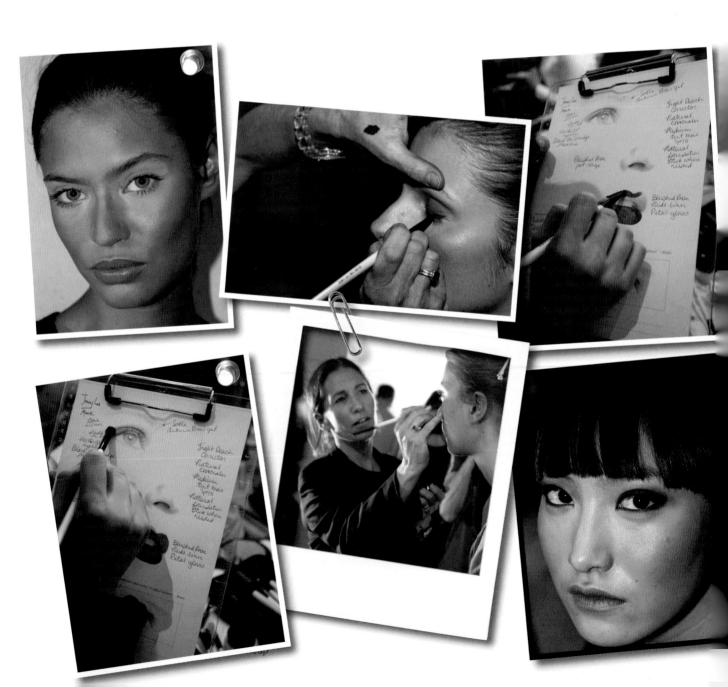

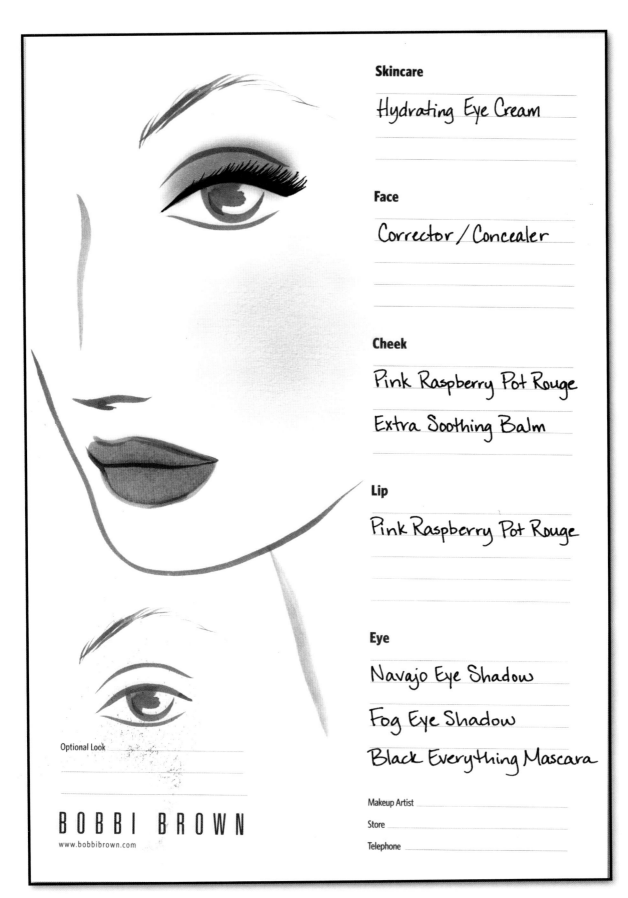

Skincare

Hydrating Eye Cream

Face

Corrector / Concealer

Cheek

Pink Raspberry Pot Rouge

Extra Soothing Balm

Lip

Pink Raspberry Pot Rouge

Eye

Navajo Eye Shadow

Fog Eye Shadow

Black Everything Mascara

Optional Look

BOBBI BROWN
www.bobbibrown.com

Makeup Artist

Store

Telephone

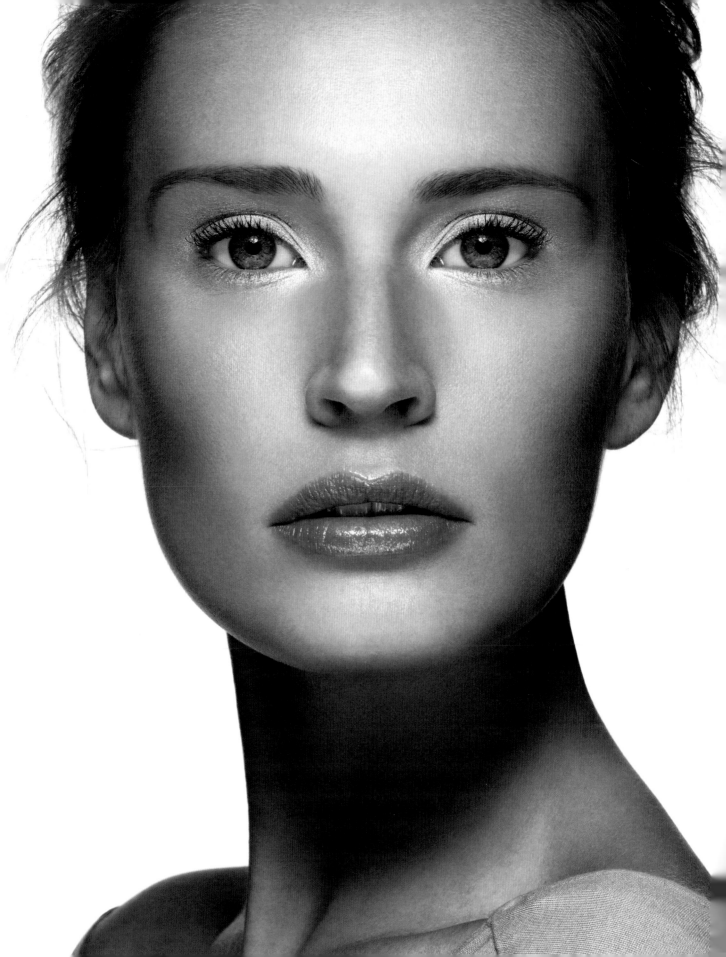

Chapter 8

SPECIAL MAKEUP APPLICATIONS

Once you master the basic techniques of makeup, **it's both fun and easy to take it to the next step for a variety of looks.** Individual beauty is about knowing what to do with your own unique skin tone and features. And it's also about being confident enough to break out of your comfort zone.

DIVERSE BEAUTY

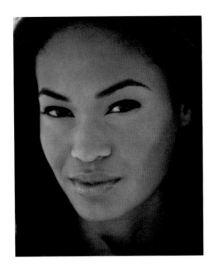

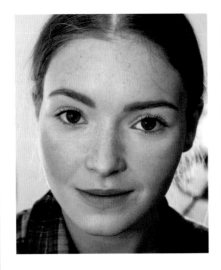

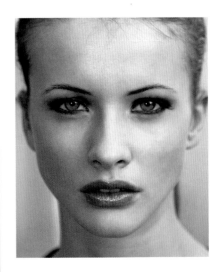

African American Beauty

For dark under-eye circles, use peach corrector and yellow-toned concealer.

Find a foundation that exactly matches skin tone. Skin tone is often uneven, with the forehead and cheeks slightly different shades. Experiment using two different tones of foundation or mixing two shades together. Undertones can be yellow, orange, red, or blue.

Some dark skin looks best with no blush or with a bit of deep bronzer. For medium-toned skin, try bronzing powder or a currant-toned blush. A range of blush tones in plum, rose, or pink look good on lighter skin tones.

Freckled Beauty

Embrace your freckles.

If you need concealer, look for a yellow-toned product that is just one shade lighter than the skin tone.

Foundation can be used to cover redness around the nose or blemishes. Tinted moisturizer gives some coverage but lets the freckles shine through.

Light tawny, coral, or pink tones of blush work well.

Sometimes foundation has to match the freckles that are a shade or two darker than the skin underneath. Do not look for coverage all over the face, only on the redness.

Porcelain Beauty

Sunscreen helps keep skin looking young and beautiful.

Use porcelain-toned foundation to cover redness, dark circles, and blemishes.

Use white face powder.

Avoid using blush with brown undertones. Go for pastels— pale pink is awesome.

Tan bronzer always looks dirty on porcelain skin.

Eye makeup in cool tones works best for porcelain skin tones. Avoid any red-toned products, which can make you look tired.

Pastel lip colors complement very light skin tones.

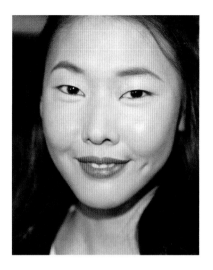

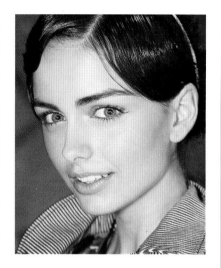

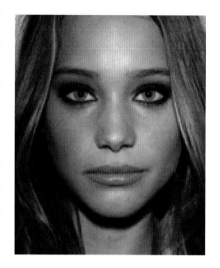

Asian Beauty

Use yellow-toned foundation. Though skin tones vary, all have yellow undertones.

Fill in sparse brows with an eye shadow powder in dark brown. Avoid using black or charcoal, even if the hair is black, because it will look too heavy.

Accentuate eyes with liner on the top only or the top and bottom. Use a stronger line on the top. Make sure it shows when the eyes are open.

Layer shadows to define the eyes. Don't make the mistake of using a very dark shadow to draw in a crease.

A pop of bright coral or pink blush on the apples of the cheeks look fresh and pretty.

Middle Eastern Beauty

Use a corrector to brighten very dark under-eye circles.

Sometimes you have to layer a few correctors (pink over peach), and then add concealer.

Find a yellow-toned foundation that exactly matches the skin. The right foundation often has a bit of orange as well.

Line the eyes with black liner or a charcoal shadow. Never go lighter than mahogany.

Use blush in deep rose and pink shades. Don't be afraid to find your pop of color.

Deep lip colors look wonderful on those with darker lip tones.

Avoid colors that turn ashy.

Latin Beauty

Skin tones vary from very fair to dark.

Use foundation with a yellow undertone that exactly matches skin.

Neutral eye shadows look best for every day. Try shades of navy, silver, chocolate, or gold for evenings or special occasions.

Accentuate natural lip color with lipstick. Choose brighter or deeper tones for evening.

Bronzers are great to add warmth and ensure foundation blends into the skin. Always finish with a pop of color.

BRIDAL MAKEUP

Bridal makeup should be special. On her wedding day, every bride should look like herself at her most beautiful. It is not a time to try a look that is very trendy or radically different from her usual style. Wedding makeup must be long lasting, look amazing in photographs, and be timeless. Every bride should love how she looks in the pictures ten years from now.

Makeup Rules

If possible, do a consultation and run-through of the makeup before the wedding day. Reserve an appointment for about four to six weeks prior to the wedding day to design and practice the look. The wedding day is also special for family and friends, so consider booking makeup appointments for the whole bridal party.

Bridal makeup needs to have enough color to compensate for the whiteness of the dress. Remember, there's a big difference between everyday clothes and a wedding dress, so there should be a difference in the makeup, too. Start by making sure the skin looks even and smooth, and then add color to give cheeks and lips a glow. Finish with eyes that are defined but not overdone. To avoid feeling rushed, allow forty-five minutes to an hour for makeup application on the wedding day.

Natural light is best for makeup application. If possible, set up your makeup station near a window, or use a superbright lamp.

Use a moisturizer that will prepare the skin for makeup. Avoid sunblocks and sunscreens that can give a "flash off" to makeup. They reflect too much light under flash photography, resulting in an overexposed shot.

Emphasize the eyes by brightening any darkness under them with corrector and concealer.

Flash photography emphasizes pink tones, so be sure to even out the skin with a yellow-toned foundation. Start around the nose and mouth, where there's redness, and then blend out to the rest of the face.

Blend well, especially at the corners of the eyes, since cameras pick up visible makeup lines.

Set concealer and foundation with a sheer loose powder. Powder applied with a powder puff assures amazing wearability and reduces unwanted shine— a must-have look for pictures.

If the wedding gown has an open neckline, warm up the neck and chest with a dusting of bronzing powder. It will ensure that the face and body have a balanced tone.

For a pretty flush that lasts, use two shades of blush. Start with a neutral shade, and apply it on the apples of the cheeks, blending up into the hairline, then downward to soften. Finish with a pop of brighter blush just on the apples of the cheeks. Balm or shimmer can be layered for a highlighting effect.

Neutral, brown, and pale lip colors look washed out in photographs, so choose a lipstick that's one or two shades brighter than what you normally wear. For those

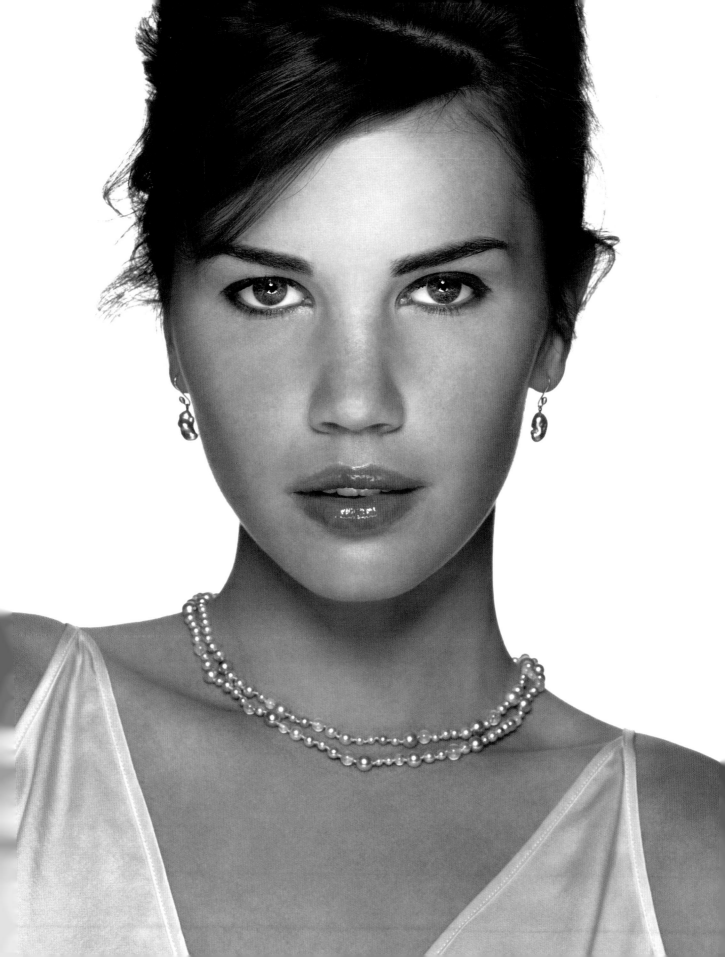

who normally wear a neutral hue, it should be worn as a base, with a pink or rose color on top. For those who normally wear dark lipstick, use that as the base, and apply a brighter pink on top to give the color a lift. Pinks, roses, and plums are great choices for brides.

To make lip color last longer, line and fill in lips with lip pencil before applying the lipstick.

Define brows with a soft matte shadow that matches the hair color.

Use a flat white shadow as a highlighter on the brow bone for those with light skin. A vanilla shade better suits deeper complexions. Use matte eye shadows, as they won't reflect light or look too shiny in photographs.

Define the eyes with a crease color, but avoid using a color that's too dense or dark, as it can detract from the eyes themselves.

Use a water-resistant liner that can withstand tears. If you prefer to line with shadow, make it last longer by applying it with a slightly damp eyeliner brush.

Use an eyelash curler before applying the first coat of mascara.

Choose mascara that's waterproof. It lasts longer and withstands tears.

After applying all the eye makeup, finish with a highlighter shade on the brow bone to make the eyes pop. Rub your finger in a light matte shade, and pat lightly on the outer corner of the brow bone.

Wedding Day Essentials

Pack a small bag with makeup essentials. Keep it simple by filling a face palette with corrector, concealer, foundation stick, pot rouge, lip color, and a soothing balm. Add a lip liner, lip gloss, tissues, Q-tips, and mints.

Include a sewing kit with pre-threaded needles and a pair of tiny fold-up scissors to fix a dropped hem or popped button.

Add prewrapped wipes to remove makeup or food stains.

Bring static spray and lint remover to get rid of static cling and lint on clothing.

Bring a small bottle of perfume in your bag.

Pre-Wedding Wellness Tips

Beauty starts on the inside.
Following these tips will help any bride prepare for her wedding day.

Eat smart.
Choose whole grains, fresh greens and fruits, and clean proteins, such as chicken, fish, and beans.

Hydrate.
Drink lots of water daily to hydrate the skin and flush out toxins.

Move your body.
Exercise at least three times a week to strengthen your body and calm your mind.

Take relaxing baths.
Add soothing Epsom salts or skin-softening powdered milk to your bathwater.

Be present.
Slow down and appreciate what's around you rather than rushing to get from start to finish.

Bridal Dos & Don'ts

Do complete a makeup trial.

Do get as much sleep as possible on the night before the big day.

Do drink plenty of water before your wedding day, and properly prepare skin with moisturizer and eye cream.

Do make sure foundation is right for the skin tone. Your color may have changed since the makeup trial.

Do buy a new mascara for your wedding day, but test it a few days before.

Don't go to a tanning bed right before your wedding. If you want more color, use a self-tanner. Test the product weeks before the date. Apply it several days before the wedding in case you need to make corrections.

Don't apply too much eye makeup. You want the eyes to stand out, not the eye makeup.

Don't use concealer on the eyelid. It causes eye makeup to crease.

Don't use a concealer under the eyes that is too light for the skin tone. It will make you look like a deer caught in headlights.

Don't experiment with eye makeup you haven't tried before.

Don't wear frosted, shiny, or sparkly shadow, as it will reflect camera flashes.

Don't apply shimmer all over the face. One or two accents are enough.

Don't tweeze or wax brows on the wedding day.

Don't wear false eyelashes if they are not 100 percent comfortable and you are not 200 percent confident that they will stay on!

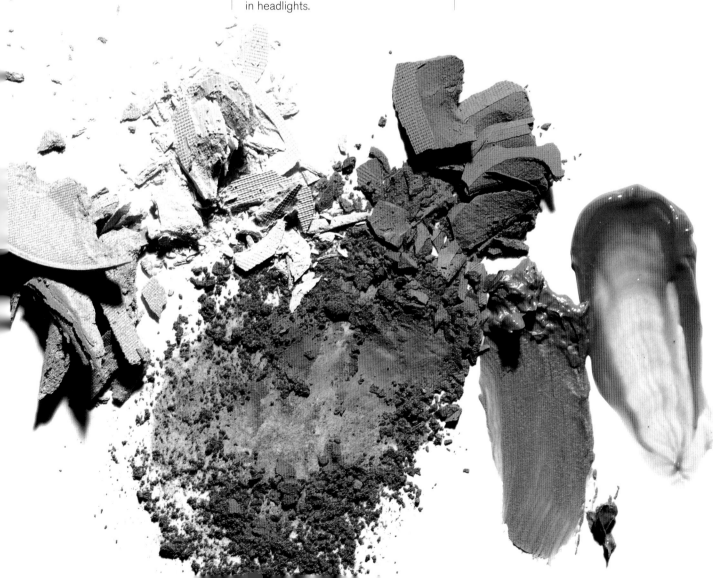

SPECIAL-OCCASION MAKEUP

Few women have the time or energy to clean their faces at the end of the workday and redo their makeup for a night out. Instead, they want a few quick tricks to make a simple transition from office to evening. Since lighting is often softer at night and the occasions are dressier, the idea is to make the face look a bit more dramatic than during the day.

Transforming a Day Face into an Evening Face

Start with a touch of eye cream to smooth out existing concealer. Reapply as needed.

Apply foundation as needed to cover any blemishes and even out skin tone, especially around the nose.

Use a blush that is slightly brighter than the one used for a daytime look. Use it alone or as a pop of color just on the apple of the cheeks.

If skin is showing on the neck and chest, make it glow with a light sweep of bronzing powder.

Use shimmer on lips, eyes, or cheeks to make the face look dressed up. Warning: Too much shimmer will look overdone, so don't use it on all three areas at the same time.

Switch to a darker shade of lipstick. Red or burgundy will add drama to your look. Or try a sheer shade paired with a more dramatic eye.

Add drama to eyes by sweeping on a darker shadow as a liner and applying plenty of black mascara. A smoky eye is always sexy for night looks. Applying white as a highlighter under the brow bone is also a great evening look.

Spritz on a warm, sensual fragrance, and put on a great pair of earrings.

Try red lips with pink cheeks and minimal eye makeup.

Pair shimmery bronzer with smoky brown eyes, bronze cheeks, and copper lips. Add shimmer to either lips or eyes, not both.

Have fun with a bright pink or orange mouth, pale pink or apricot blush, and soft eye makeup with several coats of black mascara or false eyelashes.

For very special occasions, don't be afraid to go all out. Cool colors such as white, platinum, gunmetal, and slate work on the eyes with black liner and individual false eyelashes. Using pale pink with a hint of shimmer on the cheeks and soft beige or sandy pink gloss on the lips will look great.

Use an oil-control lotion on oily areas of the face to keep it shine-free.

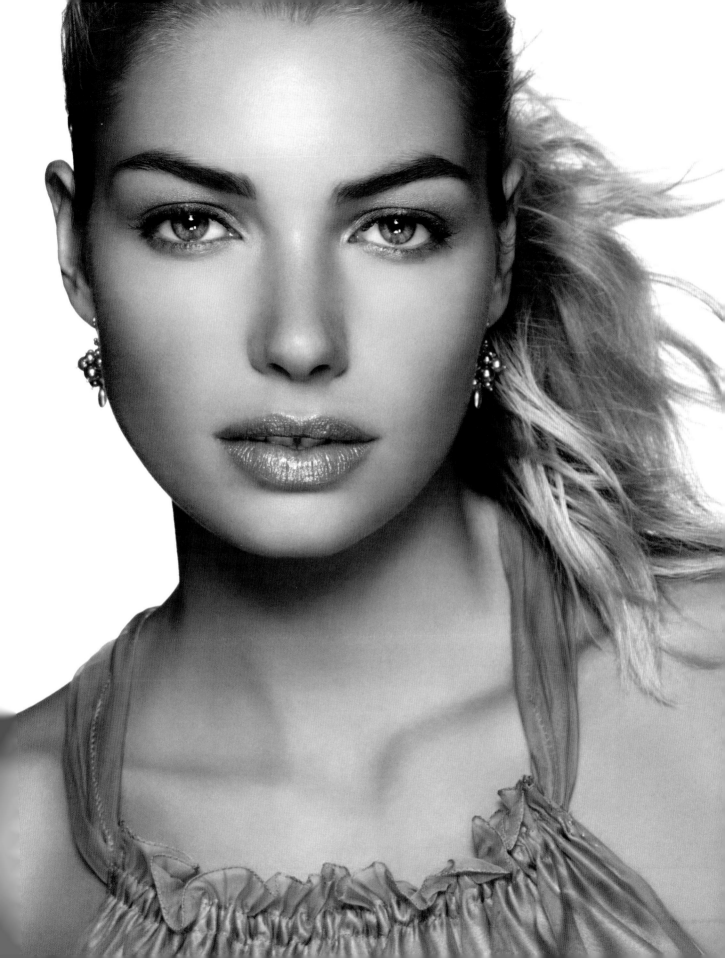

MAKEUP FOR TEENS

Most young women are obsessed with makeup, but they don't often have the knowledge, skills, or confidence to make it work. The teen years are the time to try trendy colors and textures, but a fresh young face should never be smothered in makeup.

Skip an all-over foundation application. Cover blemishes with a blemish stick. Then, apply a stick foundation to those areas that need color correction.

Do not use makeup to look older. The results look harsh and awkward.

Keep colors light and sheer. Avoid heavy, smoky eye shadow and too-bold shades for lips and cheeks.

If the skin is oily, keep blotting papers handy for touch-ups throughout the day.

To avoid drawing attention to braces, skip bright lip colors. Instead, use a moisturizing tinted lip balm or sheer gloss.

Use a clear brow gel to keep brows in place.

Master covering a pimple.

How to Cover a Blemish

1 Choose a stick foundation or concealer stick the exact shade matching your skin tone.

2 With a concealer brush, dab the product on the spot only. Wipe it away from the surrounding areas. Layer a second coat on if needed.

3 Dust a bit of skin-tone-correct powder directly on top of the spot.

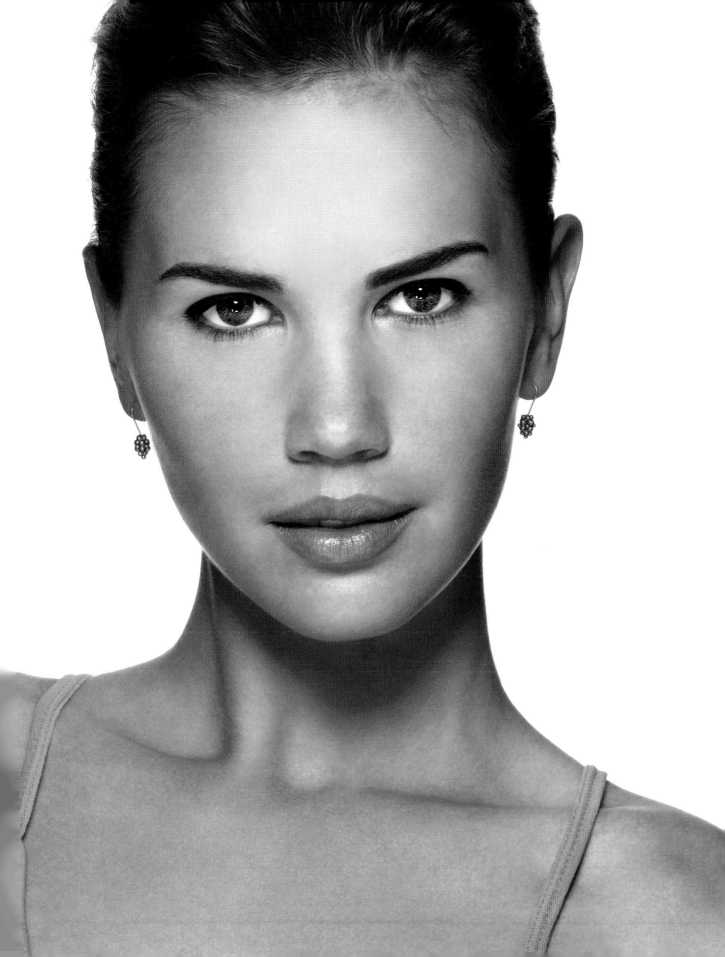

AGELESS BEAUTY

Beauty is about looking and feeling great. That means beauty depends in part on taking care of the body: drinking lots of water, eating healthy foods, using sunscreen, and getting plenty of exercise.

Good beauty routines begin with good skincare. Pamper the skin, and experiment with rich, hydrating moisturizers.

Under-eye darkness often deepens with age. Use a rich under-eye cream overnight and a lighter cream for day to hydrate and smooth the area. Use a pink or peach-toned corrector followed by a yellow-toned concealer and foundation. Lighten the upper lid with a light eye shadow.

Using moisturizers can reduce the appearance of wrinkles. Tinted balms and moisture-rich foundations help soften lines and wrinkles and don't settle into them. Match the foundation exactly to the skin tone.

Skin loses elasticity over time. Using a cream with retinoids that stimulates collagen production helps to give skin a firmer look.

Yellow-toned foundation or tinted moisturizer will tone down ruddy skin and rosacea. Bronzer helps counteract redness as well. Strong facial scrubs often aggravate ruddiness. Rosacea can be treated topically; ask your doctor.

Brown spots can be removed with laser resurfacing performed by a dermatologist or covered with the lightest pink or peach corrector and yellow-toned foundation that is set with powder.

Color will make you look pretty and fresher. Experiment.

Eye contour gives droopy eyelids a lift—the contour shadow needs to look blended and natural.

Sometimes adding a gel bronzer gives a nice boost (aka a fake tan) for a healthy look.

Smooth skin is prettier than too-tight skin.

Eyeliner is great for bringing the eyes out and making them look awake.

Crepey eyes: Make sure you moisturize at night, and stick to formulas that are not too dry.

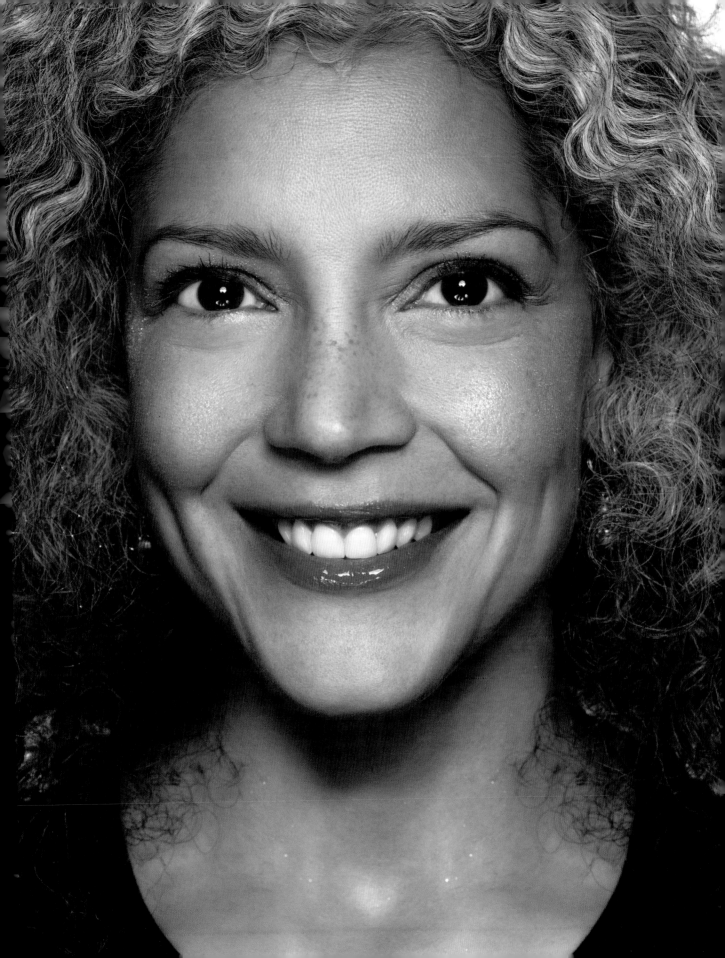

MAKEUP DURING PREGNANCY

For many women, pregnancy is a time when their bodies do not feel like their own. Hormones and physical changes caused by pregnancy create some special needs. Skin often changes during pregnancy, dark patches appear on the skin (sometimes called the "mask of pregnancy"), and some women become extremely sensitive to fragrances.

Adjust any skincare regimen for pregnancy-related changes, either by adding more moisture to combat dryness or switching to oil-free formulas if skin has become oilier.

Use sunscreen! Pregnancy hormones often leave the skin sensitive and more vulnerable to the sun. The vigilant use of sunscreen will help minimize the appearance of hyperpigmentation.

To cover hyperpigmentation, apply a corrective concealer to the area using a concealer brush. Apply foundation over the entire face, using a light touch to avoid wiping away the concealer. Use the fingers to press additional foundation into areas where needed, and then set it with powder.

For those days when there is no natural glow, fake it with a pretty shade of blush, or use a light touch of bronzer over the face.

For added glow, pat face balm over makeup or on a bare face.

Learn the quick on-the-go makeup routine and promise yourself you will do it (most days) and prepare a palette that is customized for you. Make sure you choose colors that don't need to be blended.

Minimum steps are concealer and blush.

BAD-DAY BEAUTY

Everyone, even the most gorgeous model, has the occasional bad day. These are the days when eyes look puffy, skin appears sallow, breakouts seem overly obvious, and nothing seems to help. There are many solutions to improve these situations.

Add moisture. When skin is dehydrated, it looks older and less alive. Drink plenty of water. Use a rich moisturizer to help temporarily plump up skin, making it look softer and younger.

Skip the full makeup application. Avoid the urge to apply makeup in an attempt to banish the bad-day issues. Use just a bit of concealer, a tinted moisturizer, and a pinky blush.

Curl lashes to open up eyes and make them look more awake. Do not follow with lots of eye makeup. Dark liner and shadows can make tired eyes look even more tired. Stick to light shades on the lids, and use mascara just on the top lashes.

Fake a tan. To enliven sallow-looking skin, apply a light coat of self-tanner, bronzing powder, or gel. Follow with a pinky blush.

Don't compensate for paleness with too much color. A sheer pink blush will warm up the skin without looking fake. A bit of moisturizer patted onto the skin over blush will make the skin look great.

Add sheer, glossy lip color to perk up a tired-looking mouth. The best shades match your natural lip color or add just a hint of rose or pink.

Dark eyeglass frames really come in handy on some days.

Cover bruises with a blemish stick or foundation stick.

Cover discolored scars with a blemish stick, and then apply foundation over the area to blend in with skin tone.

Ease a sunburn with a cool shower and cold compresses. Any redness still remaining can be helped with a light application of foundation or tinted moisturizer. Avoid red-colored lips. Instead, try a bronze or brown-based lip color.

Bobbi's Best Friends

Black eyeliner

Bright pink blush

Cheek glow (balms)

Bright pink scarf

Ray-Bans

PART II: ARTISTRY

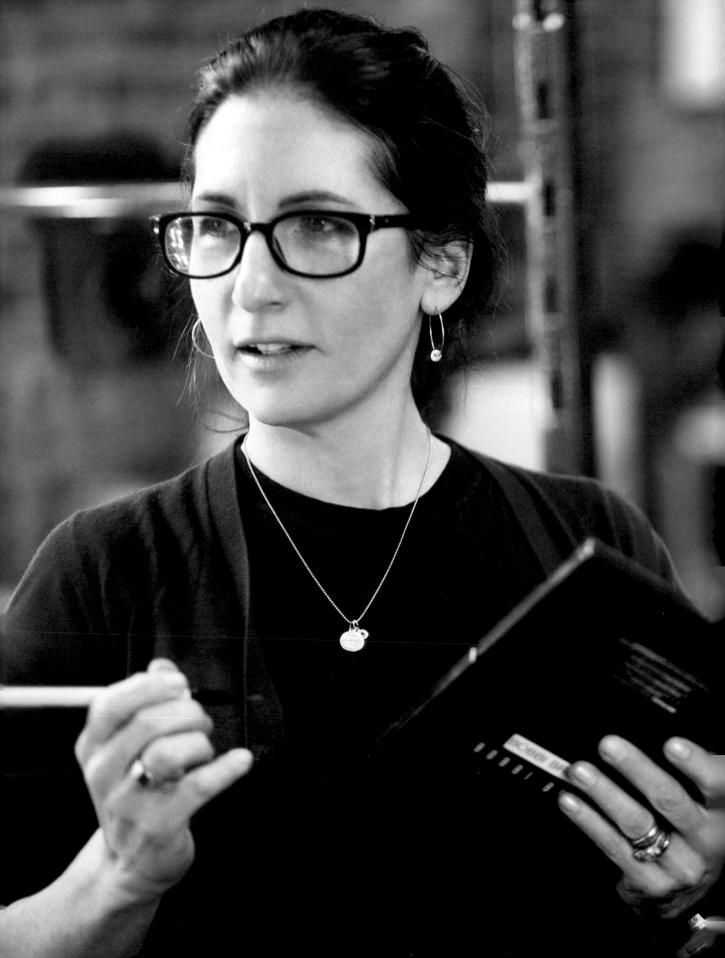

Chapter 9

ARTISTRY

What it takes to be a professional:
this chapter is all about learning to see, formulating your style, listening, collaborating, and finding inspiration.

ARTISTRY

Professional makeup artistry is a field for those who love makeup. *Makeup artists must be obsessed with both the art and business of it, and they cannot be afraid of hard work.* Makeup artists must learn to see in order to evaluate their choices and techniques. They must be open to learning and growing in their craft. Successful professionals in the field of makeup should be excellent teachers and communicators.

THE IMPORTANCE OF SEEING

The most important quality of a good makeup artist is the ability to observe. You can learn a lot about makeup and style just by observing. Look at the faces and styles of women on the street, actresses, and friends. Study women in magazines, old photos, paintings, and movies. Chances are you will begin to see some patterns emerge as to what you like. They will help you formulate your own signature style as a makeup artist. I studied photographs to discover the many ways light creates color on the skin. I love good light and brightness under the eyes, with a smooth complexion.

While your style is evolving, you can expect some trial and error. Hair color, cuts, bright lipstick, beige lipstick? Go for it. Try new things until you arrive at a look you love. You'll know you have found the right look when you feel comfortable and confident in yourself and your appearance. It's an evolution, and it's up to you to find the way.

THE IMPORTANCE OF LISTENING

Just as you have to train your eye in order to become a successful makeup artist, you also have to train your ear. Effective listening is an essential skill for all makeup artists. While it is important to have a vision and to develop your own style, a makeup artist cannot be a dictator. Your job is to take other people's ideas and visions into consideration and to collaborate with them. If the project is a photo shoot, the photographer, editor, and stylist all have input. Even though the model has no say, I believe she should feel good about the way she looks. For fashion shows, the designer usually has a vision, and it becomes your job to realize it. In theater, makeup artists collaborate with the costume designer and sometimes the wig designer to realize the director's vision.

When the subject is an actress, you have to please her and usually others, including her agent, stylist, and photographer, which is not always easy. One time I was doing Tina Turner's makeup and she requested a sexy look, which I had to balance with the photographer and stylist's request that she have a more natural, no-makeup look. And then there was the actress who insisted on black-winged eye-liner that just wasn't pretty. Or the singer

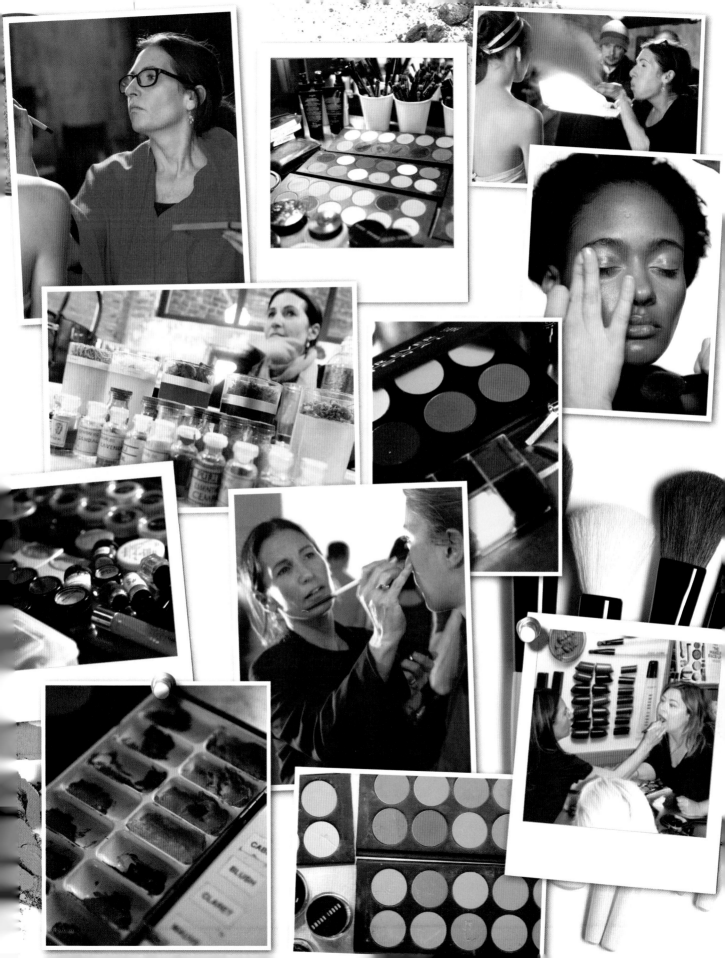

who wanted her foundation five shades lighter than her beautiful ebony skin. Just remember that in the end it is a collaboration, and if you listen well, everyone can be happy.

When your job is to make up a woman, it is important to pay careful attention to what she wants. Begin with a discussion of the woman's lifestyle and skin type. Ask about her makeup preferences, including the type of coverage and finish she likes in foundation. Before you begin any makeup application, it is important to know how much time she wants to spend on makeup on a regular basis. You want to address any concerns she has and know what is comfortable. Find out what kind of foundation she usually wears and her favorite lip color. Listen for real meaning. Sometimes what she says is not actually what she wants. One woman's idea of natural is another's evening look. Continue to ask questions at every step. Have the client watch the application in a hand mirror. Let her assess the progress at each stage, and listen to her likes and dislikes. She might find a concealer too light or dislike a darker brow. Adjust accordingly. Listening will help prevent unnecessary work (like starting over), keep the client happy, and eventually produce results that you both can love.

INSPIRATION AND CREATIVITY

One of the best ways to train your eye and encourage your creativity is to keep a scrapbook. Think of it as a visual journal for thoughts, images, and completed work. Tear any inspirational images from magazines. These could be faces, colors, or design concepts you find appealing. Sometimes even stationery, logos, or labels can inspire. Carry a digital camera to record inspirational visuals you encounter in daily life, such as colors and textures found on buildings or in nature.

The way you organize the scrapbook is up to you. Options include slipping images into plastic sleeves in a binder, taping them into a bound notebook, or tacking them onto a large bulletin board. Some artists prefer creating virtual scrapbooks, using a Web site to organize and store images and ideas. Other artists prefer to organize scrapbooks by topic rather than chronologically. They keep binders on various topics, such as bridal looks, natural looks, celebrities, color, or objects that inspire them.

As a makeup artist, you will go through dozens of scrapbooks during your career, but be sure to hold on to them. It will be helpful to reference your previous work and inspirations when preparing for a shoot or fashion show. The scrapbook becomes a historical record of your career, and reviewing old ones can be an important source of inspiration. I used to staple Polaroids into my day planner, and I still love looking back, remembering each shoot. I still have the red leather notebook I kept when starting my lipstick line. In it are the names of the women who inspired the colors and all the notes from meetings in which I discussed the line. It is a history that can reinspire me.

FINDING INSPIRATION

There are inspirations and ideas everywhere you look. I get inspiration from faces—women, men, children. I love to see how light affects different skin tones. I look at fashion magazines old and new—from the 30s and 40s up to the present. I especially love images from the 70s and 80s, possibly because that's when I became involved in the beauty industry. I shop at art supply stores, gourmet food stores, and vintage stores, looking for inspiration. I get ideas while I am exercising and listening to the music I love.

Be observant. Watch your client's reactions, and be open to change.

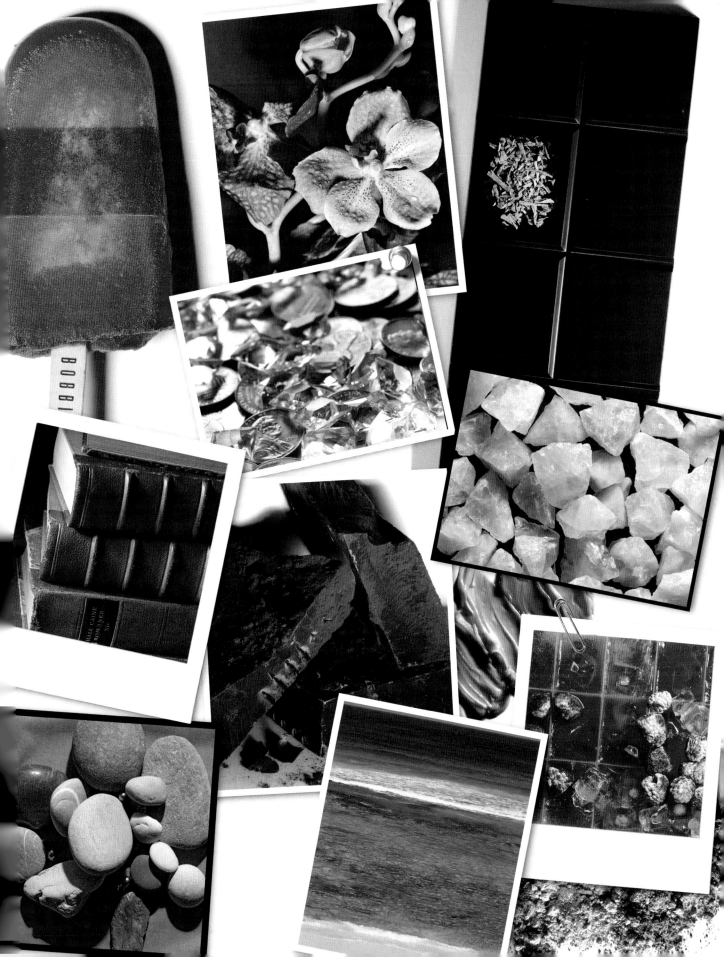

BREAKING into the BUSINESS

New artists have so much to learn about products and techniques and need to become comfortable with the basics. Beginning artists tend to do everything by the book. They often apply all the layers and don't see that a woman might not need some of the elements. *More advanced artists are confident in their product knowledge and have had time to practice their technique, so they know what works and what is not needed for different clients.* They have the ability to handle any situation that comes up. They are not afraid to reevaluate in the middle of an application. A strong knowledge base allows artists to make great choices, see when an application doesn't work, and know when to stop.

I was once hired by a big celebrity to do her makeup for the opening of a restaurant. She appeared with the biggest scratch on the side of her face. I didn't panic, but I had to try dozens of products to get the very pink scratch to blend in with her natural skin color. I was ready to handle the challenge with confidence in my ability.

It is important to stay open and eager. I received both good and bad advice when I started out. I was the pioneer of the natural, bronzy look, but I faced lots of criticism for it. I was told that I would have to change my makeup style—that nobody liked the healthy look. A hairdresser once told me that I needed to get a better hairstyle myself if I wanted to be successful.

One of the best ways to get started is to apply makeup on anyone and everyone who will let you. Practice on your friends and family until you get to the point where you feel completely comfortable working on people's faces. Practice all different types of makeup applications—natural, theatrical, bold fashion looks, bridal looks, men. Hands-on experience is invaluable.

Early in your career, experience is more important than pay. If you have the opportunity to apprentice with established makeup artists—even if it means just observing while you spend time cleaning brushes—do it. It can be a valuable learning experience. You never know whom you'll meet. Today's assistant can be the beauty editor of a major magazine in a few years.

Confident, successful artists are those who continue to train. Even top artists go back to the basics from time to time. Skills can always be improved. I learn from my artists, assistants, photographers, models, and friends. Never take a suggestion personally—it is always an opportunity. Things are always changing in the beauty industry, so you need to be open, aware, and looking for ways to improve.

Success is achieving the goals you set for yourself. Artists need to continually redefine their goals. Everyone might want to work in the fashion industry, but there are successful makeup artists working in film, television, and theater. There are those who have used their training and experience in makeup artistry to move into careers in education, marketing, merchandising, and other aspects of design.

By maintaining a clear picture of reality while seeking, creating, and fully exploiting every opportunity, artists can secure success one step at a time.

Artists are often eager to grow and move up in the industry. Patience is so important, and time is needed to perfect skills. Be happy at whatever level you are working, even if it is just observing. Look for a mentor. Work to completely understand the basics so that you can begin to make your own interpretations. Ask for help and guidance. It will be perceived as strength, not weakness.

Desire is perhaps the strongest determinant of success. When I hire a new artist, I look for someone who really wants to be doing the work. It is apparent in every aspect of the person. I want to work with people who are as passionate about beauty as I am. I look for applicants with great attitudes who are eager to work hard and to learn as much as they can. Some of the artists who assist me at fashion shows have worked for me for five to ten years. Yet they still watch carefully as I do the first model. Others seem uninterested. Guess which ones have the most talent?

ADVICE FOR BREAKING INTO THE BUSINESS

It helps to have a positive, professional attitude.

Always arrive on time.
If you plan to arrive a bit early, then inconvenient delays will not be a problem.

Be who you are.
Your appearance is an essential part of your presentation. Your personal style and makeup are reflections of your own tastes, and, like it or not, people will judge you by it.

Practice confidence.
Hold your head up, make eye contact, have a firm handshake, smile, and take a genuine interest in what others have to say.

Don't be afraid to ask questions.
Ask photographers, stylists, and models for their opinions.

Be nice to everyone.
Even when my skills were just okay, I was invited back because I was pleasant.

Never stop learning.
When I think about my own skills, I know I'm not done learning. I love watching other people do makeup. A good artist is secure enough to be open to new ideas and learning new techniques.

It's not about you.
Great makeup artists focus on the client and don't ever let their own egos get in the way. It doesn't matter if the client is a celebrity, a supermodel, or a regular woman. It is about her, not about you!

Love what you do.
Great makeup artists never lose their passion for makeup.

CAREER OPTIONS

Makeup artists have the opportunity to work in so many different areas. Career options vary from long-term jobs in television, with regular pay and benefits, to freelance jobs working on short-term runway, print, or film projects in a variety of locations and with a wide range of styles.

Department Store Counter

Artists generally work for a specific makeup line, teaching customers to choose and apply their own makeup. This job involves sales, and the compensation is often commission-based.

Bridal

Working with brides is both rewarding and very demanding. You need to do consultations and a run-through in addition to the makeup on the day of the wedding. The job usually involves traveling to the bride's location. Sometimes it will include doing makeup for the rest of the bridal party as well.

Beauty Salon

Makeup artists working in salons often find themselves in a teaching role. They do makeovers, help clients practice techniques, and are often called to do makeup for special events and weddings. Fashion and media work is sometimes booked through salons.

Television

Working on a set involves creating character looks and might include anything from doing basic makeup to designing looks for elaborate characters, aging the actors, creating the appearance of illness, replicating injuries, and much more. Artists sometimes work for years on one television show. Careers generally begin with assistant positions in the industry. Artists develop books of their work and a résumé. After gaining experience, artists are allowed to join a union, which provides opportunities, some job security, medical benefits, and a pension. Most television shows require makeup artists to have union membership.

Film

Shooting a film can take just days or several months, sometimes in multiple locations. The film industry is hard to break into, but not impossible. Any large-budget film requires makeup artists to have union membership. Which union you should join will depend on the area of the country in which you are working.

Television Commercials

Artists who work in this field are usually experienced in another aspect of the industry and have built a strong reputation either in print advertising or music videos.

Early in my career, I used to watch famous models correct the makeup I had done on their faces. The result was good—they always looked better, and I learned so much by watching them.

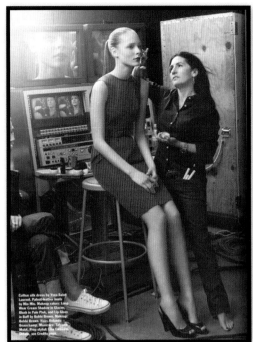

Cotton silk dress by Yves Saint
Laurent. Patent-leather heels
by Miu Miu. Makeup colors: Long
Wear Cream Shadow in Glacier,
Blush in Pale Pink, and Lip Gloss
in Buff by Bobbi Brown. Makeup:
Bobbi Brown. Hair: Melanie
Beauchamp. Manicure: Tatyana
Molot. Prop stylist: Lisa Cassara.
Details, see Credits page.

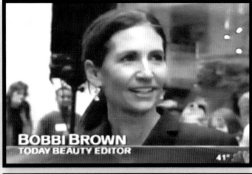

BOBBI BROWN
TODAY BEAUTY EDITOR

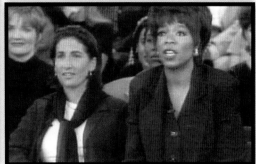

Print

Makeup artists who work in the editorial or print advertising field work with models, photographers, stylists, and editors. Collaboration is everything. Shoots take place in studios and also on location—sometimes very exotic ones. Work is obtained by sending a portfolio, or book showing your past work, to agencies that provide representation and to clients. The better the book, the higher the demand and pay rate. Print jobs include work for magazines, advertisers, catalog companies, corporate in-house publications, movie posters, and album covers.

Video

Music videos are often filmed very quickly and require flexibility, spontaneity, and simple artistry. While many videos are low-budget freelance projects, they provide opportunities for young artists to build their portfolios. Makeup artists are often hired for music videos because their print work, doing magazine and album covers, has attracted a music artist's attention. Educational and industrial video shoots also hire makeup artists and stylists.

Live Performance

This field includes work for theater, dance, and musical theater, as well as for live concerts and road tours. The artist works under time pressure and needs to maintain continuity. An artist sometimes stays with a production for months or even years.

Fashion Show

Applying makeup for the runway is both adrenaline boosting and exhausting. It involves collaboration with a designer and models. Work begins with a pretest to discuss and try out the look. On the day of the show, another pretest is completed with the actual runway lighting for final designer notes and approval. Then the work becomes incredibly hectic and fast-paced as all of the models are made-up. Makeup artists obtain work in this area by sending out their book and through reputation and connections.

Remember when I said to
be nice to everyone?
Often assistants become
editors-in-chief.

the BUSINESS of MAKEUP ARTISTRY

While makeup artists are first and foremost artists, they also need to be businesspeople. *Makeup artists need to be talented, confident, and charismatic, as well as effective entrepreneurs who are able to effectively market their talents.* To begin, you will need to find ways to gain experience, develop effective work habits, create a business system, and build a portfolio and résumé. Eventually, you will want to secure agency representation.

Your success is completely up to you. This means you need to attract and keep clients, develop and maintain several portfolios and a résumé, handle the business effectively, and stay current.

DEVELOPING A PORTFOLIO

A portfolio is a book in which you keep photographs of all your work as a makeup artist. The book can be low-cost plastic or high-end leather with your name engraved on it.

The first step in finding work is developing a great portfolio you can show to potential employers. Having professional photographs taken of your work can be prohibitively expensive and is probably not worth the investment when you are first starting out. Instead, try to find an aspiring photographer who might also like to have photos for his or her own book, and help each other out. Call every modeling agency and ask if you can do makeup for testing. Testing is when a model, photographer, hairdresser, and makeup artist all do a shoot for free to show others their work. The payment is a photo for your portfolio. It's also an excellent way to learn how to build rapport with a team at a photo shoot—an important lesson, because the same team will often work together repeatedly on jobs.

After the test, getting pictures from the photographer can sometimes be a challenge. It is up to you to confirm when the pictures will be ready to view. Set a date to pick out your own shots, and crop them if needed. Since most photographs are now digital, you can collect and store them on your computer. Prints can be made in a lab or with your own printer.

Your book should include at least fifteen amazing test shots before you show it around. Whenever possible, use professional models and photographers. Amateur work is quickly evident. Once you begin to find paid work, you will be able to include tear sheets (published work) from magazines, book covers, television commercials, and other jobs. You can begin looking for agency representation when you have at least ten to fifteen tear sheets that show a variety of work. Building a portfolio takes time. It will take at least six to nine months of consistent work to develop a book that you can show to clients. Once you have the book together, you need to show it to everyone—photographers, other artists, producers, and art directors. Get their advice, and listen to it. Thank them for their time and help.

PUTTING TOGETHER A PORTFOLIO

Presentation counts for a lot in this business, so your portfolio needs to make a brilliant first impression.

It is a representation of you as an artist.
The book needs to be neat, well organized, and an accurate reflection of your aesthetic and personal style.

Portfolio books themselves are available in a variety of sizes.
The two most popular sizes are 9" x 12" and 11" x 14". Art supply stores are a good source for portfolio books. Look for one that has plastic or acetate pages into which you can slip your photos. You will also want at least one pocket (on the inside back cover) to hold a résumé, promotional cards, and business cards. Include several of each so that whoever is looking at your book can take and keep a copy of your résumé and card. Some agencies prefer receiving portfolios on a CD rather than in book form, so always have several electronic copies available.

Keep one portfolio with all of your original photographs in it.
High-quality color copies are used in books intended for mailing. Tear sheets should be originals, so if a magazine prints your work, buy lots of copies of it. Have at least two books ready to be sent out at any time. Consider having four or even five copies. It is also not a bad idea to carry a reduced version with you in case an opportunity to show it presents itself.

From my portfolio:

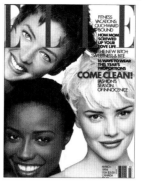
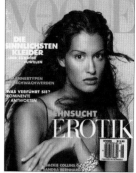
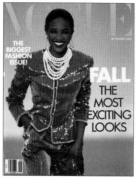
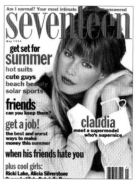
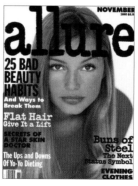
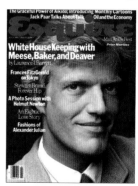
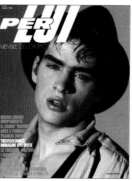
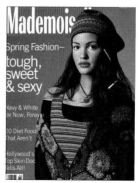

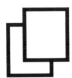

Promotional Cards

A promotional card is an essential addition to your promotional arsenal. These cards are postcard-size and have one to three photos of your work, as well as your name and contact information. Also referred to as a comp card, a promo, or a leave-behind, these cards show your artistry and style. Both print and electronic versions of the cards are necessary for self-promotion. Promo cards have four-color photographs on one side, and your contact information in black and white on the other. As photographers own the rights to their photographs, you must obtain their written permission to use any photos and credit the photographers on the card. You can send out the cards in the mail and have several in your portfolio for the editor, photographer, or agent to keep on file. That way, art directors and fashion editors always have a sample of your work on hand. Also keep the card as a PDF file on your computer, or better yet on a flash drive. This will allow you to e-mail a copy almost instantly, wherever you are, to potential employers. Carry several with you in your bag for those unexpected opportunities.

Web Sites

New artists are using the Web to promote their services. Make sure you hire a reputable Web designer to help you design and launch your site, or lease space on an existing site that will help you build your own. Some make-up agencies offer such space to their artists. Remember that the quality and style of the site, not just the content, directly reflect who you are as an artist.

On the Web site, include your promotional card and a PDF version of your résumé. Include current portfolio content. Determine how large you want the site to be and how often you will want to update it. Consider how you want people to contact you and whether you want to include links on the site. Build a site that is globally accessible.

Successfully managing your site means that it is always current and can be easily accessed. If your Web server does not automatically list you with search engines, try using Addme.com. This is a free Web site–submission engine that will add your site to the top thirty most popular search engines.

Reels

If your primary goal is to work in television, music videos, or movies, you will also want to put together a reel. A reel is a compilation of your styling work for film, television, and video on a master tape (actually a DVD), edited to several minutes that includes the best footage. Choose music for your reel that creates the perfect mood. The reel will need to be professionally edited to include transitions and titles. Make copies of the reel, and create case labels with your name, address, and phone number for identification. Most producers do not return reels, but making copies is inexpensive, and reels are great promotional tools.

Résumés

Résumés let the decision makers know the full range of your credits. A résumé needs to be complete, accurate, and professional. Pick a font that is easy to read, and print the résumé on good-quality stock. Write a clear, concise cover letter to include with the résumé when mailing your résumé or portfolio. While a cover letter and résumé are important tools in your self-promotion efforts, it is the portfolio or reel that will get you the job. In film and television, a listing of your experience in résumé form is the first thing that producers look at. They might interview and see the portfolios of only a few artists. In print work, a look at your portfolio usually precedes an interview.

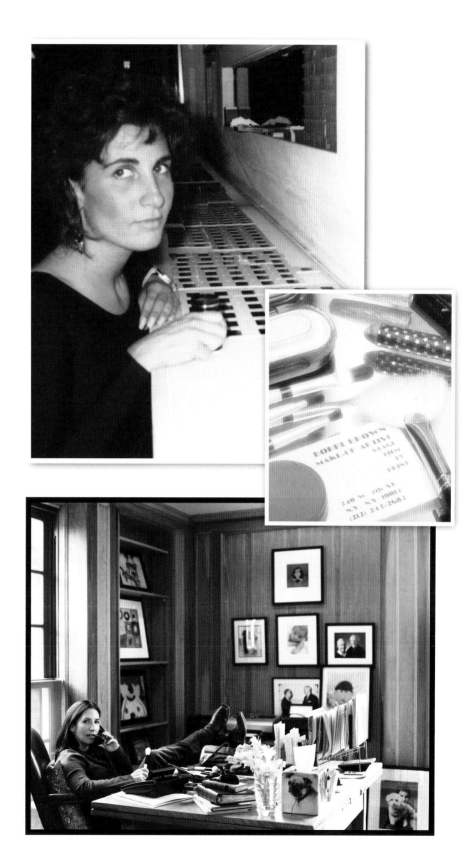

BOOKING WORK

Once your promotional tools are completed and your portfolio looks great, you need a plan. *Determine what your career goals are. Do you want to work in retail, with private clients, or for commercial clients in print or in film and television?* You might end up with a combination of work, but maintaining a focus is important. It will determine whether you spend more time developing your book or your reel. In either case, you will need to identify a group of potential clients and contact them. Follow these guidelines:

SHOW YOUR WORK
Develop a mailing list, and send out your portfolio and/or résumé. Sending promotional cards and your résumé is a quick way to remind possible employers of your work.

FOLLOW UP
Call within a week of leaving or mailing your materials.

THANK POTENTIAL CLIENTS
by sending a card thanking them for their time and advice. Ask them if there are any available opportunities.

Fashion stylists or editors are often the key to being hired on a high profile shoot. The bigger the stylist, the better the artist has to be.

Commit your goals to paper. Learn as much as you can about photographers who work in the industry, as they often decide which stylists to hire. To get print work, start bringing your portfolio to magazine editors, photographers, and other potential employers. The only way to do this is to have an appointment, so be prepared to spend lots of time on the phone. You can look on the mastheads of magazines to find the fashion and beauty editors and art directors to call. Find out the drop-off days specified by the agencies. These are the specific days and times set up for portfolio reviews. A publication called *The Black Book* lists everyone in the print world and is an invaluable resource for contact information (see Resource Guide).

Don't be afraid to explore several avenues of employment at once. Saturate the market with your card, sending it to not only magazine editors, photographers, and agents but also to local stores and salons. Contact department stores about doing fashion shows or other promotional events. Volunteer to do the makeup for fund-raising fashion shows or productions at local theaters. To help break into the more prestigious and higher paying areas of makeup artistry, do whatever you can to meet the top players in the field. Call or send a friendly personal note along with your promotional card. It will help if you keep up to date on the industry—read all the fashion and entertainment magazines to keep track of the top photographers, models, designers, and makeup

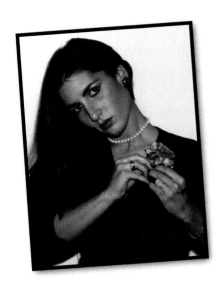
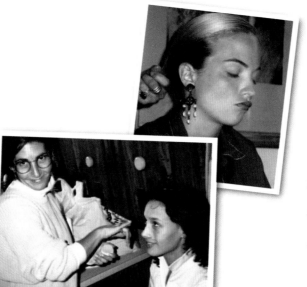
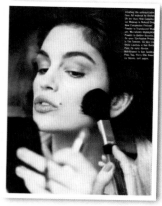

artists. Know who does which advertising campaigns, study photographers' and makeup artists' styles, and be able to recognize their work.

Remember that in the fashion industry—like any other business—people hire people. So always be nice, smile, and say thank you. Potential clients will remember you for it next time, when you come back with more experience and more photographs in your portfolio. Also, when you're just starting out, don't think too much about what you'll get out of a makeup job. Take all the jobs you can, because you never know what you might learn or what contacts you might make.

It's also worth noting that when you are getting started and looking for freelance work, there are going to be dry spells. It's important to be frugal with your money, to learn how to budget when you do get paying freelance work, and to have another source of income to fall back on (waiting tables, working retail, dog walking, etc.). And when you do have downtime between assignments, use it constructively—make calls, send out your résumé and promotional card, and do more test shoots to build your portfolio.

MANAGING YOUR BUSINESS

It is never too early to begin to develop a business plan and system. On a computer, in a planner, or directly in your current scrapbook, create a simple log of all your contacts and work completed. The log should include the date, name, company (when relevant), contact number, topic, result, and follow-up. Print your digital photographs from shoots, labeled with the date and persons involved, to include in the scrapbook or log. Networking is such a huge part of being a freelance makeup artist that it is important to keep a detailed record of all your contacts and previous work.

You will need to negotiate the terms and fees for each job, prepare confirmations to make sure that the terms and conditions are met, generate invoices, keep accurate financial records, and collect all payments. Terms might include payments for travel and per diems, materials costs, and assistant rates. You need to know the scope of the project before these terms can be set. Ask questions and take notes, only making your decision when you have all the information you need. Then send confirmation, also called a deal memo. It is a document that includes the job description, day rate, overtime rate, the flat dollar amount if overtime is not included, length of project in days, the number of assistants and pay rate, a materials budget, and for stylists, clauses regarding reimbursement for clothing damage. Create job folders for each job, with copies of receipts, any advance checks, signed vouchers, and invoices. Prepare a professional invoice form, and send it to the client at the end of the shoot. Send a credit sheet, indicating the job you worked on and how you want your credit to read, to the appropriate person. Templates of business forms used in the industry can be found at makeuphairandstyling.com.

Remember that many expenses are tax deductible. Keep a categorized record of automobile, travel, and entertainment expenses, plus records of money spent on office supplies and office equipment. Record the purpose of the expense on each receipt, and file it by category, with a copy in the job folder.

Maintaining and updating your portfolio and résumé is essential. Stay current. Know what is going on in entertainment, fashion, and beauty. Look at magazines, fashion shows, and music videos. Always dress appropriately, be prepared and on time, be decisive and efficient. If you can't say something nice about someone, don't say anything at all. Networking is a major part of the job, so make contacts, listen with interest, be positive, make phone calls, send thank-you cards, and keep your promises.

AGENCIES

Agencies provide a wide range of services, including finding work for their talent, doing promotional work, negotiating and collecting fees, and offering career management. In exchange for those services, the artist pays the agency 20 percent of his or her fee.

When starting out as a freelance makeup artist, you will undoubtedly experience frustration. You need a good portfolio to get an agent, but without an agent, it may be hard to get the jobs you need to produce a good book. Having agency representation does help you secure the best assignments. Begin with research. Take the time to learn something about different agencies. What is their philosophy? What type of work do they do? How many artists do they represent? Who are these artists? Why is a certain one the right agency for you? Interview several agencies that seem to be a good match. Ask what you can expect from them. How do they promote their talent? Bring a résumé that lists all the photographers, editors, art directors, stylists, models, etc., who have worked with you. Include all your work done for magazines, catalogs, ads, or videos. Don't be discouraged if the agency doesn't sign you on the spot. It pays to be persistent; after making the

initial contact with an agency, keep in touch. Follow up by sending additional tear sheets from new assignments, and try to make another appointment a few months later. It's also helpful to ask for constructive criticism. Find out what the agent likes or doesn't like about your book or promotional card, and take the advice to heart.

One of the best ways to get a foot in the door at an agency is to be willing to work as an assistant to one of the agency's makeup artists. Before you call, know which artists the agency represents, what projects they might be working on, and which ones you are most interested in and/or most qualified to assist on. The need for extra assistants often arises at the last minute, and whoever is available and interested may get the job.

RATES

Rates vary depending on experience and location. Rates paid in New York and Los Angeles are generally higher than rates in other places. Research the going daily and hourly rates in your area, and always charge competitively.

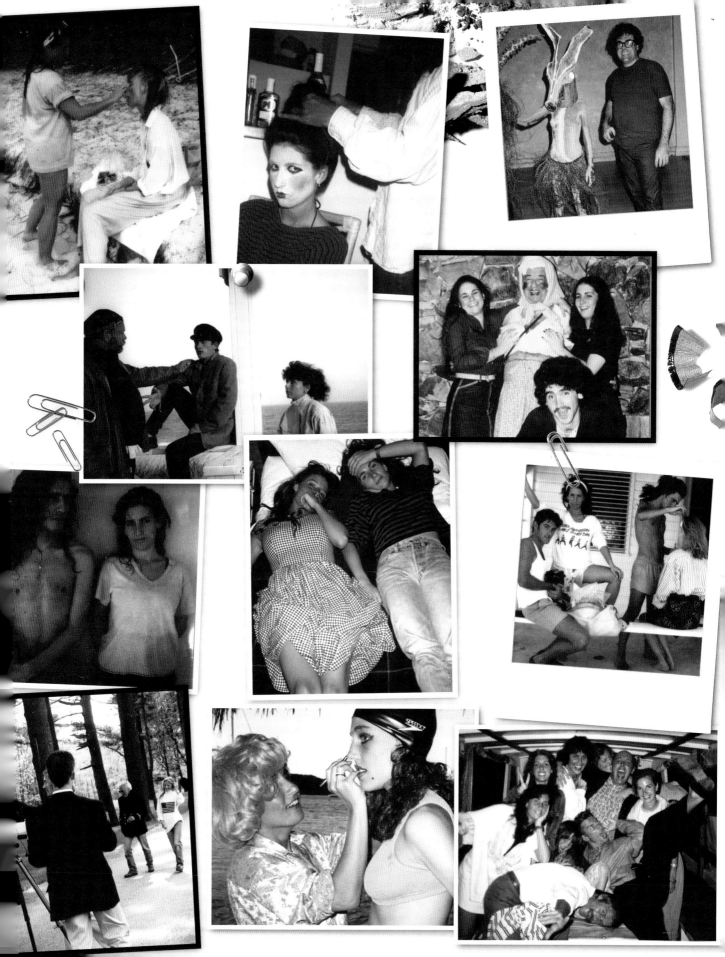

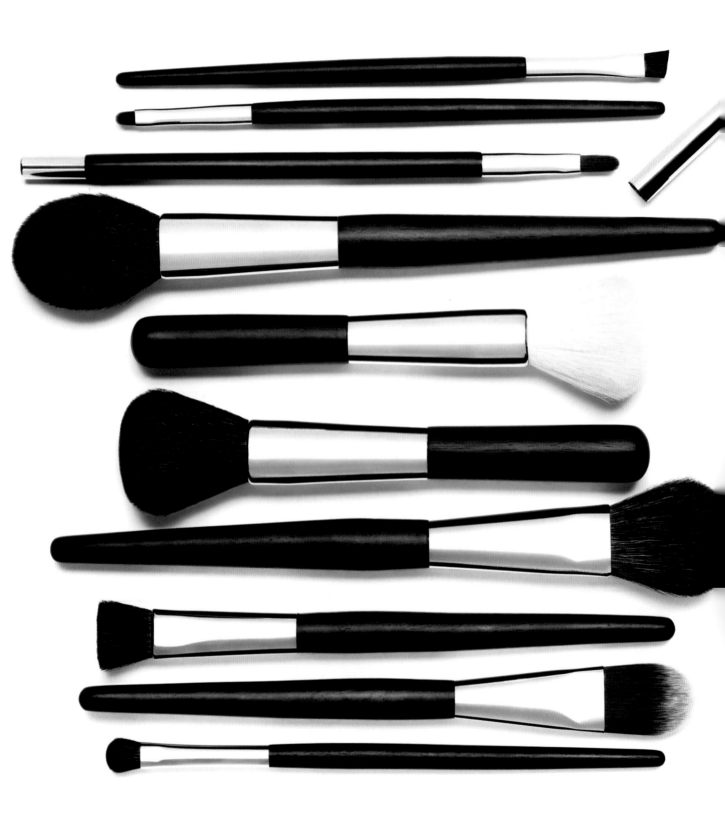

Chapter 10

ESSENTIAL EQUIPMENT for the PROFESSIONAL

DEVELOPING & STOCKING the PROFESSIONAL MAKEUP KIT

A good makeup kit contains all the products and tools you need to do your work. The appearance and organization of your kit are a big part of the first impression you make when you show up for a job. No one wants to work with a makeup artist whose kit is dirty and disorganized.

One of the best ways to carry your supplies is in a small rolling suitcase. (A shoulder bag or backpack will be too heavy and not good for your back.) Organize all your equipment and supplies in containers. Zip-top plastic bags, palettes, vitamin boxes, brush rolls, small makeup bags, and dop kits are all excellent tools for keeping everything in its place. To make it easy to find what you need, label each container clearly so you know what's inside without having to open it. A helpful trick is to transfer makeup into smaller containers to save space. Create a complete foundation palette by taking slices off your stick foundations. Pour liquids into smaller jars. Create a palette of multiple corrector and concealer shades. Arrange slices of lipsticks as well as balm in a

lip palette. The more organized your kit is, the more efficient you'll be as a makeup artist.

After each job, take the time to put everything back in its place. Clean any tools you used, sharpen pencils, spray cream products with alcohol, wipe off powder shadows, and replace products as needed. That way, your kit will always be ready to go, and you won't have to scramble when you get a call to do a job at the last minute.

You never know what you will encounter when arriving on a job, so it makes sense to have all your supplies with you. Since that means toting around hundreds of products, it pays to organize them in categories. A checklist for everything you need to complete a professional kit follows.

THE ESSENTIAL KIT
(at right)
These are the basic supplies that you should always have with you.

Skincare

Foundation palette

Lip and cheek palette

Eye shadows

Full brush kit

Lip liners

Lip glosses

Bronzer

Gel eyeliner

Mascara

Eyelash curler

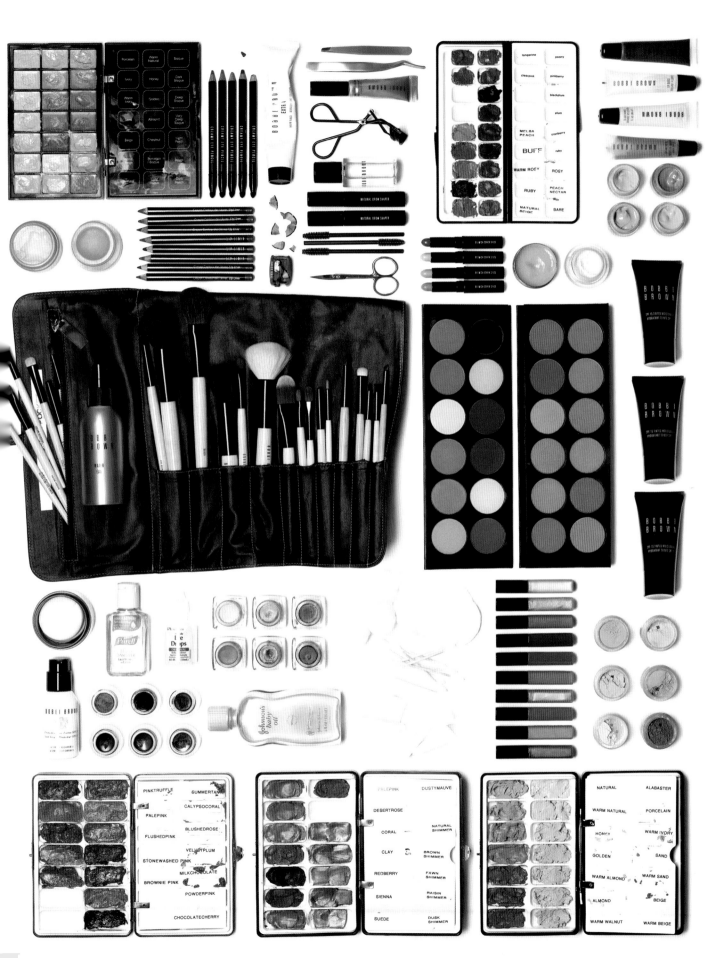

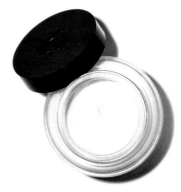

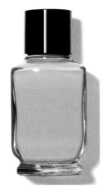

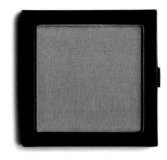

SKINCARE

Transfer moisturizers into smaller plastic jars and bottles, or purchase the smallest size container of each product. Keep all moisturizing products together in a large zip-top plastic bag or makeup bag. Appropriate skincare makes a huge difference in how makeup looks, so be prepared to cleanse and hydrate the face before applying any makeup.

Eye makeup remover, both non-oily and a product for removing waterproof makeup

Eye cream

Face lotion

Rich, moisturizing face cream

Shine-control lotion

Face balm

Lip balm

Body lotion

CONCEALER, FOUNDATION, POWDER

You will need a full range of foundation shades in order to properly match any skin tone you encounter. If using stick foundations, slice off sections, and put them into a palette; transfer your moisturizing and oil-free foundations into smaller bottles.

Five shades of corrector

At least ten shades of concealer

At least fifteen shades of foundation in a variety of formulas

Four to five shades of tinted moisturizer

Six shades of loose powder (from white, for use on porcelain skin, to dark brown)

Mix-in pigments—yellow, black, red, blue—are a help to correct wrong color foundation.

BLUSH

A complete kit includes a full range of blush in both neutrals and brighter shades in powder, cream, gel, and shimmer formulas, and a range of bronzers. Blushes are also used as eye shadow to achieve bright color in magazine work. It's also possible to mix a blush with clear lip balm for an extreme effect.

Six to eight shades of powder blush, from soft neutrals to brights

Five shades of cream blush (can be placed in a palette)

Two to three shades of gel blush

Four shades of bronzing powder

Five shades of shimmer blush or bronzer

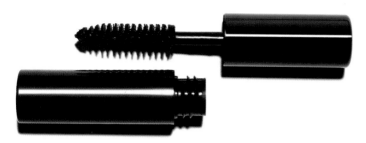

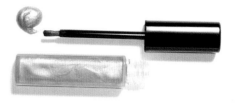

EYES

Include a wide variety of eye shadows in a range of colors and formulas, with pencils, brow pencils, and mascaras. The best way to arrange the shadows is in specially made palettes that have slots for the eye shadow containers. Arrange each palette by shade family, and label the palettes accordingly, so you can see at a glance which one you need. Making separate palettes for brights, shimmers, neutrals, and liners will help keep the kit organized.

Make sure you have all of your makeup tools, and don't forget to include cotton swabs or a non-oily eye makeup remover as well as a waterproof one. It's always better to be overprepared, than underprepared.

Four shades of all-over shadow color, such as white, bone, toast, and banana

A wide range of shadows to use as a lower lid color, include at least twelve choices

Three to six shades of shadow to use as liner, such as black, navy, medium brown, dark brown, dark green, and plum

Twelve shimmery shadows in a range of shades

Six to ten bold shadow and liner colors

Tinted and clear brow gels

Brow pencils in brown, blond, reddish brown, gray, taupe, and ash

Eye pencils in dark gray, brown, black, dark green, plum, and navy

Gel eyeliner in black, dark gray, and dark brown, optional extra colors could include violet and dark green

Black and dark brown mascara in both a thickening and a waterproof formula (colored mascaras are optional)

False eyelashes, both strips and individual

Eyelash glue; precolored glue in black helps fill the lash line

LIPS

It's easy to carry an extensive selection of lipsticks, because slices can be arranged in a palette. Using lipstick is the quickest and easiest way to change both a model's face and the feel of a photograph. In addition to the everyday colors, I like to keep an array of more unusual lip colors as well as other creamy pigments from the color wheel. It's amazing what a black lipstick does.

At least twenty different shades in a wide range of colors. These can be mixed to create dozens more. Essential colors include pale beige, pale pink, light orange, bright pink, bright orange, bright red, deep red, deep wine

At least ten shimmery lipsticks in a wide range of colors

At least ten lip glosses in a wide range of colors

At least ten lip pencils in a wide range of colors

A cream-based color wheel for blending

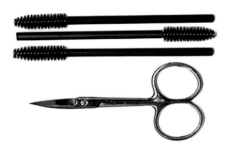

TOOLS

A complete set of brushes stored in a brush roll

Spray-on brush cleaner

Disposable makeup sponges

Cotton swabs

Cotton pads

Tissues

Tweezers

Eyelash curler

Baby scissors (for trimming unruly brows)

Disposable mascara wands

Water spray bottle

Makeup artists keep backups. Keep an extra set of brushes and all the products you can't live without in your home or office so you can access them if anything happens to your kit.

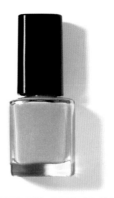

ESSENTIAL EXTRAS

Keep these things in your kit because you just never know when you might need them.

Hand disinfectant

Baby wipes

Mints

Baby oil

Eyedrops

Sheer, red, and chocolate nail polish

Nail polish remover

Extra zip-top plastic bags

Hand mirror

Protein bars, almonds, or other snacks—you will often be working through lunch and other meals

Paperback book for downtime, notebook for writing down inspirations

Business cards, as you never know whom you'll meet

TRICKS FOR PACKING YOUR KIT

Slice any product that comes in a stick (foundation, lipstick, bronzers, blushes), and put the slices into palettes. That way, you can have a whole array of shades in front of you at once.

Use zip-top plastic bags to store things and rubber bands to hold lip glosses and pencils together.

Use a label maker to label every bag, box, and palette neatly.

It's important for makeup artists to have a system. Pack your kit the same way each time, so you can find things in a hurry.

THE FUN KIT (at right)
These are the extra things you won't need very often, so store them all together in a separate plastic bag or makeup kit.

Sparkle and glitter powders

Nail polish in an array of colors

Intense theatrical eye shadow shades and blushes

Lip lacquers and matte stains in bold colors

Self-tanner and/or bronzing gel for the body

Body paints

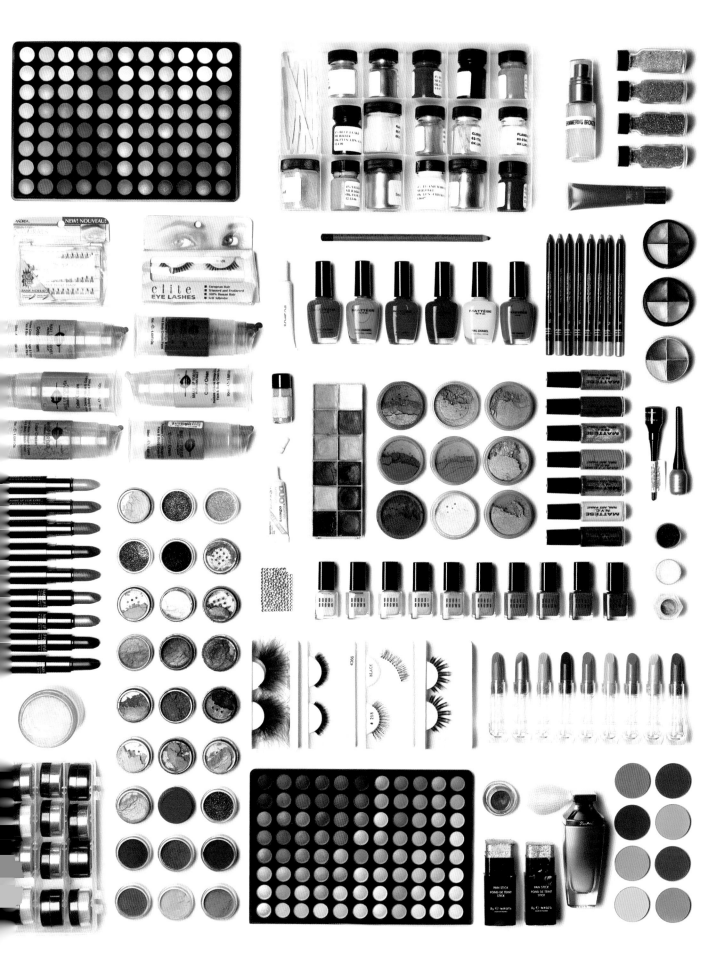

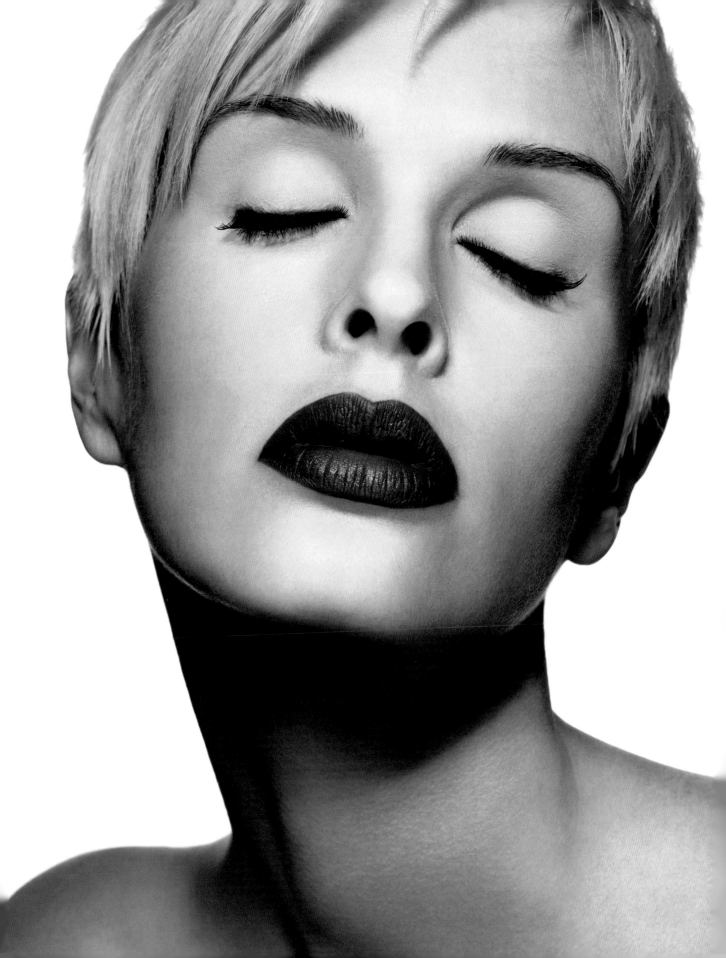

Chapter 11

ADVANCED MAKEUP APPLICATIONS

Every artist needs to learn skills to successfully apply makeup on subjects for photography, fashion shows, film, and television. These opportunities allow an artist to express her or his creativity. **There are no limitations when working in advanced artistry.**

MAKEUP for PHOTOGRAPHY

Applying makeup for photo shoots involves specific techniques that depend on a number of factors: *Lighting: Indoors or outdoors? Film or digital technology? Color or black-and-white? Style: What image does the photographer want?*

The makeup will differ depending on the purpose of the photograph—whether it is a passport photo, a wedding shot, a model in a natural outdoor setting, a corporate portrait, or a highly stylized fashion or beauty shoot. There is no one rule for how to do makeup that will be photographed. But the lighting in which you do the makeup is very important. I often do makeup with the model facing a window or, better yet, on the photo set with the lighting that will be used in the shoot.

Some guidelines follow that will help you understand the process and develop just the right look each time.

THE ROLE OF A MAKEUP ARTIST AT A PHOTO SHOOT

Making a photograph is a collaborative effort. As the makeup artist, you are part of a team that includes the photographer, the stylist, the hair stylist, the dresser, and the editor (if it is a magazine shoot), publicists and handlers (if the subject is a celebrity), and the subject being shot. Your job is to be true to your own style, yet be open; to understand the requirements of the stylist, editor, and model; and to create a makeup look that works.

The only way to accomplish that is to communicate with everyone on the set and be observant. Don't ever be embarrassed to ask questions or to give your opinion. Throughout the process, ask the photographer, stylist, editor, and subject for feedback. After you have applied the model's foundation, let her look at it in a mirror to see if she thinks it looks right. It is much easier to change things at that stage than to wait until the whole face is done. When analyzing the first shot, get the photographer's opinion on how the makeup is working—or isn't—with his or her lighting. Adjust accordingly. Once the shooting starts, don't think that your job is done. You need to stand by the set with your tools—powder, blush, lipstick, etc. Watch the model through a pair of mini binoculars to keep a close eye on how the makeup is holding up and what might need fixing. And be ready to jump in and try something that just might make the shot great. When a photographer teams up with a makeup artist, magic can happen. They understand each other's style and needs. They can work in sync to get the best results.

I have had a handful of collaborations with different photographers, and my work really grew as a result. I was able to be comfortable with them and try new things, and saw the results the next day. Each photographer moved my work in a different direction and I am grateful to all of them.

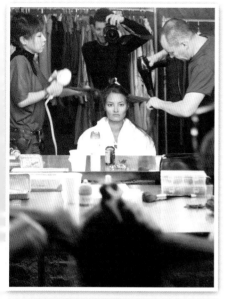
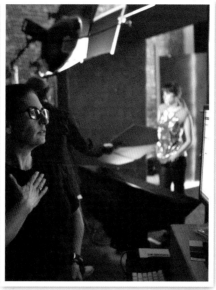
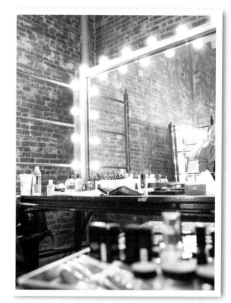
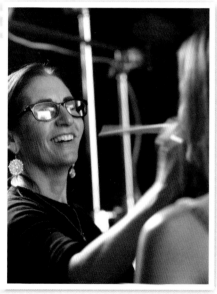
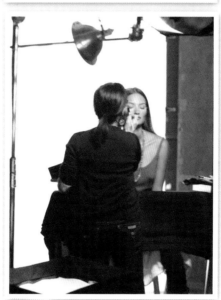
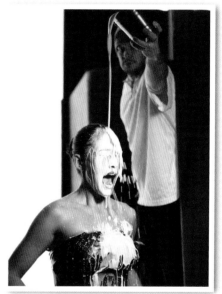
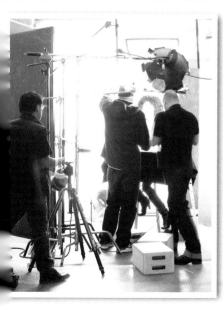
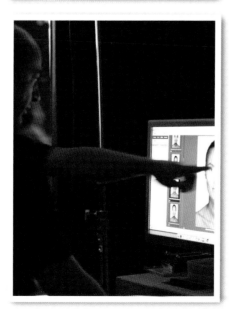
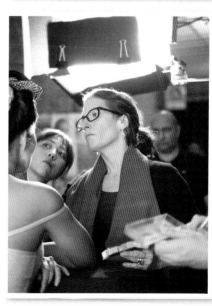

WHAT THE PHOTOGRAPHERS SAY ABOUT MAKEUP ARTISTS

It's important to adapt the makeup to the girl. You can't just decide what makeup you want to do and put it on, like a mask, on the model. It has to be adapted to suit the person you are working on. Working with celebrities can be difficult, because they have a very strong idea of what they want to look like, and it's harder to get them to change their look. You have to really work with them and be gentle.

—Patrick Demarchelier

The lighting that I use is strong, very revealing; therefore, I require perfection from a makeup artist. A makeup artist that I will want to have on my set must have that innate ability to enhance a woman's face and do it quickly. It seems that time is always of the essence, we are always under pressure, and the subject can't see the makeup artist hesitate. She needs to exude complete confidence. This helps put everyone at ease. A great makeup artist needs to inspire the women seated in front of the mirror in my studio. She needs to build up their egos, make them feel truly beautiful, give them the confidence to stand in front of my lens and feel proud about who they are. These elements are the first steps in a great collaboration and capturing an incredible visual. The makeup artist needs to be able to make women not only look beautiful but feel beautiful. That's what makes my photograph. I love shooting women who feel beautiful; you can really feel that in a photograph.

—Walter Chin

When I look at a makeup artist's work, first and foremost, I look for creativity. I look for someone who can think outside the box and who is able to look at a face and see what not to do, how much makeup not to apply. As a portrait and fashion photographer I am always interested in the geography of the face, and people's so-called flaws are often the most interesting things about them. I would never want to hide any of that. A makeup artist should always look for inspiration anywhere and everywhere and not just in their immediate realm. Museums, exhibits, nature, history: it's all there for the taking. Never become complacent; always be excited.

—Henry Leutwyler

I rely on the makeup artist's input from the beginning. I will always trust her opinion of which model we should use. Especially when you're doing close-up beauty shots, the less you have to do, the better it looks. So if we choose the model that already has great skin or long lashes, the less work it takes to nail it. We shoot so much digitally now, and that's really changed the way both the photographer and the makeup artist work. It's so easy to retouch and remove a blemish that usually I tell the makeup artist not to even bother trying to cover it up. But the most important thing for the makeup artist to know is that for beauty shots, you really have to exaggerate the effect you're trying to create. Film has a tendency to neutralize, so the color needs to be much stronger than what it would be in real life. You need to overdo it, and then assess it not by how it looks to your eye, but how it looks on camera.

—Troy Word

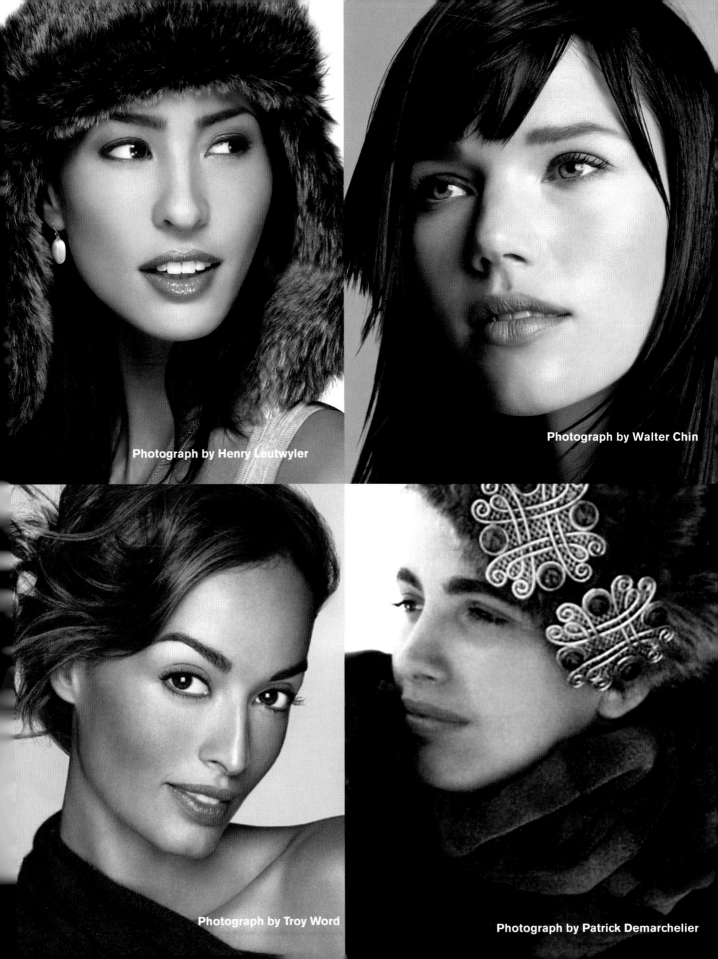

Photograph by Henry Leutwyler

Photograph by Walter Chin

Photograph by Troy Word

Photograph by Patrick Demarchelier

INDOOR OR OUTDOOR PHOTOGRAPHY

Whether photographs are being taken indoors or out, the most important rule is that foundation must exactly match skin tone, and the face has to match the body. Sometimes that means bringing the foundation lower on the neck or using some bronzing powder on the neck and chest to help eliminate any obvious color difference between the face and the body.

With outdoor photography, what you see is what you get. Outdoor lighting is very unforgiving. Use little foundation and a very light hand with blush. Everything has to look great to the naked eye, and makeup has to be well blended.

For indoor photography, the amount of makeup you apply depends on lighting. Define the features and determine if the lighting will wash out the skin tone or enhance it. Extremely strong lighting requires a heavier hand and more definition. But there are many variables in determining the style you want, so you have to be open to trying varying degrees of coverage and definition.

MAKEUP FOR PHOTOGRAPHS

Keep in mind the type of photo being taken. You use different techniques for a simple portrait than for a shoot for a high-end European fashion magazine.

Portrait
Keep the look simple, and make sure the subject is comfortable with the look.

Athlete
Do what's right for the person, and stick to his or her own style.

Musician
Unless the subject asks for a change, take your cue from his or her style, and don't stray too far from it.

Actor
Always ask before you start working. Actors like to evolve and try new things.

Fashion
When working with designers, it is important to be a good observer. Look carefully at the clothes. Ask about the designer's vision for the makeup.

Magazine
This kind of work varies tremendously. It is important to understand the style of the magazine and to get the input of the photographer, editor, and stylist on the shoot. I always befriend the photo assistant. That person has the best view and lets me know when something is not quite right.

BLACK-AND-WHITE OR COLOR PHOTOGRAPHY

In general, black-and-white photography is more forgiving than color photography, but both call for careful makeup application in order to get the best results.

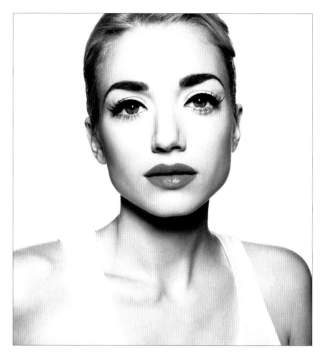

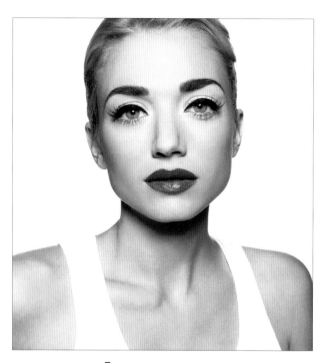

For Black-and-White Photography

Define the features. **That means a precise application of eyeliner and lip liner, as well as perfectly applied blush.**

Avoid using very shimmery shades **on the eyes, and don't use bronzer, as it can look dirty.**

Less is more. **Smooth out skin and conceal any imperfections, especially under the eyes, with bright concealer that blends perfectly, but don't go overboard with too much foundation or color.**

Lighting will dictate **how much makeup you need.**

For Color Photography

Foundation must match **the skin exactly.**

Never use translucent powder; it can make the face look masklike in a photograph. Instead, use warm, skin-tone-correct shades.

Don't overdo powder. **Especially in close-up photography, too much powder will call attention to any peach-fuzz facial hair.**

Skin needs to have even texture. **Coverage depends on many variables.**

Check Polaroids or digital monitor **to see if any corrections have to be made.**

A DYNAMIC DUO:
Gail Hadani & Paul Innis

The photographer Gail Hadani began painting and exhibiting her work at the age of ten, but her love of singing led her to a career in opera. After years of travel and life on the road as an opera singer, she discovered her passion for photography. Paul Innis, an artist, illustrator, and makeup artist, saw her ad in *Le Book*, loved the lighting and composition, took a chance, and called her. They now work as a team almost exclusively.

My career really began when I teamed up with Gail Hadani. Gail allows me to be completely creative with no limits. Having the support of a great photographer and friend is the best tool for success in this industry…

I believe in makeup as an art form. It's wonderful to do pretty makeup, but there has to be a little art to set you apart from everyone else. You have to find that thing that is creative and beautiful. For me, it is color and three-dimensional objects. I love to glue objects to the face, making what I call beautiful art with a model's face.

"Candy Land" (photos at right) all started when Gail bought some colored sugar at Dean & DeLuca, not knowing how she could incorporate it into an interesting photograph. At the time, Gail asked me what I thought we could do with this sugar, and, at the time, I was stumped.

A year and a half later, I realized what I could do with colored sugar, and Candy Land was born. I have developed a love for using common materials to create works of art on models' faces. In this project, I started with the colored sugar, gradually adding other bright and powerful candy-inspired colors (photo at lower left). I immediately thought of Life Savers, inspiring the Life Saver–like striped lips, which became one of my pride and joys as a makeup artist (upper right photo).

I have also always been a fan of making my lashes by chopping up different types of lashes, and then combining those pieces to make different shapes.

The lashes in the shot in the lower right hand corner were four pairs of lashes stacked together to create a unique shape. The lashes were custom fitted to the model's eyes, but unfortunately, they were also very heavy. So, the model was made to keep her eyes closed in between each shot.

As an artist, I believe you can use almost any products to transform a face into a work of art. Whether it is candy sprinkles, sugar, feathers, or rhinestones, it is all about thinking outside of the box to create spectacular and unique images!

—Paul Innis

Meeting Paul changed the course of my life. If it weren't for him, I would not be in this business that I have come to love with the same passion I used to have as an opera singer. We developed a distinctive style and worked so frequently together that we learned the art of making a powerful image. Both of us understand the basics of a great painting: composition, shape, light, color balance, emotion, and expression. The camera, lighting, and makeup are the paintbrushes. The set becomes a stage, where as director, I can mold the performances…

Our advice to young makeup artists: practice, practice, practice. Look, learn, create relationships, and put yourself out there.

—Gail Hadani

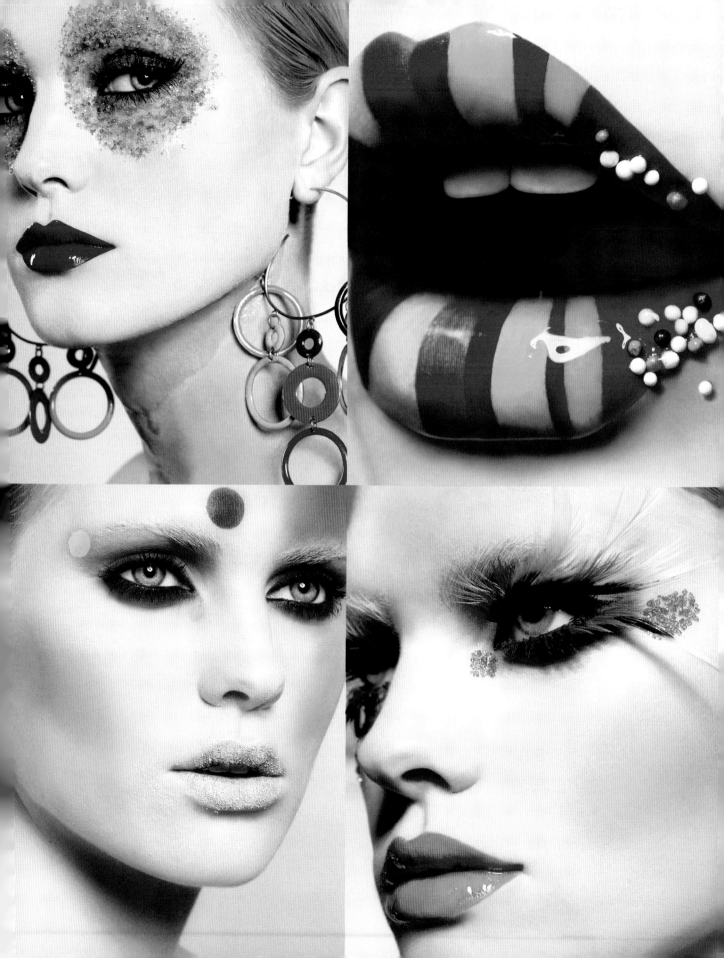

MAKEUP for MAGAZINES

The difference between doing basic makeup and doing makeup that is over the top for highly styled fashion shows or magazine work is thinking outside the box. ***Doing the unexpected*** — whether it's as simple as not putting on mascara or brows to a finished face or strengthening the brows to become a full blown experimental piece — is the difference between "basic" beauty and editorial freedom. It's all about being confident enough to experiment outside of your comfort zone.

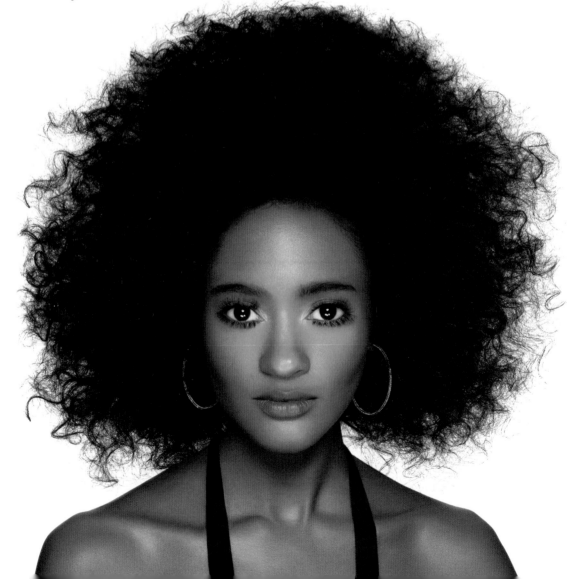

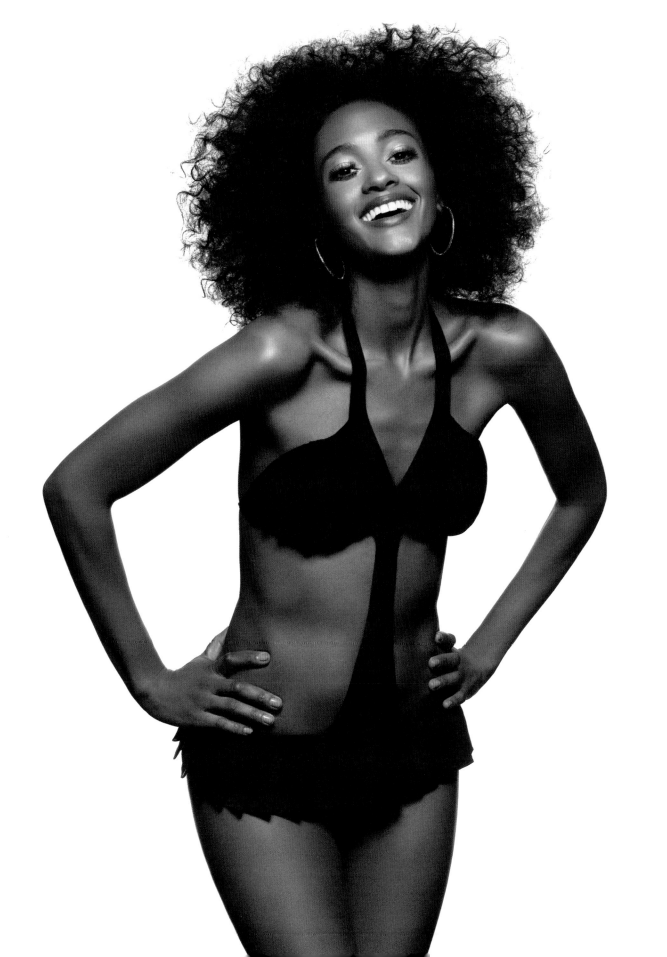

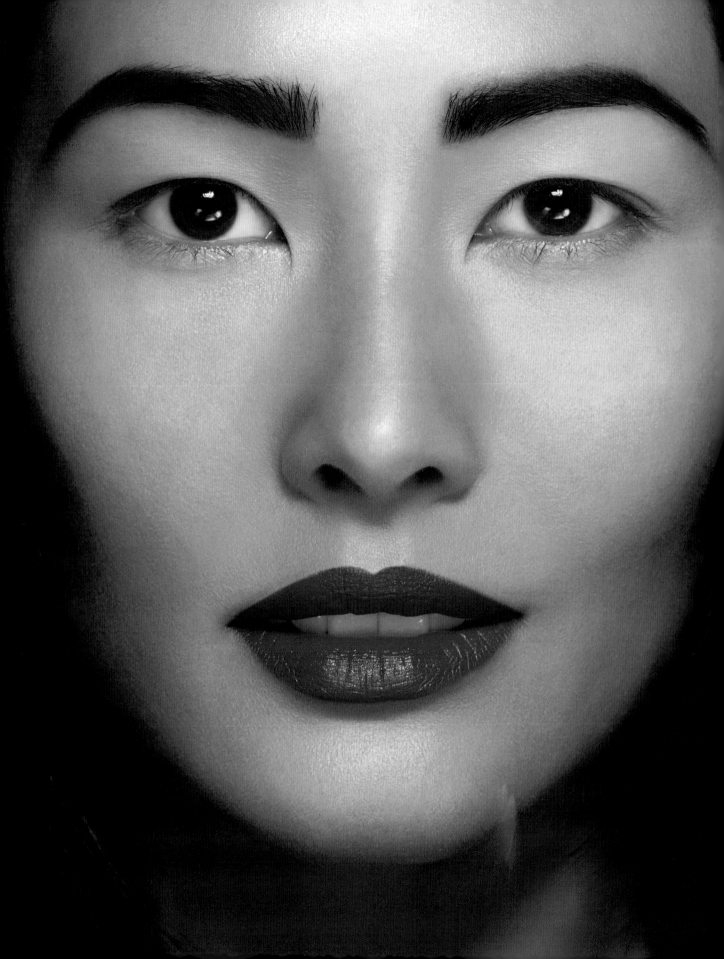

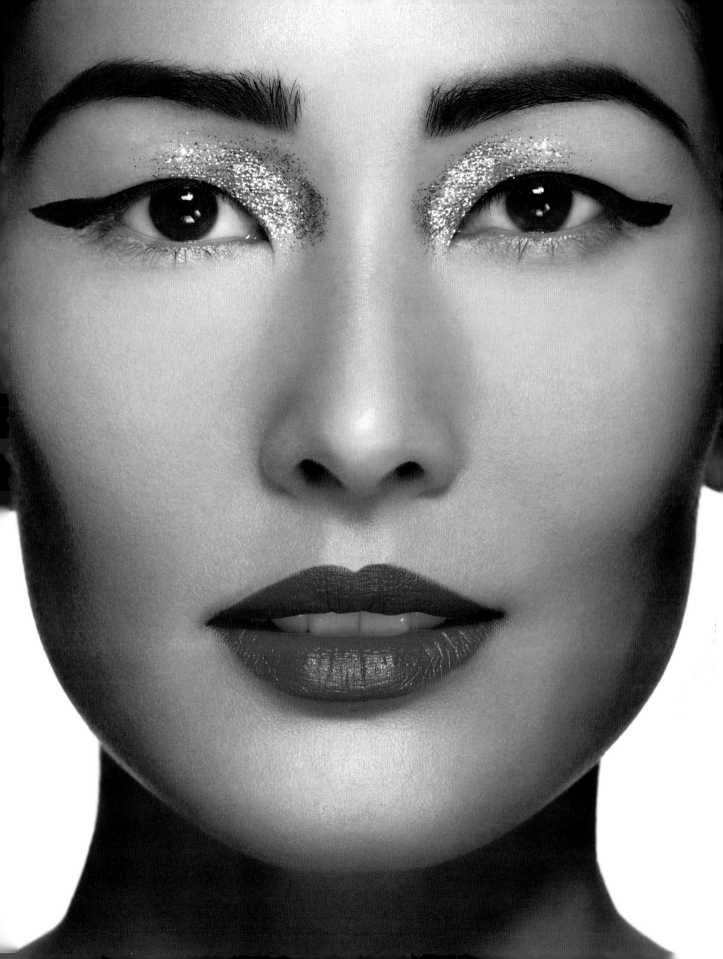

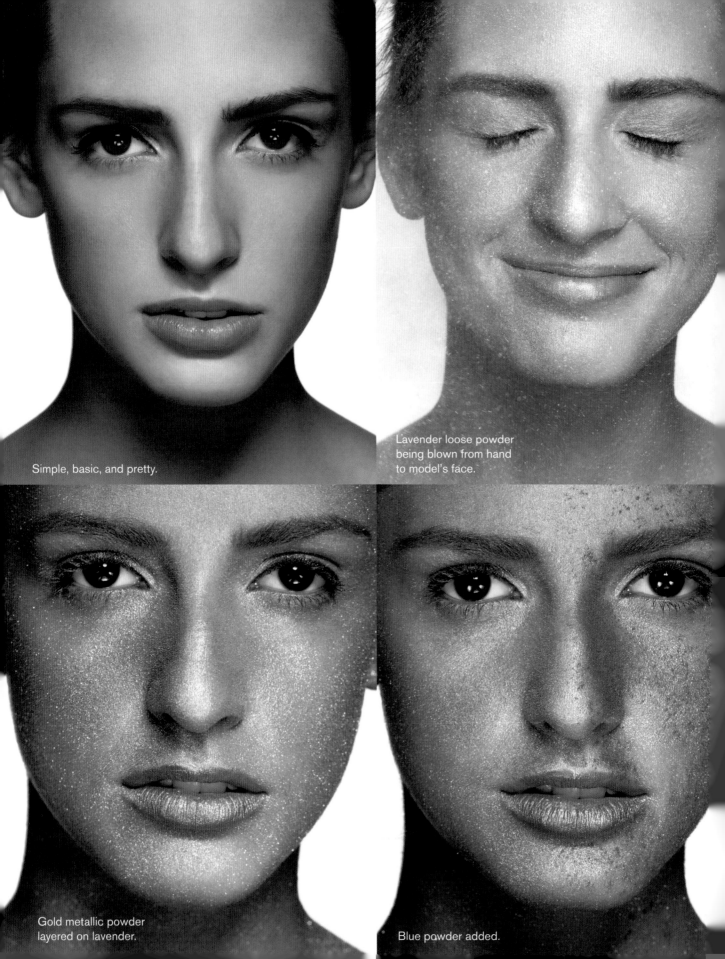

Simple, basic, and pretty.

Lavender loose powder being blown from hand to model's face.

Gold metallic powder layered on lavender.

Blue powder added.

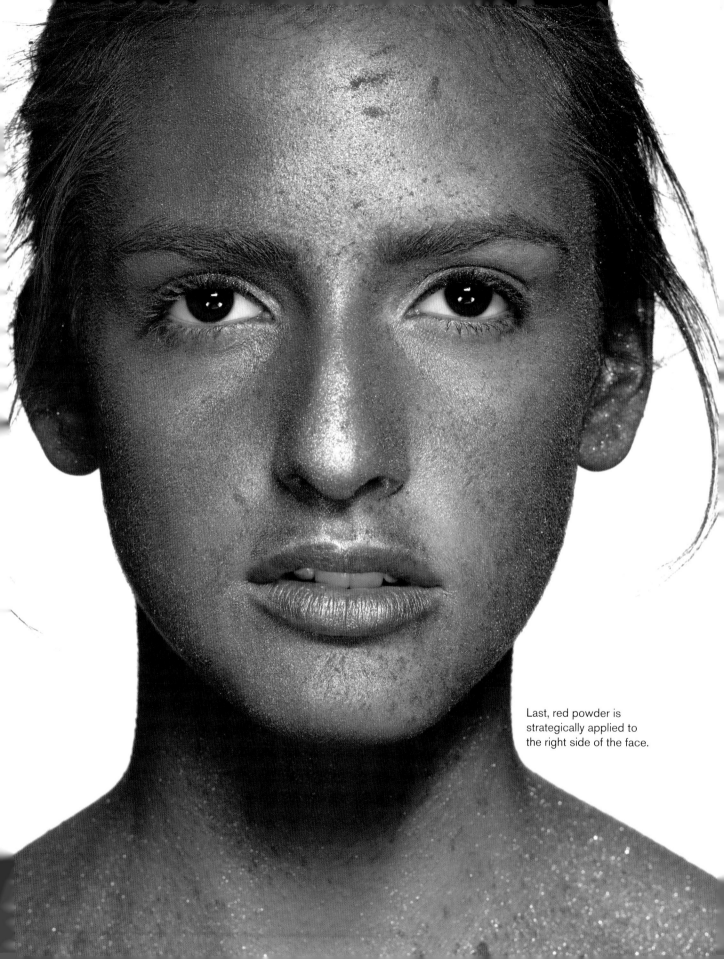

Last, red powder is strategically applied to the right side of the face.

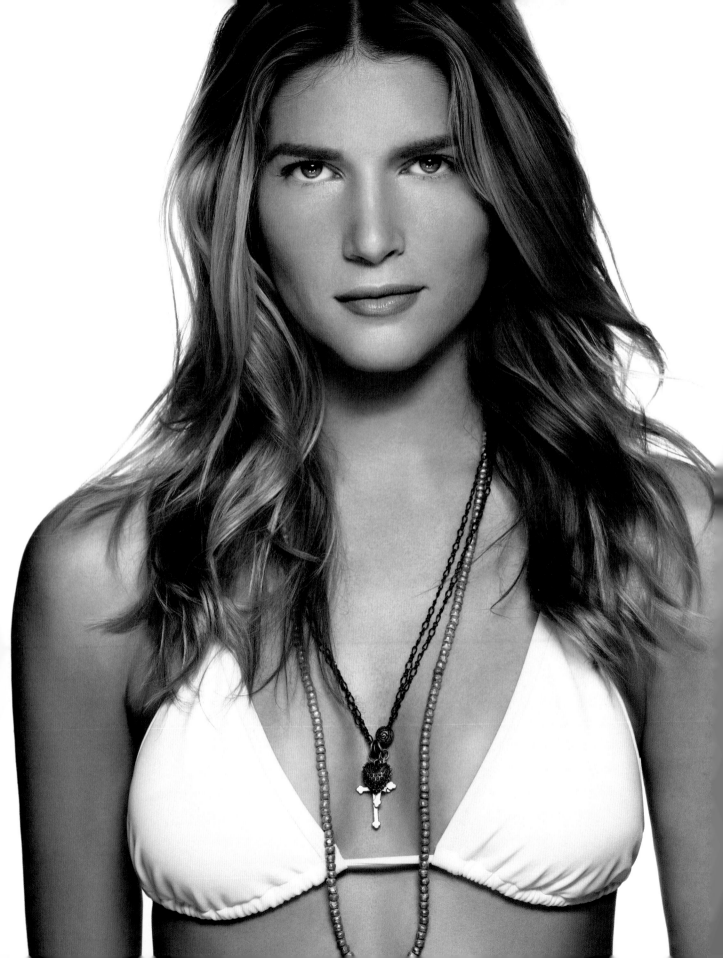

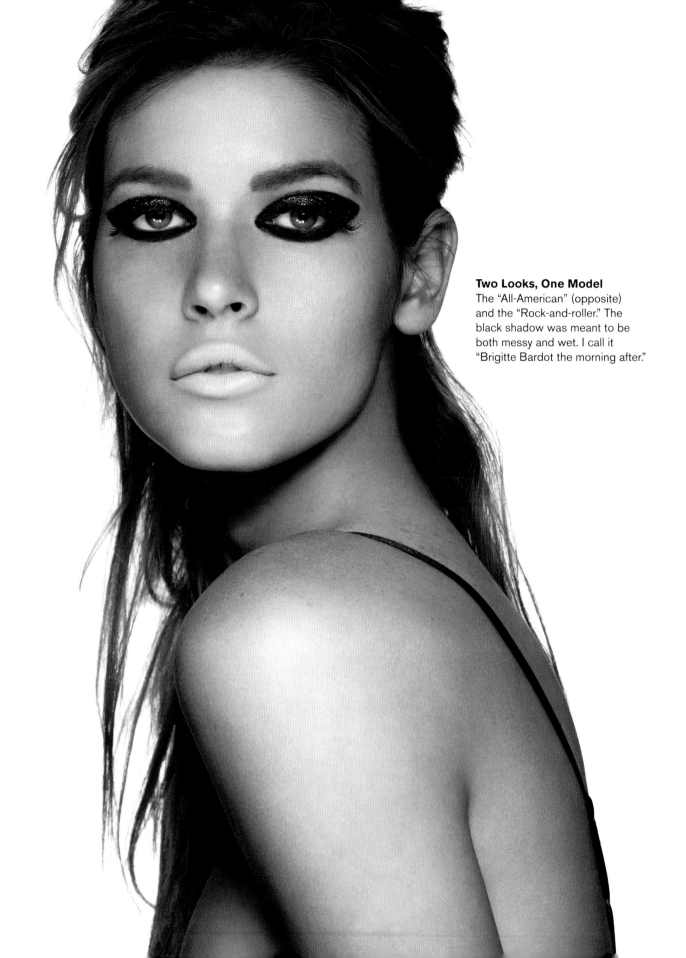

Two Looks, One Model
The "All-American" (opposite)
and the "Rock-and-roller." The
black shadow was meant to be
both messy and wet. I call it
"Brigitte Bardot the morning after."

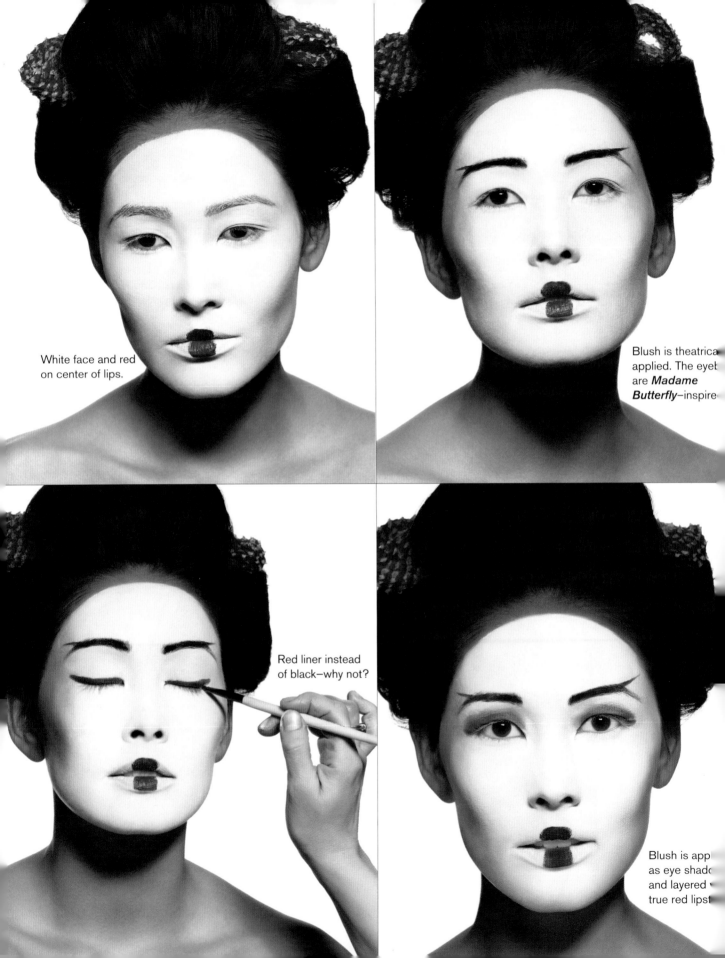

White face and red on center of lips.

Blush is theatrica[lly] applied. The eyeb[rows] are *Madame Butterfly*-inspire[d].

Red liner instead of black—why not?

Blush is app[lied] as eye shado[w] and layered [with] true red lipst[ick].

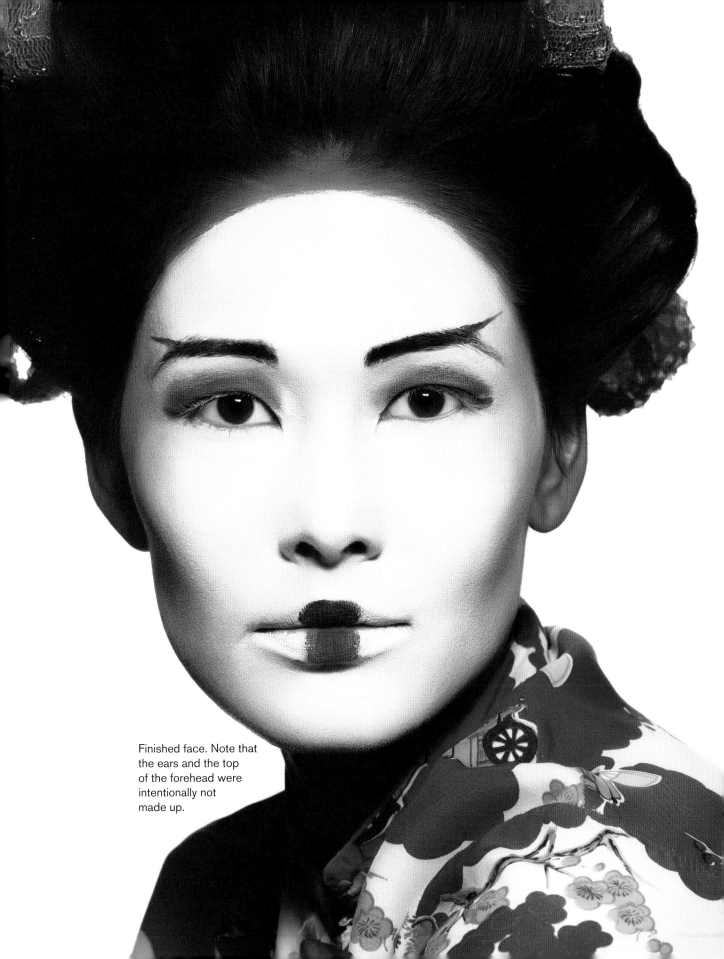

Finished face. Note that
the ears and the top
of the forehead were
intentionally not
made up.

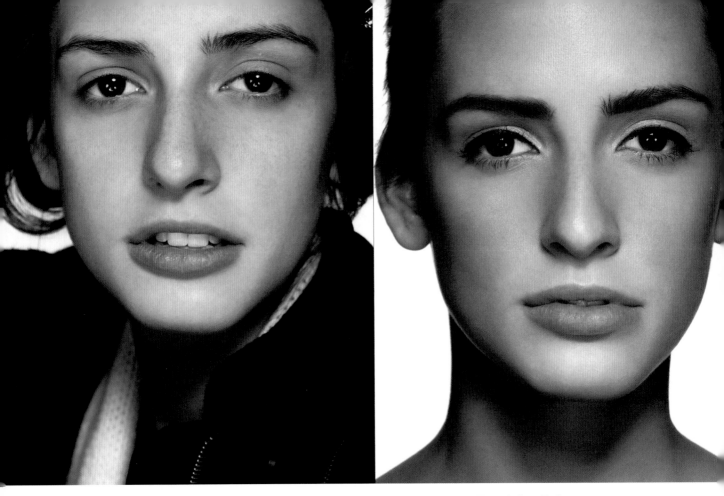

I've always loved unusual beauty.
This is not a before photo. To me this
face is a blank canvas.

The model looks like a Joffrey Ballet
dancer. Pretty, pink, and elegant.

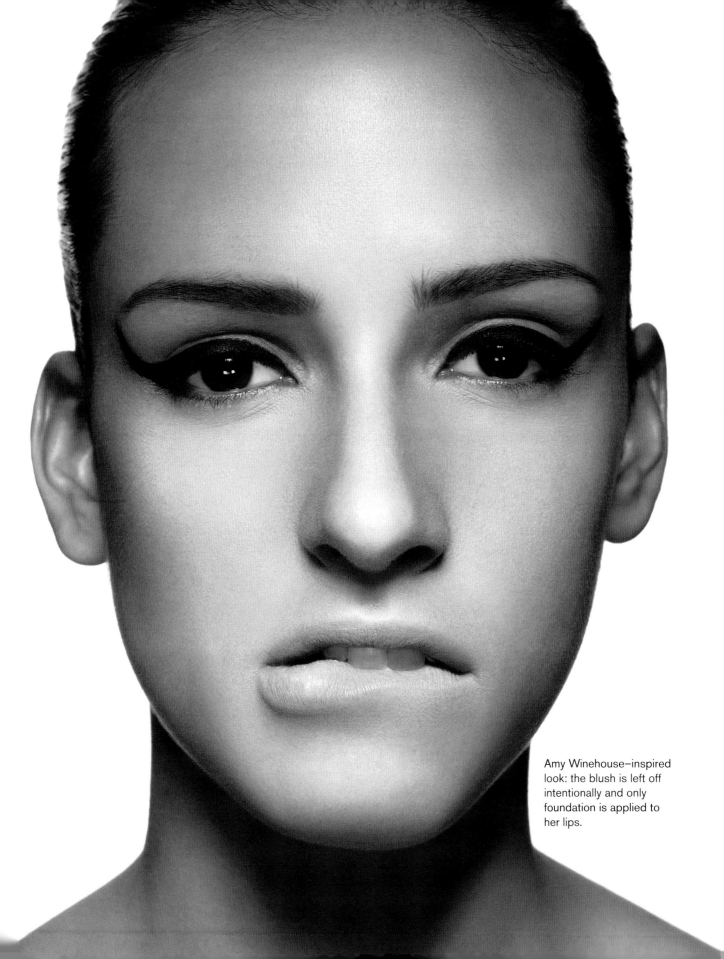

Amy Winehouse—inspired look: the blush is left off intentionally and only foundation is applied to her lips.

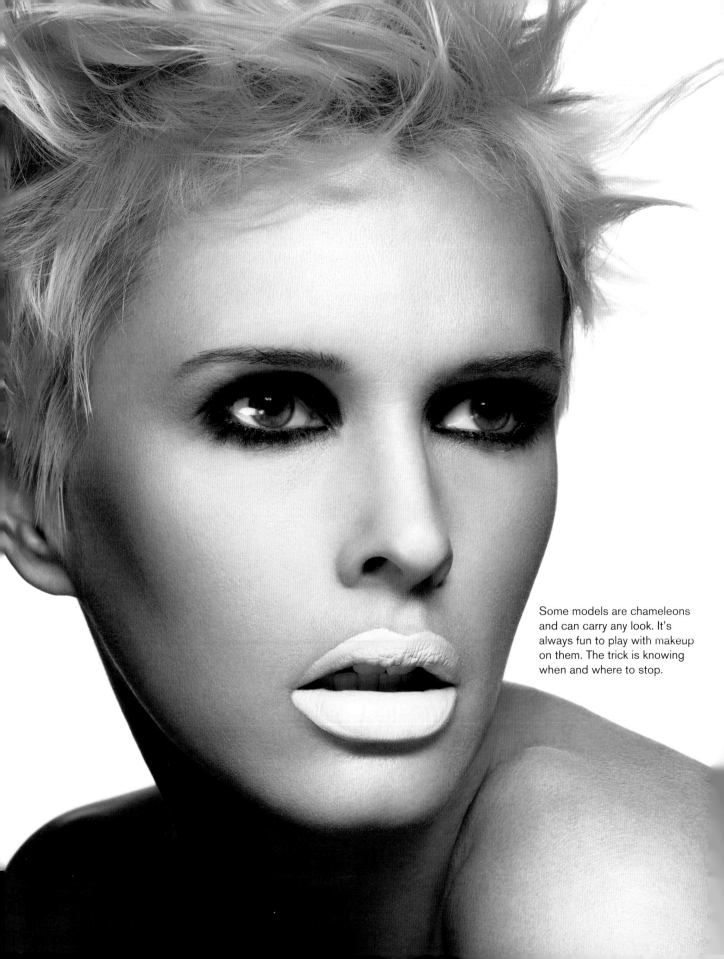

Some models are chameleons and can carry any look. It's always fun to play with makeup on them. The trick is knowing when and where to stop.

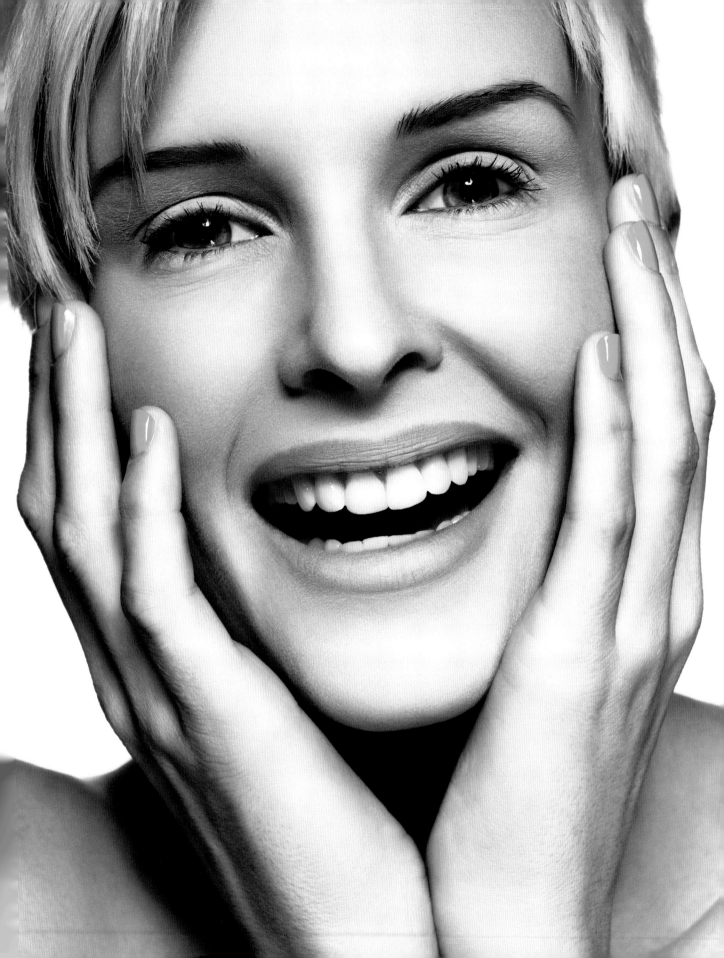

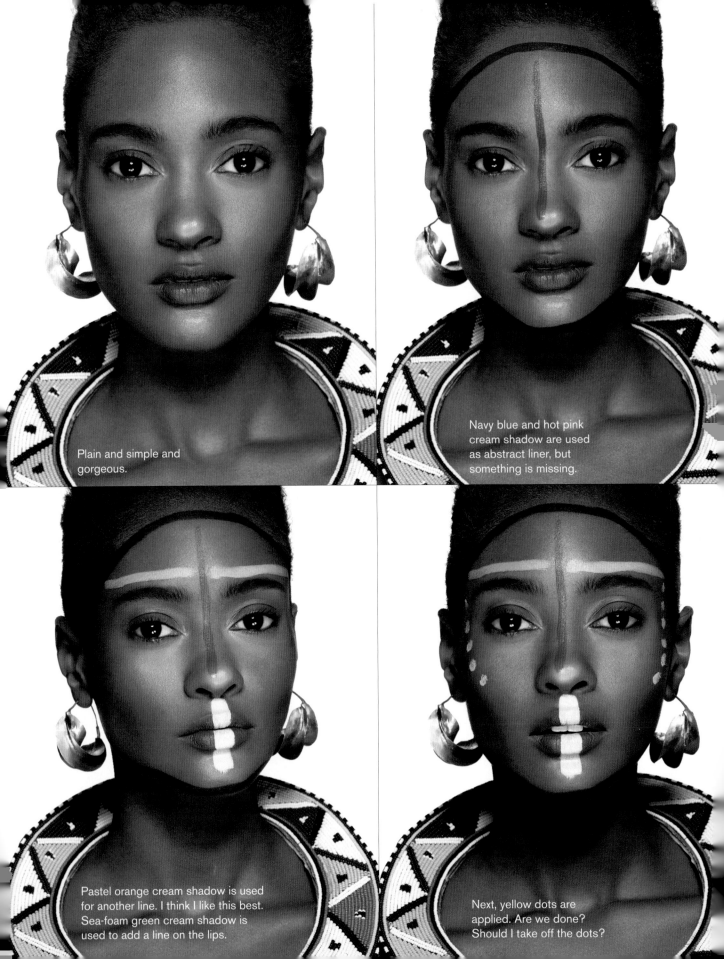

Plain and simple and gorgeous.

Navy blue and hot pink cream shadow are used as abstract liner, but something is missing.

Pastel orange cream shadow is used for another line. I think I like this best. Sea-foam green cream shadow is used to add a line on the lips.

Next, yellow dots are applied. Are we done? Should I take off the dots?

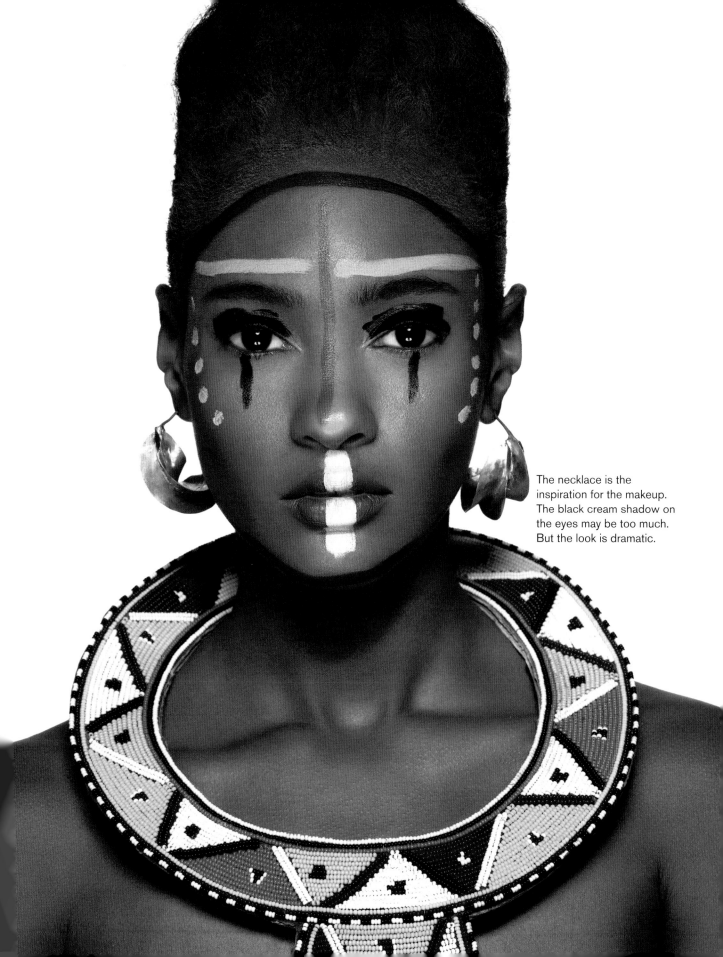

The necklace is the
inspiration for the makeup.
The black cream shadow on
the eyes may be too much.
But the look is dramatic.

MAKEUP for TELEVISION & FILM

TELEVISION

There is a misconception that makeup done for television has to be heavy. That is not the case. The bright lights of television studios can wash out makeup colors, but don't overcompensate with too heavy a hand. Use the same products you would use for day. Just make sure they are pumped up a notch, and perfectly blended.

Brighten the under-eye area **by layering pink-toned corrector under yellow-toned concealer. Then set it with loose powder applied with a powder brush or puff. This step is an absolute necessity as television lights increase shine.**

Use full-coverage foundation **followed by powder to keep it matte. Sheer tints are too subtle for television.**

Even if a glow is desired, **it needs to be added to the cheeks at the end of the makeup application.**

Color tends to wash out, **so always use two shades of blush—one natural shade followed by a brighter pop of color. Correct blending is a must.**

Avoid lip colors that are too light **unless the subject's lips are so full that you want to downplay them. Television tends to wash out natural tones.**

Define lips with pencil.

Make sure hands, arms, neck, and ears **all match the face.**

Bronzer is a great help, **especially on the neck.**

High-Definition Television

High-definition television is extremely unforgiving. (It definitely wasn't invented by a woman over twenty years old.) It conveys very sharp contrast with great detail. The makeup you apply has to be both fluid and perfectly blended. Foundation that is not correctly applied will look like it's melting off the face. Remember two words: *coverage* and *blending*.

Always check makeup in the monitor **to see how it reads with lighting.**

Blemishes **need to be expertly covered.**

FILM

Directors, lighting, and scripts dictate what style of makeup needs to be done. Communicate with everyone involved, ask lots of questions, and do lots of testing. The real makeup challenge, when working on films, is maintaining continuity. Scenes are often shot out of sequence, and part of a makeup artist's job is to make sure the character looks the same in each scene. It can be a slow process, so always have a digital camera and a notebook handy to keep track of the shots. Lighting and style dictate what the makeup should look like.

NINE MEMORABLE WOMEN

These women are all icons and their looks have inspired many makeup artists to recreate them either in movies or editorial work. Whether it's a direct period piece or just an element—these are the looks that inspire editors and photographers.

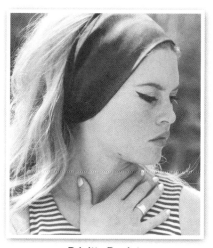

Brigitte Bardot
Light foundation and blush, extra pale lips, and classic medium-thick eyeliner.

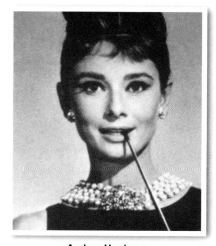

Audrey Hepburn
Her look was all about the strong squared-off brow, a matte powdery face, and natural colors.

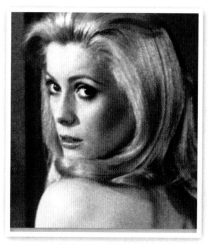

Catherine Deneuve
Sexy kitten, smoky eyes, and medium lips.

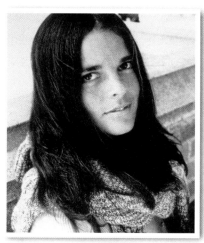

Ali McGraw
The icon of the natural American look. Brown eyeshadow, simple dark brown liner, naturally strong brow, clean skin, tawny cheek, and nude lip.

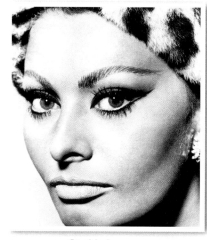

Sophia Loren
Classic Italian, sexy yet understated. Her strong features don't need a lot. Strong brows, medium lips, clean black eyeliner, and a little blush.

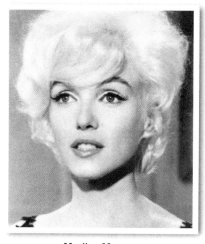

Marilyn Monroe
Her makeup was all about a sexy face. Strong brows, white eyelids, smoky contour, false eyelashes, and strong eyeliner, often with a red lip—classic 50s.

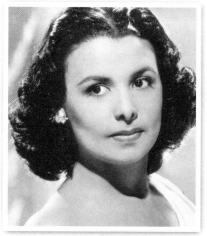

Lena Horne
40s glamour—burgundy lips, eyes lined on top, shadow artfully applied, strong brow, and visible black false eyelashes.

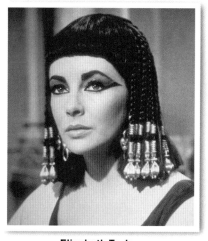

Elizabeth Taylor
Whether playing the title role in *Cleopatra* or Martha in *Who's Afraid of Virginia Woolf*, she always had her violet eyes rimmed with black shadow, eyeliner, and lashes.

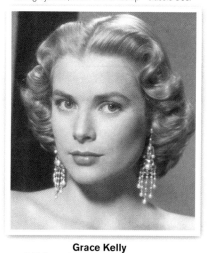

Grace Kelly
A Hollywood princess: classic blonde and "Ralph Laurenesque" at a black-tie ball.

MAKEUP for FASHION SHOWS

Working as a makeup artist at a fashion show is similar in many ways to doing the makeup for a theatrical production. Just as theatrical makeup has to represent the vision of the director or the playwright, *the final look you see on the runway is a collaboration between the designer, the makeup artist, the hairstylist, and the model.* As fashion shows have increasingly become a media circus, with television cameras and photographers recording every aspect of the event both on the runway and backstage, the makeup artist's role has become even more important. It is not enough to make a model look beautiful; a makeup artist must be able to speak about the designer's vision and the current style trends.

Working with models is like working with a blank canvas. You can experiment and try things that would probably look horrible on a real woman but look great on the runway or in a photo. I do believe that if the model likes her look, the shoot will go better. I have had to apologize for creating a severe look that the model hates but is required by the designer or photographer. *All of these situations take confidence, patience, communication, and a willingness to take risks.*

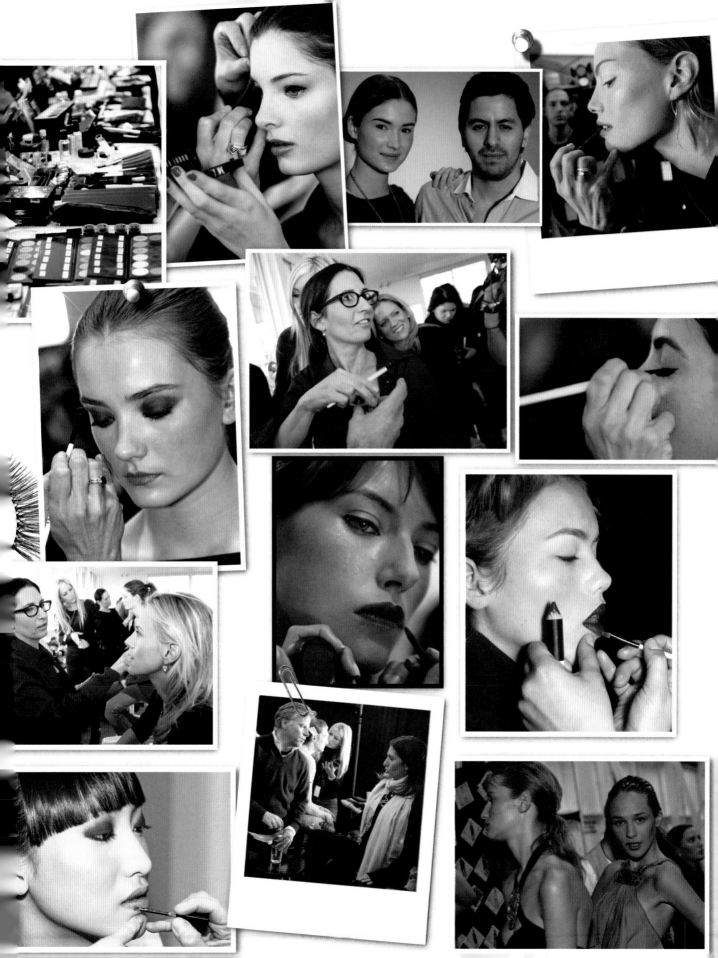

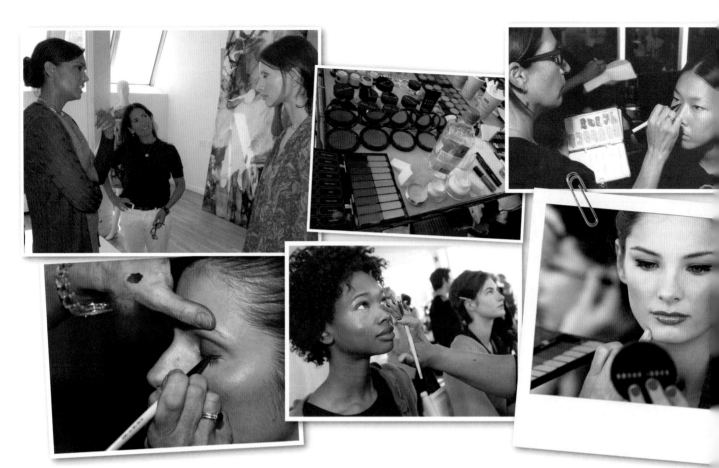

WHAT HAPPENS BEFORE THE SHOW

The Makeup Test

If it's the first time you've worked with a designer, research his or her design style and history. This will give you an idea of the aesthetics of past shows.

About a week before the fashion show, the makeup artist and designer meet to discuss the look. After viewing the clothes, the designer will give you his or her vision for the collection. Designers are very visual, but aren't always able to communicate what they want. Your role is to interpret their vision. Most designers have photos of inspirational objects to help you with the interpretation. Ask a *lot* of questions. If the designer mentions he wants a strong eye, ask if he's thinking Sophia Loren in the 60s or the modern Gucci eye. Keep asking until you feel confident that you have the right vision in your head.

Next, do some trials and experiment with some options to show the designer and stylist your interpretations of the look. You may get the right look quickly, or it can take quite a long time. Sometimes makeup is done on a pretty assistant, but show makeup works best on a model. There is a reason models are models: they showcase makeup better than other people.

Once the final look is approved, sketch it. Purchase anything you think you will need that is not already in your kit, and complete a face chart that includes all of the products, with color identification, location on the face, and any special information needed to complete the look. You will need a makeup team. Find out how many models will be walking and hire one artist for every two to three models.

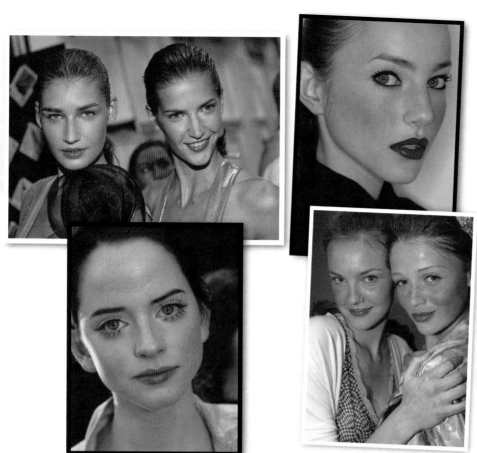

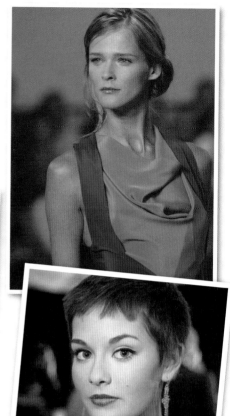

WHAT HAPPENS DURING THE SHOW

Stay calm. This is the key to working on a fashion show. There will be plenty of chaos, lots of distractions, and last-minute emergencies. You also have to be flexible; sometimes makeup is completely changed thirty minutes before the show.

On the day of the fashion show, you need to arrive two to four hours before the show is scheduled to begin.

Start by using one of the models to do a trial run of the makeup. When her face is done, bring her out onto the runway so you and the designer can check the results under the lights. If you have assis-tants working with you, bring them out as well so they hear what you and the designer decide.

Once the look gets approved, the team begins to work. Adjust the colors for each model's skin tone. Even if the designer says he wants pastel pink on everyone's cheeks, remember that the exact same color won't work on differ-ent skin tones.

Many of the models will arrive backstage from another show. They will already have a full face of makeup on, and you will have only minutes to change their look completely. To save time, hand the model a tissue covered in non-oily makeup remover, and instruct her to wipe off her lipstick and eye shadow. You can have her leave the foundation and mascara on, but you must check it carefully to determine whether it will work with the look you're try-ing to create. No matter how little time you have, if the foundation isn't right, you must take it all off and start from scratch.

Right before the show begins, you need to check the models for refreshing or additional powder to combat shine.

Even after the models start heading down the runway, your job is not done. As the models change clothes, they might mess up their lips, or they might need a touch-up with powder. Your job is to continue standing by, ready to fix whatever might need fixing.

WORKING with CELEBRITIES

Working with celebrities is fun and challenging. Just like every woman, they want to find a look that is right for them while looking beautiful. *Whether you are doing their makeup for an early-morning television appearance, a movie premiere, a photo shoot, or the Oscars, you have to adapt the look to suit the clothes, lighting, and occasion.* And as with any relationship, if it's your first time working with a certain celebrity, go slowly, ask a lot of questions, and hand her the mirror frequently to avoid getting big surprises at the end of the application. If it is a celebrity you've worked with regularly, just ask a few quick questions about what she's going to be wearing and the look she wants.

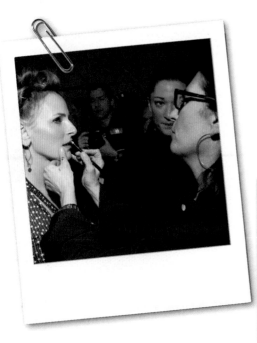

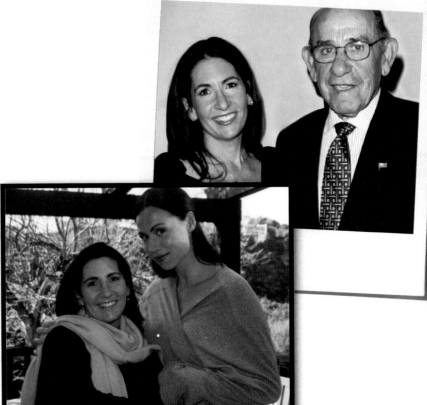

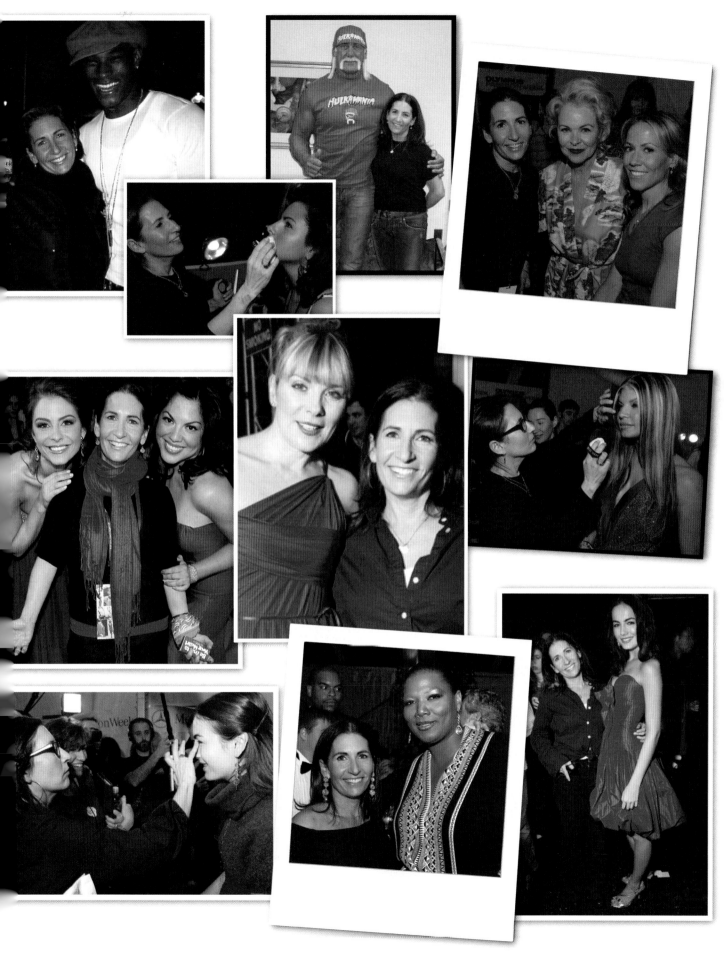

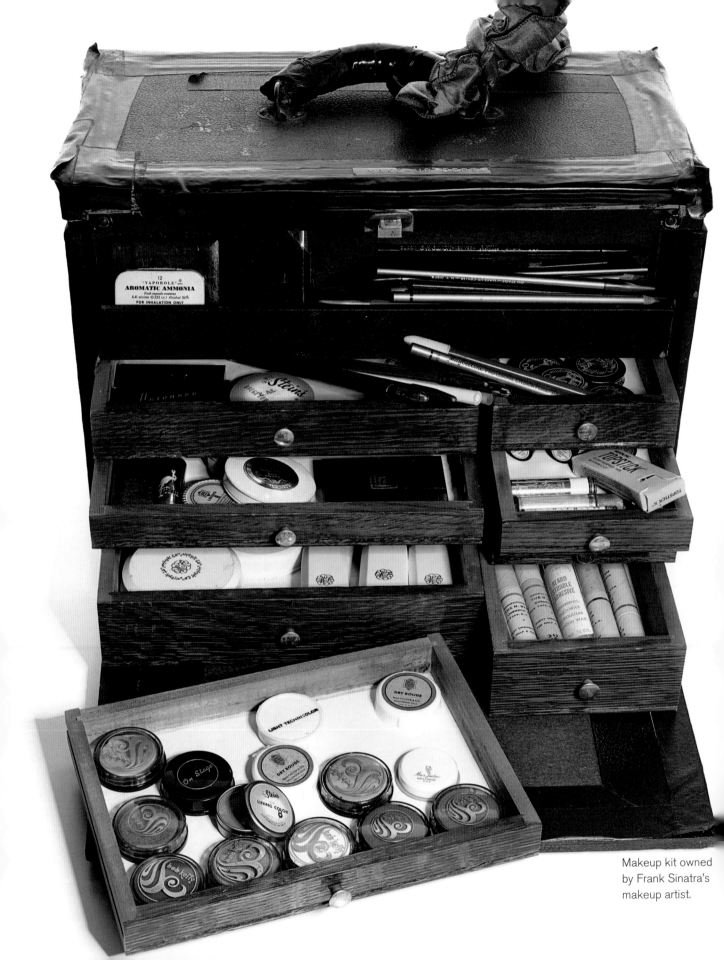

Makeup kit owned
by Frank Sinatra's
makeup artist.

Chapter 12

MEMORABLE MAKEUP MOMENTS & LEGENDS

the HISTORY of MAKEUP

c. 500,000 B.C.E. Cave dwellers in Africa and South America cover their bodies with mud applied in decorative patterns. The mud also functions as an insect repellent.

c. 3000 B.C.E. Egyptians use more than thirty different types of cosmetic balms and ointments made from ingredients such as beeswax, vegetable oil, and animal fat. Moisturizers are considered so essential, they are routinely distributed to workers and farmers.

Egyptian women have elaborate makeup chests, equipment, and products. They give themselves egg white facials, use complexion cream, and apply perfumed oils. Women paint their faces with a (deadly) powder made from lead carbonate and water. Nails are painted with henna, and lipsticks are available in several orange-based shades. The use of red is banned, as it is considered magical. To outline the eyes, they use either powdered kohl or crushed ant's eggs. Eye shadows in red or green are created using plant stems. Other makeup tools include stone pestles for grinding, bronze or silver mirrors, ivory or alabaster spoons, bronze jars for holding face cream, linen, razors, ivory combs, and pumice.

c. 2000 B.C.E. An Egyptian papyrus includes formulas for removing wrinkles, pimples, age spots, and other blemishes. One mixture includes bullock's bile. Egyptians who want to get rid of wrinkles are told to apply a mixture of incense, olive oil, crushed cyperus, and wax to the face and to leave it on for six days.

Overseers stop all work on the pyramids until makeup supplies (kohl, green malachite, and galena) that help to protect the eyes of workers from the sun are delivered.

c. 2500 B.C.E. Sumerians invent the first tweezers to get rid of unwanted hair and use a flat bone to push back cuticles.

c. 1800 B.C.E. Gold dust is used by Babylonian men to powder their hair.

c. 1500 B.C.E. Egyptian women use body oils scented with frankincense and myrrh to moisturize and protect their skin from the dry, dusty climate.

Mesopotamian soldiers are paid in bottles of oil and perfume, which are more highly valued than cash.

c. 1200 B.C.E. Egyptians of this era are wearing a full face of cosmetics. They create eye shadows out of malachite, a copper ore that has a greenish tone, to line their bottom lids. Eyelashes and upper lids are darkened with powder made from lead ore.

c. 600 B.C.E. Makeup and lavish clothing is worn by all Babylonians of rank. An ambitious warrior named Parsondes was said to have complained to King Nebuchadnezzar about the governor Nanarus's focus on beauty rather than on government. When word got back to the governor, Nanarus ordered that the warrior shave all his hair and wear makeup and perfumed oils.

c. 400 B.C.E. Women from various cultures use powders made from crushed minerals, such as ocher, hematite, and white lead, to color their skin.

FIRST CENTURY B.C.E. Roman women use saffron or wood ash as eye shadow and antimony to darken their lids, lashes, and brows. Fucus, a purple pigment, is mixed with saliva and used for rouge and lip color. Blue paint is used to outline veins, which are seen as a sign of beauty. Nails are buffed with sheep's fat. Pumice is used to whiten teeth.

SECOND CENTURY A.D. Women in Palestine apply a mixture of starch, white lead, and crimson dye to their faces as an early form of blush.

THIRD CENTURY A.D. Talmudic law forbids Jewish women from applying makeup on the Sabbath.

636 The first glass mirror is invented. Women hang them, placed in elaborate cases, on a chain from their girdles, and men keep theirs under their hats.

1370 Charles V of France receives a gift of Hungary water, a body rub made of an alcohol base with rosemary, cedar, and turpentine. Soap is a luxury, but the use of these waters sweetens the smell of the body.

c. 1400 Cosmetics, including a white paste made of flour to cover the face, become increasingly popular among the French aristocracy. Women pluck their hairlines and even remove their eyebrows in the name of beauty.

c. 1500 Renaissance women use a mixture of honey and egg whites to condition their skin. White lead is applied to reduce the appearance of wrinkles. Mercuric sulphide is used for rouge. To keep complexions clear, some wash their faces in urine or a mixture of rose water and wine. To reduce ruddiness, raw veal soaked in warm milk for several hours is placed on the affected area.

c. 1550 Catherine de Médicis uses a skin tonic made from crushed peach blossoms mixed with almond oil.

1597 *Gerard's Herbal* is published. This is one of the first printed publications to include recipes for various skin creams, including one for acne.

c. 1600 To soothe chapped lips, it is recommended that sweat from behind the ears be applied to the affected area.

1603 Queen Elizabeth I dies and is rumored to have an inch and a half of makeup on her face at the time of her passing. This is not uncommon in an era when no one washes their faces, and makeup is used to cover the horrible scars left by smallpox.

LATE 1600s A doll-like look with a pure white face and scarlet cheeks is all the rage. A foundation of white ceruse, which contains lead, is mixed on a palette with water or egg white and applied to the skin. Rouge is commonly applied by rubbing a piece of Spanish felt or wool that has been dyed scarlet onto dampened cheeks.

LATE 1600s TO 1700s Silk taffeta or thin leather patches in shapes like flowers, stars, and moons become a popular product to temporarily conceal smallpox scars on the face. More than just cover-ups, however, the patches signal a woman's availability if placed near the lips. Engaged women wear them on the left cheek and switch to the right after marriage. Some even carry small patch boxes with them to social events to replace any that fall off. Small scenes are sometimes pasted over an eyebrow, and profiles of family members are sometimes worn on the face.

c. 1830 Women put a few drops of belladonna into their eyes to dilate the pupils, creating a dreamy look. Belladonna is a plant extract used since ancient times as a poison.

1846 Pond's Extract, a commercial cold cream, is introduced.

1867 The department store B. Altman and Company opens a "making up" department to teach women to apply rouge, powder, and eyebrow pencil.

1886 Avon, the door-to-door cosmetics line, is founded by David Hall McConnell, a former door-to-door book salesman.

c. 1900 Guerlain introduces the first lip colors to come in stick form.

1891 Polish-born Helena Rubinstein opens the world's first modern beauty salon, in Australia. She sells a simple face cream inspired by her mother's beauty cream. The product is an instant hit among Autralian women. In 1902 Helena expands her business to London, followed by Paris in 1906 and New York in 1912.

1908 Actresses are the only people who know much about makeup, as it is used exclusively for the stage. No woman dares to go out in public with more than the lightest dusting of rice powder. Rice powder makes the face appear lighter but also swells up in the pores of the skin, enlarging them. Helena Rubinstein starts to produce a tinted face powder that is more natural looking, does not have harmful side effects, and has a broad appeal.

1909 Rubinstein's lifelong rival, Elizabeth Arden, opens her Fifth Avenue salon.

1909 The Russian immigrant Max Factor opens his first makeup studio in Hollywood.

1909 Eugène Schueller, a French chemist, opens the French Harmless Hair Dye Company, selling the first safe commercial hair dye product. A year later, he renames his product L'Oréal.

c. 1910 The first pressed compact powders—complete with mirrors and puffs—are introduced.

1910 *The Daily Mirror Beauty Book* is published. The makeup hints and recipes for homemade lotions reflect the fact that cosmetics have become publicly accepted for the first time in almost one hundred years. The little booklet includes references to a device that curls lashes, a homemade eyebrow darkener, and astringent lotion, and it suggests using a pencil line to elongate the eyes.

1910 Tattoos are extremely popular in Britain. George Burchett, a famous tattooist, practices his art on men and women alike. His card indicates that he can tint and shade complexions and remove moles, blemishes, and other marks.

1914 After seeing his sister Maybel apply petroleum jelly to her lashes, T. L. Williams formulates the first mascara. He forms a company, named Maybelline after his sister, to manufacture the new product.

c. 1920 Coco Chanel makes tans chic, calling a suntan an important "fashion accessory."

1920s The flapper Clara Bow is everyone's favorite "it" girl. Her look includes heavy eyeliner and ultrathin eyebrows.

The opening of chain stores, in which products and prices can be examined by all, make inexpensive cosmetics available to everyone.

1922 Elizabeth Arden opens a salon on Bond Street in London.

1930 When she finds that her new cream can heal and improve the skin in a matter of hours, Elizabeth Arden names the product Eight Hour Cream. It remains a best seller to this day.

1932 Revlon launches its first nail enamel.

1939–1945 World War II restricts the manufacture of cosmetics. Petroleum and alcohol, two principal ingredients used in makeup, are needed for war supplies.

1940s Joan Crawford's heavily penciled-in, arched eyebrows become the trademark look for the 1940s career woman.

1943 Estée Lauder launches her company with a line of six products.

1952 Revlon's Fire and Ice, an all-out sexy red lipstick color, is launched and becomes an instant success.

1960 The Color Additive Amendment requires that coloring ingredients in cosmetics be tested for safety and approved by the FDA.

1967 Estée Lauder launches a new line called Clinique, which emphasizes scientific skincare and cosmetics.

1967 The supermodel Twiggy popularizes a dramatic eye look; she draws lashes around the eye with a pencil and applies numerous false lashes, creating a doe-eyed effect.

1970s Natural makeup is all the rage.

Models to know: Veruschka, Marissa Berenson, Lauren Hutton, Margaux and Mariel Hemingway, Cheryl Tiegs, Christie Brinkley, Beverly Johnson.

Beauty icons: Jacqueline Kennedy Onassis, Bo Derek, Farrah Fawcett, whose poster was the top-selling poster in history.

1972 Ilana Harkavi, a former professional dancer, launches Il Makiage. The line is positioned as "the makeup artist's makeup."

1974 Lauren Hutton becomes the first model to sign an exclusive cosmetics contract. Revlon signs her for $100,000.

1975 Trish McEvoy launches a line of makeup brushes to fill the demand for high-quality makeup tools.

1977 Calvin Klein launches a line of cosmetics, which relaunches in 2005.

1980s Makeup is strong and exaggerated. Color trends are bold—lots of blues and fuchsias. Avon and Mary Kay create palettes to take the guesswork out of choosing a color scheme.

Models to know: Rosemary McGrath, Pat Cleveland, Esme, Lisa Taylor, Jerry Hall.

Beauty icons: Madonna, Grace Jones, Jane Fonda, Pat Benatar.

1984 Canadians Frank Toskan, a makeup artist and photographer, and Frank Angelo, a hair salon owner, launch Make-up Art Cosmetics, or MAC. Their line, which is originally designed for use in fashion photography, wins a wide following with its socially conscious motto: "All ages, all races, all sexes."

Make Up For Ever is launched by Dany Sanz and Jacques Waneph to meet the unique needs of the stage and fashion industries.

1985 Paulina Porizkova signs on as the face of Estée Lauder for six million dollars.

1990 Hollywood makeup artist Carol Shaw launches LORAC, a line featuring oil and fragrance-free foundations.

1988 Ultima II relaunches the Naked Collection.

1990s Makeup is all about looking natural.

Models to know: Linda Evangelista, Christy Turlington, Naomi Campbell, Cindy Crawford, Tatjana Patitz.

Beauty icons: Jennifer Aniston, Jennifer Lopez.

1991 New York makeup artist Bobbi Brown launches Bobbi Brown *essentials* with ten brown-based lipsticks at Bergdorf Goodman.

1994 Kate Moss appears on Calvin Klein Obsession perfume ads and billboards

Jeanine Lobell launches Stila cosmetics.

Fashion model Iman launches IMAN, a line of cosmetics for women of color.

François Nars launches NARS with twelve lipsticks at Barneys New York. In 1996 he shoots his first advertising campaign for his brand, and continues to do so today.

1995 Frustrated by the lack of bold, vibrant colors, Vincent Longo launches his own line.

1996 Crème de la Mer, a potent cream developed by aerospace physicist Max Huber, is relaunched.

Laura Mercier launches her line of cosmetics.

1999 Sonia Kashuk launches the Sonia Kashuk Professional Makeup collection for Target. This marks the first partnership between a high-profile makeup artist and mass-market retailer.

2000s–Present Fake tans, sun beds, and tanning products are all the rage, mineral-based makeup enters the marketplace, and makeup brands explode.

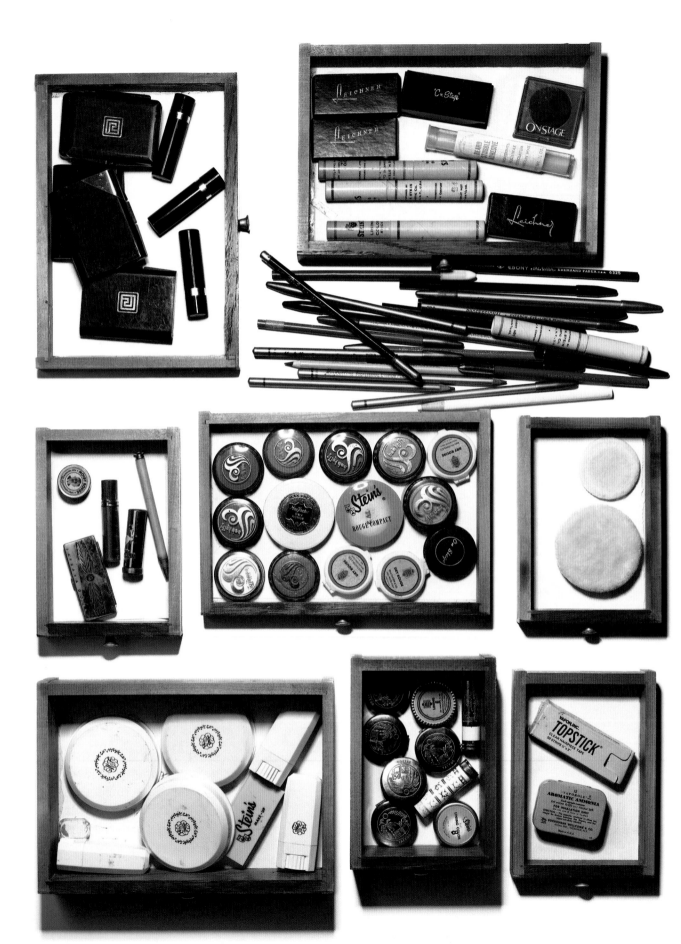

WHO'S WHO in MAKEUP

These are the pioneers *who helped shape the beauty industry* and also greatly influenced me as an artist.

Helena Rubinstein
(1870–1965)

Born in Poland, she was the eldest of eight daughters. After immigrating to Australia, she opened the world's first modern beauty salon. She later relocated to the United States, opened a salon in New York City, and became a lifelong rival of Elizabeth Arden. In 1962, Rubinstein's salon was the first to introduce the concept of a "day of beauty." It consisted of an exercise class, massage, lunch, facial, shampoo, hairstyling, manicure, pedicure, and makeup session and cost $35.

Max Factor
(1877–1938)

Born in Poland as Max Faktor, his name morphed into Factor in 1904, when he went through Ellis Island on his way to becoming an American. In Los Angeles, he began selling his lotions and makeup, and soon he had developed a new type of makeup formulated specifically for the movies. It was called "flexible greasepaint" because, unlike standard film makeup, it didn't crack. In 1920, Factor introduced his cosmetics to the public, giving the average woman a chance to buy a little bit of Hollywood glamour at her local drugstore.

Coco Chanel
(1883–1971)

Although primarily remembered as a fashion designer, Chanel also created some of the world's most memorable perfumes. In 1922, she introduced Chanel No. 5, which to this day is a worldwide best seller.

Elizabeth Arden
(1884–1966)

Born in Ontario, Canada, as Florence Nightingale Graham, she moved to New York in 1908, where she worked as a bookkeeper at E. R. Squibb Pharmaceuticals Company. Whenever possible, Graham spent time in the company's lab, learning the skills she would later use to create her own skincare lotions. She jumped at an opportunity to go to work for a "beauty culturist" doing skin treatments. There she met Elizabeth Hubbard and, in 1909, the two opened their own Fifth Avenue salon. When the partnership ended, Graham retained her partner's first name, Elizabeth, and chose the last name Arden, from the Tennyson poem "Enoch Arden." Thus, Elizabeth Arden was born. She quickly expanded her repertoire from giving skincare treatments to creating makeup colors. She worked tirelessly for her self-made company into her eighties.

Charles Revson
(1906–1975)

In 1932, Revson went into business with his brother and a chemist named Charles Lachman. They founded a company called Revlon and launched it with the introduction of a nail polish. Revlon became known for nail polishes in a wide variety of colors. Eventually, they marketed matching lipsticks, including the legendary Fire and Ice shade of bold red.

Estée Lauder
(1908–2004)

As an enterprising young woman, Lauder began selling the skin creams created by her uncle, a chemist. In 1948, she convinced the managers at Saks Fifth Avenue to give her counter space to sell her line. She is credited with pioneering the concept of "gift with purchase," giving away free samples to her customers. In 1953, she introduced her first fragrance, Youth Dew, a bath oil meant to be lavishly splashed over the entire body. By 1984, annual sales of that product had reached $150 million.

Mary Kay Ash
(1918–2001)

Born in Hot Wells, Texas, Mary Kay Ash worked in direct sales until 1963, when she retired to write a book to assist women in business. The book turned into a business plan and by September 1963, with only five thousand dollars, she founded Mary Kay Cosmetics with her son, Richard Rogers. They developed a line of skincare products and color cosmetics, initially sold out of a storefront in Dallas, Texas. With the Golden Rule as the founding principle of her company, she insisted that her employees keep their lives in balance. She authored a total of three books, all of which became best sellers. Her book on people management, has been included as a text at the Harvard Business School. At the time of Ash's death, Mary Kay Cosmetics had over 800,000 representatives in 37 countries, with total annual sales of more than $2 billion at retail.

Shu Uemura
(1928–2007)

The founder of shu uemura cosmetics, he was the first to merge makeup and art through makeup performances on stage and his seasonal Mode Makeup collections. His career began in Hollywood in 1955 and it took off when he was called to substitute for Shirley MacLaine's makeup artist. His first product, Unmask Cleansing Oil, came out in 1960. His first makeup school opened in Tokyo shortly thereafter. His first open workshop/concept cosmetics boutique opened in 1983. The Tokyo Lash Bar, with a huge variety of false-lash concepts, was launched in 2007.

Way Bandy
(1941–1986)

Bandy was one of the best-known freelance makeup artists of the 70s and 80s. He created Calvin Klein's first cosmetics collection, which featured burgundy packaging. His best-selling books are a great source of information and inspiration to makeup artists today.

George Newell
(1954–1992)

George Newell began his career as a model and makeup artist in Houston. He moved to New York in 1977 to work as a freelance makeup artist, and became famous for a Halston layout he did for *Vogue* in 1979, where he served as both a fashion model and a makeup artist. In the early 1980s he established George Newell, Inc., a management and talent agency in Los Angeles, representing photographers, stylists, makeup artists, and hair stylists. During his career he designed many *Vanity Fair* and *Vogue* covers.

Frank Toskan & Frank Angelo
(1948–1997)

In 1985, these two Canadians joined creative forces to form MAC (Make-up Art Cosmetics). Toskan was a makeup artist and photographer, and

Angelo operated a chain of beauty salons. Toskan was frustrated with the available cosmetic offerings, all of which had glossy finishes that he thought reflected too much light in photographs. The company marketed an expanded color line (to suit more skin tones) and products with matte finishes. Today, MAC is known as much for its ethical policies and good works as it is for its products.

Kevyn Aucoin
(1962–2002)

As a child growing up in Louisiana, Aucoin studied fashion magazines and tried to duplicate the looks he saw on his younger sister, Carla. After attending beauty school, he moved to New York in 1983. His big break came when a beauty editor at *Vogue* asked to see his book. In 1986, he did his first *Vogue* cover shoot with the photographer Richard Avedon. During his career, he worked with countless A-list celebrities and showcased his work in three books: *The Art of Makeup*, *Making Faces*, and *Face Forward*.

Ariella

Ariella is best known for her longtime collaboration with the photographer Richard Avedon. She did the makeup for countless American

Vogue covers as well as the iconic photo in 1981 featuring Natassja Kinski entwined with a boa constrictor.

Serge Lutens

Serge Lutens is a French photographer, filmmaker, hair stylist, perfumer, and fashion designer. In 1962, he moved to Paris, where *Vogue* magazine hired him to create makeup, hair, and jewelry looks. During the 60s he worked with photographer greats such as Richard Avedon, Bob Richardson, and Irving Penn. He created a makeup line for Christian Dior in 1967. In 1980, he was hired by Shiseido to develop its image internationally and to create the fragrance Nombre Noir. Both the fragrance and its packaging were considered ahead of their time. In the early 90s he designed Les Salons du Palais Royal, a perfume boutique, and in 2000, launched his own brand.

Alberto Fava

Alberto Fava began his career as a makeup artist in Rome in 1970, assisting Gil Cagne. In the 1970s he collaborated with fashion magazines, started to design makeup for fashion shows, and worked with several prominent photographers. As beauty editor for *Mirabella* magazine, he helped envision

and plan the style and content of beauty stories.

Sandy Linter

Sandy Linter is a legendary makeup artist in New York City. Linter has spent the past thirty years working with celebrities and models. She is recognized throughout the beauty community for her age-defying techniques, which have been known to take off more years than cosmetic surgery. A frequent contributor to the country's leading fashion and beauty magazines, Linter's work has appeared in *Vogue*, *Harper's Bazaar*, and *Vanity Fair*.

Linda Mason

Linda Mason reinvented the role of makeup on the runway in the late 70s. Her artistry was an integral part of signature looks for designers such as Gaultier and Mugler and for the label Comme des Garçons. In 1987, she started Linda Mason Elements, Inc.

Mary Quant

Working as a fashion designer in London in the 50s, Mary Quant was on a mission to make youthful fashion affordable. Her King's Road boutique became a Mecca for girls in search of the mod look and Quant's famous miniskirts. In the 60s she expanded her line to include paintbox makeup—a collection of bold, fun colors in a compact container.

Bonnie Maller

New York–based freelance makeup artist Bonnie Maller is best known for introducing the natural makeup look in the late 70s. She created looks for Ralph Lauren, Perry Ellis, and Calvin Klein, and her work was showcased in magazines around the world. She collaborated frequently with the photographer Bruce Weber.

Stéphane Marais

Stéphane Marais is a French makeup artist and entrepreneur whose quirky imagery has earned him global attention. He is widely known for his collaboration with Peter Lindbergh, his consulting work for Shiseido, and his ability to be understated and dramatic at the same time. He opened a flagship store in Paris in 2002.

Linda Cantello

Linda Cantello's career began in the early 80s, and since then she has worked in high-luxury advertising campaigns, collaborated with top photographers, and worked with some of the best fashion and beauty publications. She was commissioned by MAC and Kanebo to recast their color lines and recently launched her signature makeup and skincare line.

Mary Greenwell

Mary Greenwell began her career in the 80s in Paris. She has since worked with every big-name photographer, and trained many of today's makeup artists. Her eye for detail and color led to a contract with Shiseido, where she created new colors, taking the collection in a new direction. She is a regular artist at fashion shows and has a large celebrity clientele. Her work has been seen in all the leading magazines, in editorial, and in ad campaigns for Yohji Yamamoto, Valentino, DKNY, Estée Lauder, Guerlain, L'Oréal, Max Factor, and Comme des Garçons.

Barbara Daly

British makeup artist Barbara Daly began working in the 1960s and is popularly known for her work on the 1971 Stanley Kubrick film, *A Clockwork Orange*. She was called on by Diana, Princess of Wales, to do her wedding day makeup. And she is the creator of a makeup line available at the UK retailer Tesco.

François Nars

Born in the South of France, François Nars attended the Carita makeup school in Paris. In 1984, he began working with fashion's top publications, collaborated with top designers, including Dolce & Gabbana, Marc Jacobs, and Karl Lagerfeld, and with legendary photographers, such as Richard Avedon, Patrick Demarchelier, Steven Meisel, Helmut Newton, Irving Penn, and Bruce Weber. Frustrated with the cosmetics lines available, Nars developed and successfully launched NARS, a cosmetics and skincare company, in 1994. He is also a professional photographer and the author of *X-Ray* (1999) and coauthor of *Makeup Your Mind* (2002).

Joey Mills

Joey Mills was widely known in the 70s and 80s for his classic American style. His work appeared in countless magazine covers, editorials, and advertising campaigns.

Reggie Wells

A veteran in the makeup industry, Reggie Wells has worked with countless actresses, painting his iconic, glamorous sculpted faces. Reggie is also widely known for his work with Oprah Winfrey as both a guest and behind-the-scenes makeup artist. He is an Emmy Award winner and author of *Face Painting*.

Tom Pecheux

Tom Pecheux lives and works in Paris. He is a beauty designer and key makeup artist for some of the top makeup brands, including Shiseido and MAC. His work on fashion shows for Prada, Karl Lagerfeld, and Alberta Ferretti, among others, has won him a loyal following in the fashion industry. He's also worked with countless musicians including Madonna and Avril Lavigne on music videos, collaborating with the top fashion designers in the business.

Dick Page

This British makeup artist has a reputation as an industry leader. He is known for his editorial, advertising, and runway work. Since 1997, he has worked with Shiseido in Japan on its premier domestic line of cosmetics, and in 2001, he was made artistic director of the makeup line. He redesigned and relaunched the line in August 2002 as Inoui ID. In March 2007, he was named artistic director of Shiseido The Makeup. Page frequently contributes to *Allure* with his own insider's page of tips and ideas entitled "The Makeup Guy." He currently acts as the key makeup artist for the runway shows of Michael Kors, Narciso Rodriguez, Marc Jacobs, Marc by Marc Jacobs, and United Bamboo.

Pat McGrath

Pat McGrath is a British makeup artist known for her wide range and inventive use of materials: her makeup is often handmade, and she works mainly with her fingers rather than with brushes. McGrath's big break came while working with Edward Enninful at *i-D* magazine in the early 90s. She became known for her dramatic, stylized designs, including bodies drenched in paint and petals glued to faces. She designed Armani's cosmetics line in 1999 and in 2004 was named global creative-design director for Procter and Gamble, where she is in charge of Max Factor and Cover Girl cosmetics, among other brands.

Laura Mercier

Raised in Provence, Laura Mercier trained at the Carita school, where she specialized in makeup application. In her early career, she began working closely with Thibault Vabre, a well-known French makeup artist. In 1985, Mercier moved to New York to join the team to launch American *Elle*. She soon began working for advertising campaigns for major corporations, editorial spreads for magazines, and multiple cosmetics and clothing companies, and worked with Madonna to create looks for print, television, and film. She then contracted with Elizabeth Arden to design the makeup looks for advertising campaigns and worked on Chanel's advertising campaigns in France. In 1996, Mercier developed her own line, which is now in four hundred stores in twenty-one countries.

Sam Fine

Sam Fine began his education in makeup behind the cosmetics counters of department stores. He studied art in New York while continuing to work in the cosmetics department of a large specialty store. His transition to freelance artist occurred when Naomi Campbell's makeup artist was unavailable for a show and she called Sam. He is known especially for his work with African American women and as the author of *Fine Beauty*.

Joanne Gair

Joanne Gair is an artist and image maker who has emerged as the premiere makeup artist/body painter in the world. From New Zealand, Gair has an interest in art photography. Her work as a makeup artist and body painter has appeared in editorial covers, layouts, fashion campaigns, advertising, music videos, commercials, and motion pictures.

Heidi Morawetz

Heidi Morawetz was the creative director of Chanel's makeup

studio in Paris for over thirty years. Morawetz created the "face" of each season for the runway shows. She developed Chanel's famous Rouge Noir nail polish (Vamp) in 1994; the blood red shade is still Chanel's best-selling nail polish color. She began as a freelance makeup artist and stylist until Dominique Moncourtois discovered her work and brought her into Chanel. Together with Moncourtois, Morawetz built the Chanel makeup business into the success it is today.

Dominique Moncourtois

Dominique Moncourtois spent thirty-six years as the director of Chanel's Makeup Creation. As a child, he spent holidays in Paris with his great aunt, a former model who introduced him to the art of makeup. From 1963 to 1967 he worked as a makeup artist and wigmaker in the film industry, and in 1968, he joined Chanel. He continues to create and develop new looks and technology for makeup.

Fulvia Farolfi

Fulvia Farolfi's work appears in *Vogue*, *Harper's Bazaar*, and *W* magazines, to name a few, and she works regularly with top photographers including Irving Penn, Bruce Weber, and Raymond Meier. She's a fixture at the runway shows in New York and Europe and has developed makeup lines for Emporio Armani and Shiseido.

Charlie Green

Charlie Green began her career in London, working on music videos for talents like Kylie Minogue and Bryan Ferry, then headed to Paris where she made her name collaborating with photographers David LaChapelle and Michael Thompson, and designers like Vivienne Westwood and Chloé. Now based in the United States, Green is a celebrity and editorial favorite.

Paul Starr

Paul Starr is a Los Angeles–based celebrity-makeup artist whose clients include Jennifer Garner, Salma Hayek, Michelle Pfeiffer, Angelina Jolie, and countless others. He has worked with photographers such as Patrick Demarchelier, David LaChappelle, and Annie Leibovitz. Starr has worked over twenty years in film, music videos, and print, and he has also worked with Estée Lauder on a makeup collection.

Gucci Westman

Gucci Westman studied makeup in Paris, then headed to Los Angeles, where she focused on special-effects makeup. She was "discovered" when photographer Annie Leibovitz called on her for a 1996 *Vanity Fair* cover shoot. In addition to working regularly with the beauty and fashion industry's top magazines and designers, Gucci has lent her expertise to the cosmetics company Lancôme.

Scott Barnes

Scott Barnes came to New York City at the age of seventeen to begin a career as a painter. A graduate of Detroit's Center for Creative Studies, and New York's Parsons School for Design, he began to find work on fashion photography shoots. Scott used his painting skills to model faces for fashion and soon secured an agent for his work. His work is known for its sexiness with a global sensibility and has been published by *Vogue*, *InStyle*, *Elle*, *Vanity Fair*, *Rolling Stone*, and *Premiere*. He works regularly with celebrated photographers such as Herb Ritts, Patrick Demarchelier, Annie Leibovitz, and Matthew Rolston, as well as many A-list celebrities.

Joe Blasco

Joe Blasco began his study of the art of makeup at the early age of seven. He was awarded a scholarship to cosmetology school, and after graduating in 1964 at the age of eighteen, he arrived in Hollywood to work for the Max Factor cosmetics company. In 1967 he set out to pursue a career in Hollywood as a makeup artist. He took a job as an instructor with a small makeup school and recognized the need for a course that taught motion picture and television makeup artistry. He became known for his work in special makeup effects. In 1976 he opened the first of two renowned makeup training centers.

Diane Kendal

Diane Kendal's signature look—one that's rock and roll but gorgeous and approachable—has made her an industry favorite. She collaborates regularly with Catherine Malandrino, Jean Paul Gaultier, Balenciaga, Carolina Herrera, and Calvin Klein. Her work appears frequently in *W*, *Vogue*, and *Vanity Fair*. Additionally, she regularly represents MAC at Fashion Week and designed Calvin Klein's cosmetic line from 2002 to 2003.

RESOURCE GUIDE

Theatrical Makeup Stores

ALCONE 235 West 19th Street, New York, NY 10019; alconeco.com; 212-633-0551,

BALL BEAUTY SUPPLY 416 North Fairfax Avenue, Los Angeles, CA 90036; 323-655-2330

CINEMA SECRETS 4400 Riverside Drive, Burbank, CA 91505; 818-846-0579

FREND'S BEAUTY SUPPLY 5270 Laurel Canyon Boulevard, North Hollywood, CA 91607; 818-769-3834

THE MAKEUP SHOP 131 West 21st Street, New York, NY 10011; 212-807-0447

NAIMIE'S BEAUTY CENTER 12640 Riverside Drive, Valley Village, CA 91607; www.naimies.com; 818-655-9933

RAY BEAUTY SUPPLY 721 8th Avenue, New York, NY 10036; 800-253-0993

RICKY'S 590 Broadway New York, NY 10012; 212-226-5552 / 1574 Third Avenue, New York, NY 10079; 212-996-7030 / 107 Montague Street, Brooklyn, NY 11201; 718-522-5011

SALLY BEAUTY SUPPLY Locations nationwide; sallybeauty.com; 800-ASK-SALLY

Makeup Artist Agencies

NEW YORK AGENCIES

THE ARTIST LOFT 580 Broadway, Suite 606, New York, NY 10012; www.aartistloft.com; 212-274-0961; Attn: Sara Mouzianni

ARTISTS BY TIMOTHY PRIANO 131 Varick Street, Suite 905, New York, NY 10013; 212-929-7771; Attn: David Kelley

ART + COMMERCE 755 Washington Street, New York, NY 10014; www.artandcommerce.com; 212-206-0730; Attn: Joshua Hiller

BRIAN BANTRY AGENCY 4 West 58th Street, Penthouse, New York, NY 10019; 212-935-0200

JED ROOT 61A Walker Street, New York, NY 10013; www.jedroot.com; 212-226-6600; Attn: Kelly Obaski Hass

MAGNET: 270 Lafayette Street, Suite 901, New York, NY 10012; www.magnetla.com; 212-941-7441

MAREK 508 West 26th Street, New York, NY 10001; 212-924-6760

NEW YORK OFFICE 15 West 26th Street, New York, NY 10010; www.nyoffice.net; Attn: Julianne Hausler

OLIVER PIRO 128 West 26th Street, 3rd Floor, New York, NY 10001; www.oliverpiro.com; 212-925-2112; Attn: Massu Nedjat

R. J. BENNETT REPRESENTS 530 East 20th Street, Suite 2B, New York, NY 10009; www.rjbennettrepresents.com; 212-673-5509; Attn: Rose Bennett

CALIFORNIA AGENCIES

ARTISTS BY TIMOTHY PRIANO 8447 Wilshire Boulevard, Beverly Hills, CA 90211; 323-782-0021; Attn: Jared Franco

ARTIST UNTIED www.artistuntied.com; 323-933-0200

ATELIER MANAGEMENT 543 South Spring Street, Los

Angeles, CA 90013; 323-933-2983; Attn: Brian

CELESTINE 1548 16th Street, Santa Monica, CA 90404; www.celestine.com; 310-998-1977; Attn: Frank Moore

CLOUTIER 1026 Montana Avenue, Santa Monica, CA 90403; www.cloutieragency.com; 310-394-8813; Attn: Imari McDermott

LUXE 6442 Santa Monica Boulevard, Los Angeles, CA 90035; 323-856-8540; Attn: Nadia

TRACEY MATTINGLY LLC/AVANT GROUPE 1617 Cosmo Street, Loft 402, Los Angeles, CA 90028; 323-467-0000; Attn: Tracey Mattingly, Cale Harrison, or Jessica Johnson

ZENOBIA 130 South Highland Avenue, Los Angeles, CA 90036; www.zenobia.com; 323-937-1010; Attn: Keith or Heidi

Creative Directories

ASSOCIATION OF FILM COMMISSIONERS INTERNATIONAL www.afci.org. Published annually. This directory has listings for film and television productions globally.

THE BLACK BOOK www.blackbook.com. Published annually in December. It is a directory of advertising photography—an excellent resource for finding photographers to send your work.

LA 411 www.la411.com. Published annually in January. It lists the names and contact information of professionals in the television, video, and film industries in Los Angeles. The book includes rate tables and information on union rules.

LE BOOK www.lebook.com. Published annually. It is an international guide to the fashion world. It includes contact information for designers, modeling agencies, catalog companies, and photographers.

MIAMI PRODUCTION GUIDE www.filmflorida.com. Published annually in December. It lists film and television production resources in Miami.

SELECT www.select-magazine.com. Published six times a year. Issues focus on different cities and provide information including clubs, agencies, and more. It is a good source for finding catalog and entertainment photographers.

THE WORKBOOK www.workbook.com. Published annually, in January. It is a resource for the graphic arts industry and is great for finding photographers, stylists, makeup artists, costumers, etc., who work in advertising. Select a target group for a mailing. The Workbook will give you a count, and for a small fee will send you labels for your promotional mailing.

Suggested Reading

Designing Your Face by Way Bandy (Random House, 1984)

Face Forward by Kevyn Aucoin (Little, Brown & Co., 2001)

Making Faces by Kevyn Aucoin (Little, Brown & Co., 1997)

Make-up Artist magazine http://makeupmag.com

Stage Makeup by Richard Corson (Prentice Hall, Inc., 1990)

Other Books by Bobbi Brown:

Bobbi Brown Beauty (Harper Style, 1997)

Bobbi Brown Beauty Evolution (Harper Resource, 2002)

Bobbi Brown Living Beauty (Springboard Press, 2007)

Bobbi Brown Teenage Beauty (Cliff Street Books, 2000)

ACKNOWLEDGMENTS

This book was a labor of love and could not have been done without the talented and hardworking team that made it possible. First I want to thank Jill Cohen, who managed this intricate process and worked with me every step of the way. A special thank-you to my editor, Karen Murgolo, whose hard work and patience were invaluable—and to the rest of the publishing team at Hachette Book Group, including Jamie Raab, Matthew Ballast, Tom Hardej, Dorothea Halliday, Pamela Schechter, Melissa Bullock, Nicole Bond, and Peggy Boelke.

I'm grateful to my creative director, Ruba Abu-Nimah, who always surprises me with her aesthetic. Thanks also to designer Eleanor Rogers, and everyone else who brought this book to life: writers Debra Bergsma Otte and Sally Wadyka, Matthias Gaggl, John Cassidy, Jason Nakleh, Billy Jim, Daymion Mardel, Kellie Kulton, Gail Hadani, Nicolai Grosell, Maxine Tall, Brian Hagiwara, Bret Baughman, Sydney Wicks, John Eaton, Guy Aroch, Joy Glenn, and Rosanne Guararra. Thank you to Henry Leutwyler for the stunning photos, to Lise Varrette for the beautiful and perfect step-by-step shots, and to Ben Ritter for the behind-the-scenes reportage. Thanks to the photographers who contributed advice, including Patrick Demarchelier, Walter Chin, and Troy Word. My heartfelt appreciation goes to my makeup artists who worked on this book, including Kimberly Christine Soane, Elizabeth Keiser, Sarah Sugarman, Tanya Cropsey, Ellice Schwab, and Waltaya Culmer. And thank you to hair stylist Yannick d'Is and his assistant, Mako, to hair stylist Mario Diab, and to manicurist Roza Israel.

Thanks to everyone at Bobbi Brown Cosmetics. A shout-out to my support team, including Matthew Riopelle, Joe Pinto, Kristen Boscaino, and Ron Hill. And big thanks to my incredibly fun and tireless PR team, including Veronika Ullmer, Gretchen Berra, Jay Squire, Ashley Badger-Wakefield, Elizabeth Just, Samantha Bailye, and the HL Group. Thank you also to the creative team, including Dorothy Mancuso, Marie Clare Katigbak, Nicole Kirkitsos, and Sarah Honeth, and to the product development team, including Sarah Robbins, Sotiria Cherpelis, and Gabrielle Nevin. And as always, my deep appreciation to Maureen Case, president of Bobbi Brown Cosmetics, my friend, biggest supporter, and all around great human being (breathe!).

PHOTO CREDITS

Guy Aroch: 89; **Walter Chin**: 175 (top right); **Patrick Demarchelier**: 175 (bottom right); **Nicolai Grosell**: 2; **Gail Hadani**: 179; **Brian Hagiwara**: 8, 11, 12, 13, 14, 18, 19, 37, 66, 68 (compact), 84 (lip pencil), 90 (brush), 91 (brush), 93, 98 (makeup), 99 (brush), 112 (brush), 133, 166 (jar, bottle), 167, 168 (nail polish); **Henry Leutwyler**: endpapers, ii, vii, viii, 6, 9, 10, 16, 17, 21, 22, 24, 25, 26, 27, 28, 29, 31, 35, 40 (cigarettes), 42, 44, 46, 48, 49, 51, 53 (Darker Peach), 54 (brush cleaning), 57 (makeup), 58, 61, 63, 65, 67, 69, 70, 71, 73, 74, 75, 76 (makeup), 77 (makeup), 78, 81, 82, 83 (lipsticks), 85 (makeup), 86, 95 (eye shadow), 97 (makeup), 100, 101, 104, 105, 110, 111, 114, 116, 124, 126, 131, 135, 137, 139, 142, 149, 157 (Bobbi with feet on desk), 162, 165, 166 (blush), 168 (tools), 169, 170, 175 (top left), 180, 181, 182, 183, 184, 185, 186, 187, 188, 189, 190, 191, 192, 193, 194, 195, 204, 210, 222, 223, 224; **Patrick McMullan**: v, 202 (Bobbi with Yogi Berra); **Ben Ritter**: 144, 147, 173; **Lise Varrette**: 40 (model), 52, 53 (Corrector Application for Asian Eyes), 54 (model), 55, 57 (three models), 59, 68 (model), 72, 76 (model), 77 (model), 83 (model), 84 (model), 85 (model), 90 (model), 91 (model), 92, 95 (model), 96, 97 (model), 98 (model), 99 (model), 102, 103, 106, 107, 108, 109, 112 (model), 113, 115, 118, 119, 120, 121, 122, 123, 177; **Troy Word**: 175 (bottom left).

Face Chart (125): Illustrated by **Tobie Giddio**.

Nine Memorable Women (197): Brigitte Bardot: MPTV.net; Catherine Deneuve: MPTV.net; Audrey Hepburn: MPTV.net; Lena Horne: © 1978 **Maurice Seymour** / MPTV.net; Grace Kelly: Photo by **Bert Six** / MPTV.net; Sophia Loren: MPTV.net; Ali MacGraw: © 1978 **Ken Whitmore** / MPTV.net; Marilyn Monroe: MPTV.net; Elizabeth Taylor: MPTV.net.

Fashion week and special event photography courtesy of: **Berit Bizjak**, **Dan Lecca**, **Patrick McMullan**, **WireImage**: 128, 129, 153, 199, 200, 201, 202, 203.

Other photography from Bobbi Brown's personal collection: 5, 157, 159, 161, 202, 203.

All photographers retain their copyrights, except Lise Varrette, whose photos are © Bobbi Brown Evolution, LLC.

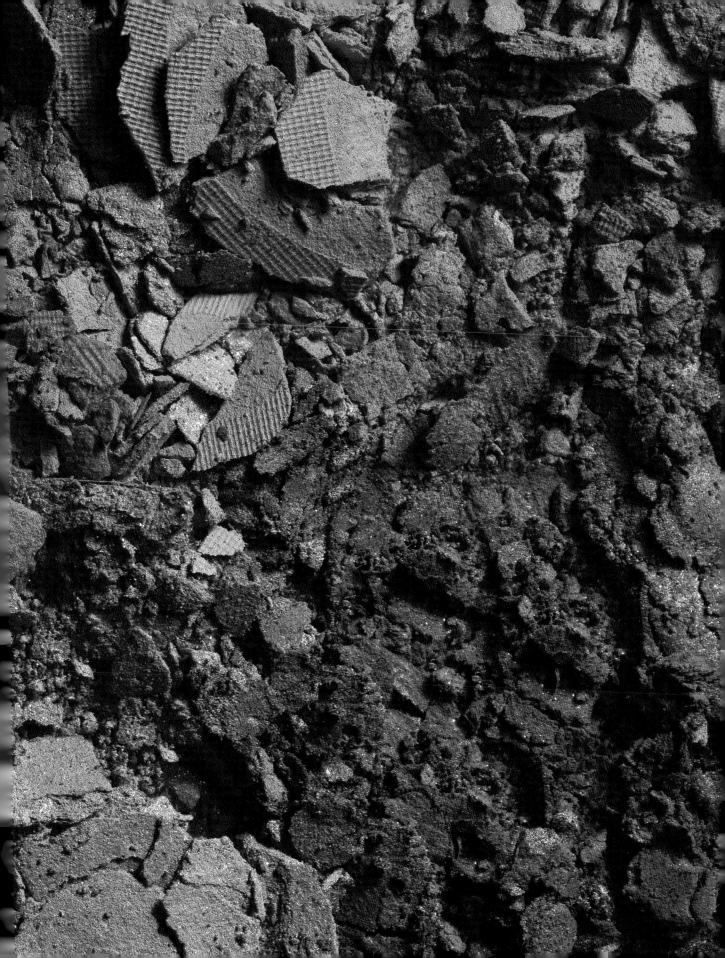

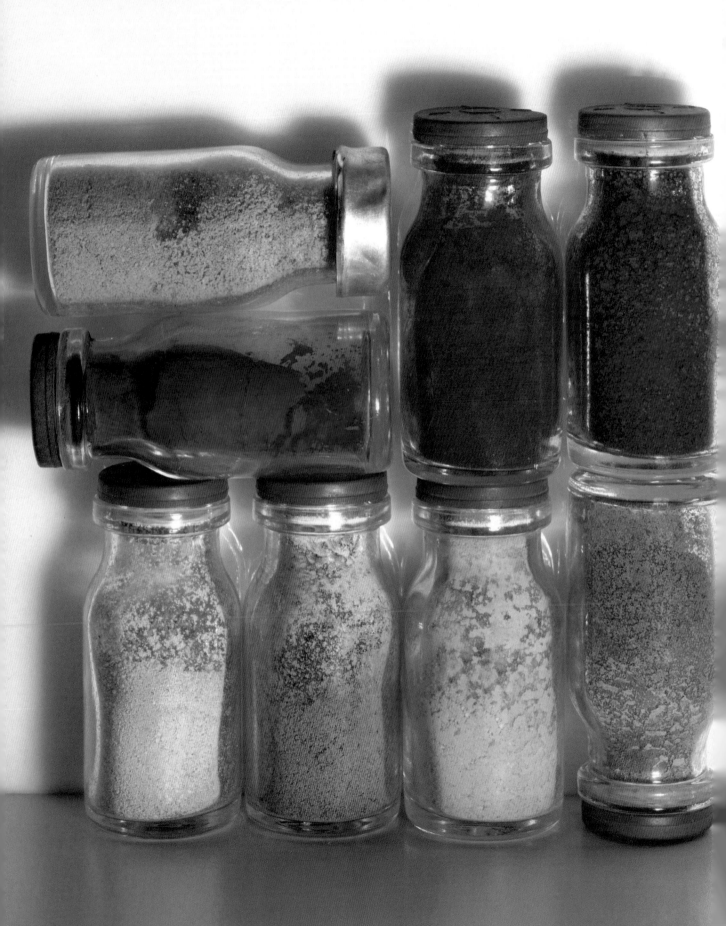

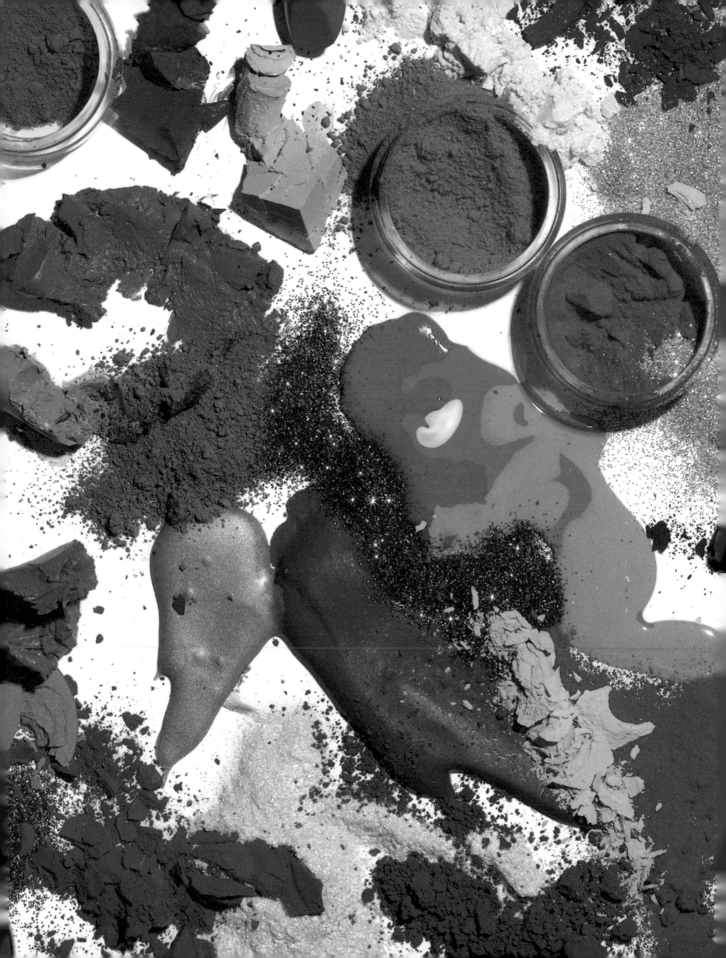

WAT

T-381-340

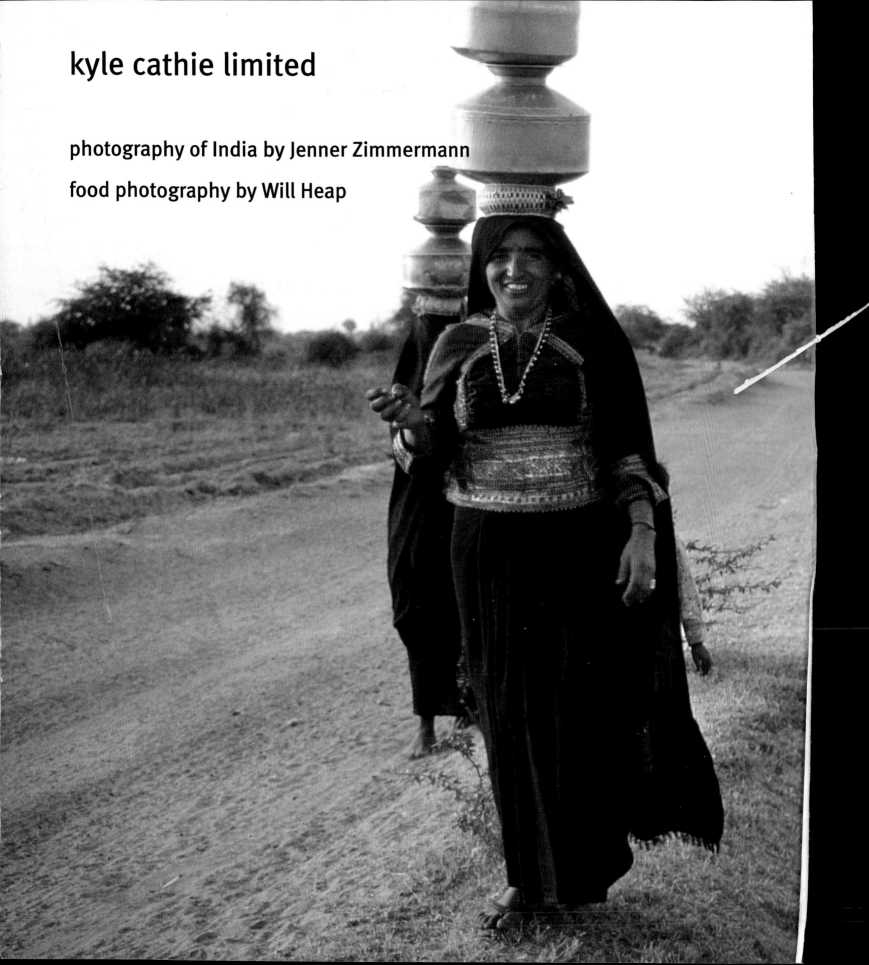

kyle cathie limited

photography of India by Jenner Zimmermann

food photography by Will Heap

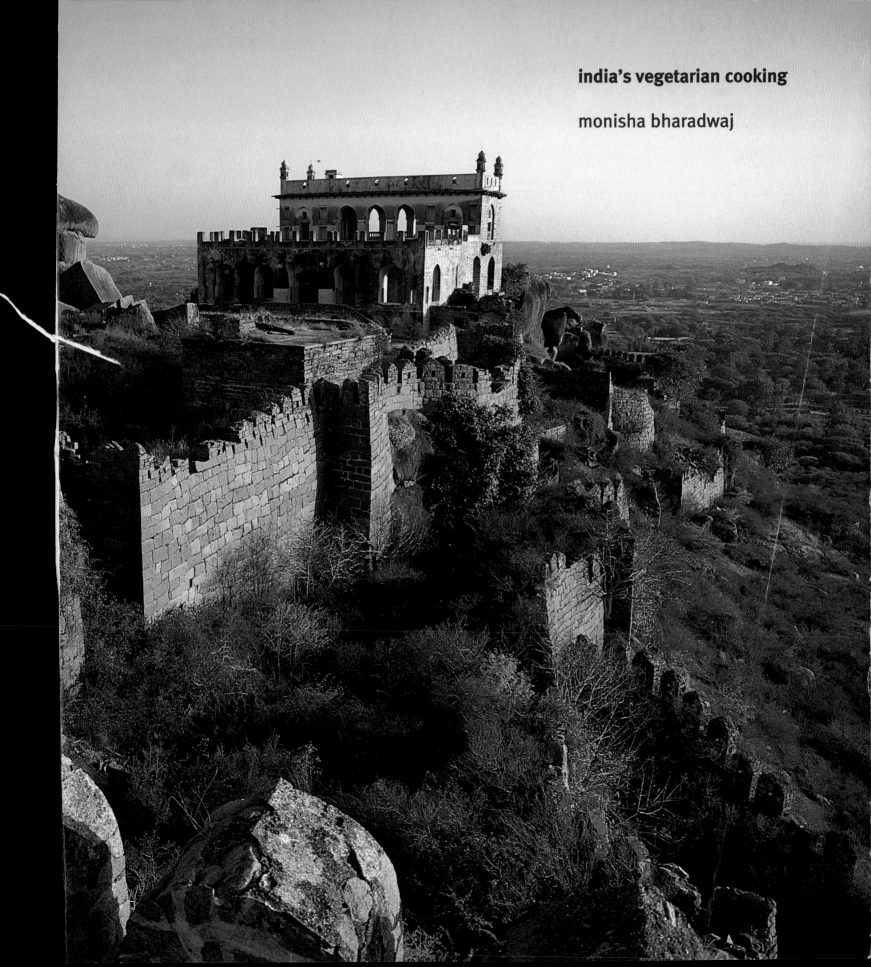

india's vegetarian cooking

monisha bharadwaj

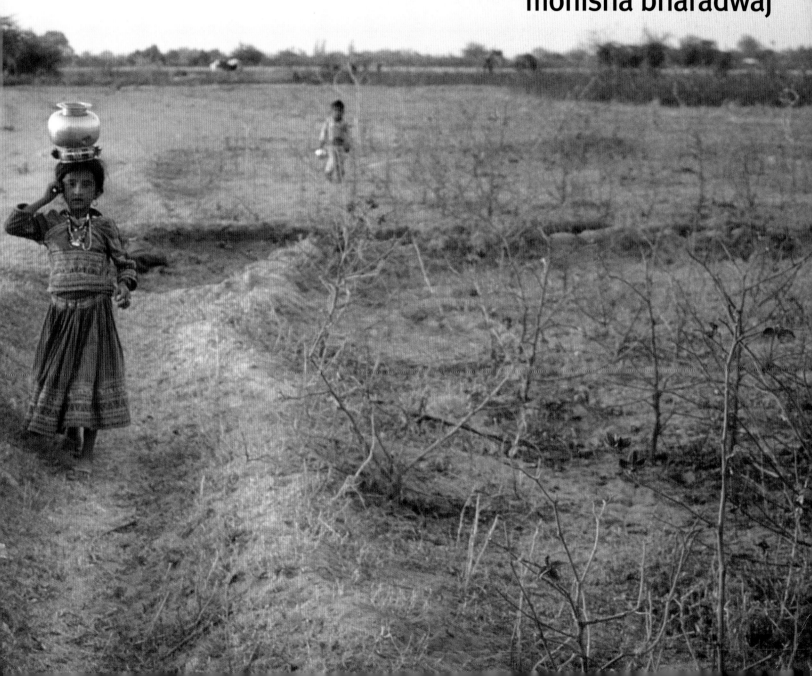

india's
vegetarian
cooking

monisha bharadwaj

First published in Great Britain in 2006 by
Kyle Cathie Limited
122 Arlington Road
London NW1 7HP
general.enquiries@kyle-cathie.com
www.kylecathie.com

ISBN 1 85626 661 3
ISBN (13-digit) 978 1 85626 661 1

Designer Geoff Hayes
Proofreader Sarah Epton
Indexer Alex Corrin
Production Sha Huxtable & Alice Holloway

Monisha Bharadwaj is hereby identified as the author of this
work in accordance with Section 77 of the Copyright, Designs and
Patents Act 1988.

A Cataloguing in Publication record for this title is available from
the British Library.

Colour reproduction by Colourscan
Printed in China by C&C Offset Printing Co., Ltd.

contents

introduction

My introduction to regional cookery began at an early age. As children, my parents took my brother and me travelling around India at every given opportunity. Aged six, I had eaten the finest Gujarati thali in Rajkot, by eight I had tasted the choicest tandoori foods in Amritsar and by twelve, we had covered most of south India with its steaming hot Kanjeevaram idlis and chutneys. Of course the extensive range that I was exposed to was not something to wonder about at the time. I sort of took it for granted and slowly my love of food and cooking developed. It was almost like a bud opening into a flower, the myriad taste sensations gradually becoming more and more distinct as I grew up.

Later I went to the Bombay Catering College, the finest in the country at the time, and was taught about the theory as well as the practical side of cookery – classic recipes, quantity cooking, nutrition and how to standardise recipes. Here again regional cookery was important. The nuances of Kerala cuisine were set apart from those of Kashmiri cooking and the history, traditions and rituals associated with food, which are all so essential in India, began to come alive.

Having grown up in Mumbai, arguably India's most cosmopolitan city, meant that I had friends from every state in the country. Their families had moved to Mumbai (or Bombay as it was then called) for work or education and I remember us spending a lot of time at each other's homes. Often this was to share a family meal which meant that, almost every weekend, I was eating delicious south Indian, Parsee, Gujarati or Punjabi food. They in turn loved the Maharashtrian and Goan delicacies at my home. I never failed to ask their mums and grandmothers for special recipes and, by the time I was sixteen, I had a formidable recipe collection of my own. Later I would enchant my family with delicious lentils and curries from around the country. When I joined the Catering College, I began practising classic French cooking at home because it formed a large portion of our syllabus. My friends and relatives were often willing volunteers for tastings and adventurous cooking.

Little has changed. I still ask for recipes when I have had a fantastic meal and most cooks are flattered. And I still have many volunteers willing to come over for dinner when I do recipe trials.

Much of my own home cooking is vegetarian because that was how I was brought up. All my favourite foods are from the vegetarian world. I also feel happier, healthier and more energetic after a vegetarian meal.

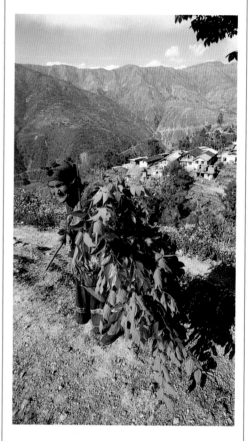

Indian cookery is an art form, subtle, delicate and beautiful. The variety is endless and, in a country that is home to billions of people, there is a new way of cooking as you travel every few miles. I have often said that it is almost like living in many countries at the same time so great is the variety of food, language, dress and custom. Even within particular regions, each household will often have their own recipe for the same dish, one that has been passed down the generations in that home. Over time, it will have been adapted so that hundreds of recipes exist for the same dish.

deeper knowledge
about food

Having said that, original recipes do exist and every variation is still true to this original. Cooks are taught, as I was, to use their senses while cooking. I can only cook if I smell, touch and see my ingredients and appreciate all the qualities of the food I am working with. Often an Indian cook will know what amount of seasoning to add simply by the aroma of the dish. It is important to know exactly when a fruit is ripe, what it will taste like when cooked and also, very importantly, how it will nourish and heal the body.

That food is perfectly balanced, is a large part of Indian cookery. As children we are told that certain foods cool us in the summer or that particular food combinations make us feel lethargic or dull. Ayurveda, the Indian system of holistic healing, is a natural inclusion in the everyday process of eating and cooking. Knowing when to cut open a melon or how to dry its seeds to make a nutritious snack for the children are skills that are passed down as fact. There is also a vast body of knowledge that tells us how foods affect our moods and feelings and we are taught to eat for positive well-being.

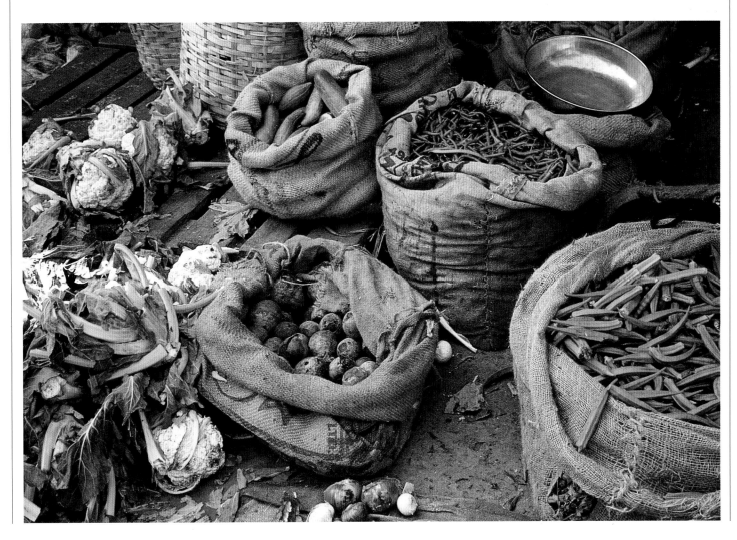

short history of vegetarianism in india

Almost 85 per cent of India is Hindu and, because of religion, vegetarian. Not all Hindus are vegetarian, as caste and community also affect this choice. Some of my strict Brahmin ancestors ate fish simply because they lived near the coast around Goa. Most non-vegetarians will eat meat or fish a few times a week or even just once, firstly because it is expensive and secondly because the choice of vegetables, lentils, beans and dairy products is so vast that there is an endless variety for each day of the year. Vegetarian food is also considered healthier than meat because it is easier to digest. Few people today believe that a vegetarian diet is lacking in protein; in fact, the lentils and beans that are an essential part of the Indian diet provide an extremely good source of protein.

India is already well-known for its tradition of vegetarianism which has a history going back almost two millennia. During the Vedic period, almost 5,000 years ago, animals were hunted for food and meat was eaten regularly by the warrior community of Kshatriyas. The anti-meat eating sentiment began to be felt at the end of the Vedic period. This coincided with the rise of Buddhism and Jainism whose founders, the Buddha and Lord Mahavira respectively, taught their followers the doctrines of non-violence. As more and more people began to convert to these newer beliefs, Hindu priests, fearing that a great number of their people would convert, also began preaching against the killing of animals. They adopted 'ahimsa' or non-violence and followed a vegetarian diet, regarding it as superior to the older Brahminical ideas of animal sacrifice.

essentials of indian vegetarian cooking

What binds the cuisines of the different regions of India is the use of spices. Used originally to preserve foods, they are now added in extremely complex combinations to bring out the best flavours and textures in a dish. Grains and rice provide the carbohydrate element. Many types of rice have been known in India for the past 5,000 years and references to them can be found in the ancient texts. Protein is eaten in the form of lentils and beans and every Indian kitchen will have a myriad of jars full of colourful lentils and pulses.

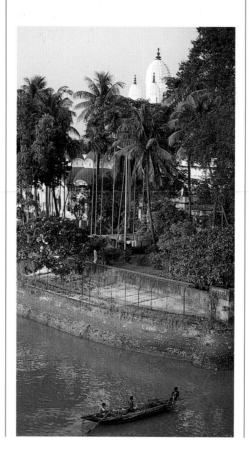

influences

Over the centuries, several dynasties came to India and built new empires. With these foreign powers came an amazing variety of cooking styles and ingredients. New world ingredients such as tomatoes, chillies and potatoes became everyday food in many parts of India. English cookery influenced areas such as Calcutta and Madras, which were strongholds of the Raj. French cooking became a part of the daily diet in Pondicherry and Goan food showed influences of the Portuguese style. The Parsees who came from Iran brought their own unique food combinations and became a part of the local population as did the Jews. North Indian cookery was vastly influenced by the Afghani rulers who founded the Mughal Empire. It is this ability to absorb all influences, turn them around and take ownership of the new styles that makes Indian cookery so fascinating and vibrant and a constantly evolving mélée.

Spices which today signal the advent of cooking are found in abundance in India. Most of the world's spices are grown here and many have been studied not just for their culinary uses but also for their healing powers. Spices and fresh herbs are very intricately woven into Indian life, featuring in food, prayer and medical treatments. For example, turmeric is revered as an antiseptic, asafoetida helps with flatulence, carom counters nausea and ginger is an aphrodisiac. Fenugreek and cumin seeds are given to nursing mothers to aid secretion. How a spice is used and when it is added to the pot can easily reveal what province of India the food is from and for whom it has been cooked.

equipment

A rural Indian kitchen and an urban one are quite different in the way that they function, but some functional tools and utensils are essential to every Indian kitchen, throughout the world. A spice-box is a must; this handy box has small compartments and tiny individual spoons for the main spices used in everyday cookery, including turmeric, chilli powder, cumin, coriander, black mustard seeds and asafoetida.

Most Indian cooks prefer to use a selection of stainless steel, aluminium, brass and iron utensils and, due to the intense heat, the bases of these pots and pans are reinforced with a thick layer of the same metal or one of copper. A kadhai, or heavy Indian wok, is found in every kitchen. Ideal in shape and thickness, it can be used for stir-frying or deep-frying and ensures even, non-stick cooking. Kadhais are available in many sizes and qualities. Look for a thick, heavy aluminium one with a handle that makes it easier to work with. Highly decorative, kitchen-to-table kadhais look pretty but they are not very heavy and can heat up too quickly. Other popular utensils are rimmed, straight-sided, upright vessels called degchis. No Indian kitchen can function without a grinder of some sort. The vast panorama of spice pastes and powders, chutneys and masalas demand a heavy-duty method of reducing whole spices, fruits, herbs and nuts to a smooth blend. Stone slabs with a heavy, rounded grinding stone are still used and are actually preferred by many cooks as the pastes made on them need less water and are often more concentrated. However, these are being rapidly replaced by powerful electric blenders, which

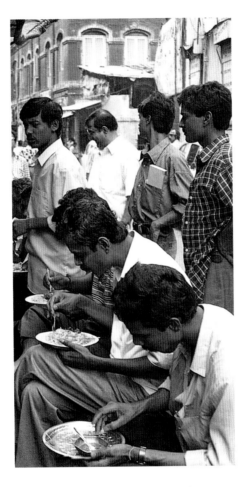

have various attachments for dry and wet grinding and can reduce the hardest spices to a fine, soft powder. They make an invaluable investment. You can also use a coffee-grinder to grind small quantities of spices very effectively. However, remember to wash it well afterwards or you might end up with coriander-flavoured coffee the next time you use your machine! Very small amounts of spice seeds, made brittle by dry-roasting, can be ground in a mortar with a pestle and I use mine to make fresh garam masala and other

spice blends; I need the spice powders to be fine for some dishes and coarse for others. Food processors that can grate, chop and knead are also becoming more and more popular in Indian kitchens, though many cooks genuinely believe that traditional methods produce tastier food.

In India, where coconut inspires the cuisine of many states, there will be a coconut-scraper in the majority of southern and eastern homes. This is a flat, wooden base to which a sickle-shaped blade is attached. It has a serrated fan at the end, which is used to scrape out the white flesh from the coconut shell. The blade is also used to chop meat and vegetables. This whole device is placed on the floor and one has to sit on the plinth to use it. Coconut can also be grated effectively in a food processor after breaking open the shell and prising away the flesh. Small stainless steel or brass graters are used for grating ginger and garlic and you can always use a garlic press.

One of the most versatile tools available to an Indian cook is a pressure cooker. Although they seem to have gone out of fashion in the West, they are used to make everything from curries to puddings. As they reduce cooking times drastically and give a perfectly finished product, they are invaluable to anyone who wants to rustle up a meal in minutes.

Another must is a refrigerator. As Indian food retains its flavour even after freezing, it can be prepared well in advance and stored for later use. In very hot weather, along with the usual meat, milk and vegetables, flour goes into the fridge too.

what is a curry?

Many people in my demonstrations ask me whether 'curry' is an anglicised dish that does not exist in India. I have to say that hardly any Indian meal is complete without a curry. The word comes from the Tamil 'kari' which means gravy or vegetable dish. In south Indian curries it is based on a blend of coconut and tamarind, while in the north it is made from a range of mild spices. There is really no such thing as a Madras curry or even Madras curry powder as the terms seem too general for the hundreds of variations that exist.

Many things are important when judging a curry. Firstly think of the consistency: is it too thick or too watery? A good curry should be fairly thick and, as I have often said in this book, like custard. A thin curry will not support an even blend of spices whereas too thick a one will not moisten the accompanying rice or bread sufficiently.

Secondly think of colour. Turmeric, chillies, tamarind and coriander are some of the ingredients that add colour to a curry. They add flavour and aroma as well. Generally curries can be white (as in a Kashmiri yoghurt-based yakhni), red (as in a makhani), yellow (as in many kormas) and green (as in a south Indian nilgiri). The oil used also varies from region to region giving each curry a unique fragrance. Many parts of the south use peanut oil or coconut oil. In Bengal, it is mustard oil. Over most of the country it is ghee although younger cooks are now choosing healthier options such as sunflower oil.

All good curries begin with patience. In the north, a basic curry starts with the heating of the oil. Then the seed spices are added to release their aromatic oils. The onions, ginger, garlic and tomatoes go in next to add moisture. The pan is now ready to receive the powdered spices so that they do not burn. The main ingredient, salt and a little water are added next to obtain the right consistency. Controlled heat and an eye for the right texture and colour are equally important.

Thus curries are made in steps, almost like building blocks. The blocks can be moved around and rearranged in countless ways to give never ending recipes that tease the tastebuds and create a burst of complementary flavours.

and finally

I have enjoyed writing this book immensely because it is really the way I cook and eat on a daily basis. I truly believe that vegetarian food can be immensely exciting, infinitely diverse and wonderfully fresh and healthy. I hope that my readers discover the many pleasures of Indian regional vegetarian cooking through this book, as I have done through the years.

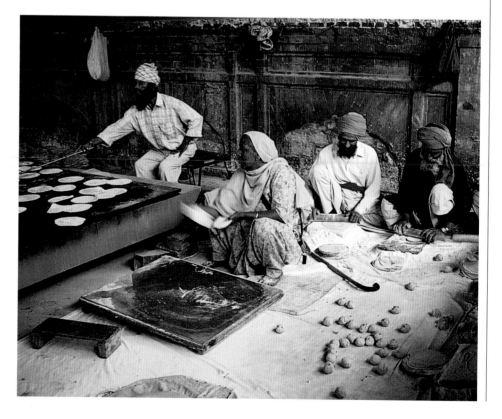

basic recipe

Ginger-garlic paste

These are almost always used together in Indian cooking. To make the ginger-garlic paste used in this book, take equal quantities of each and whiz in a blender until smooth. I usually make this paste in big batches and freeze it in thin sheets between plastic. Of course you will have to put the frozen sheets of ginger and garlic in big freezer containers or else everything from your ice cream to ice cubes will smell weird! Just break off bits when you need them and add straight into the pan.

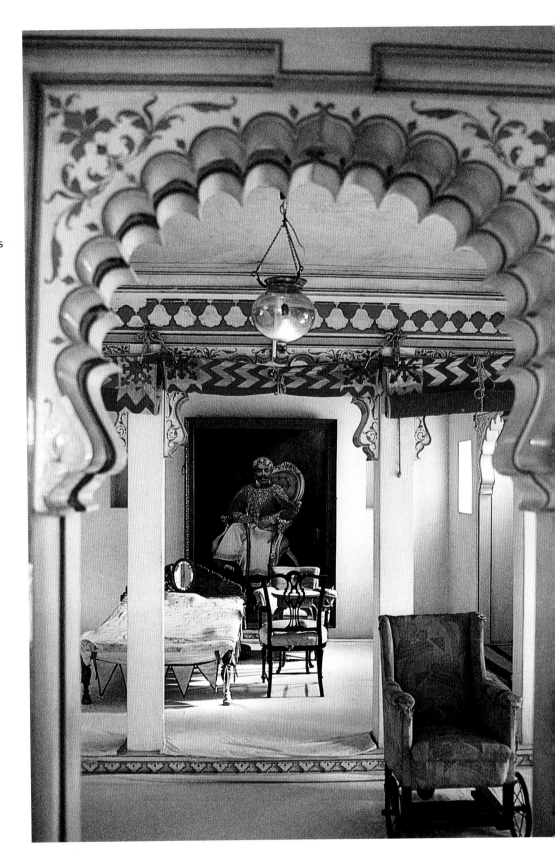

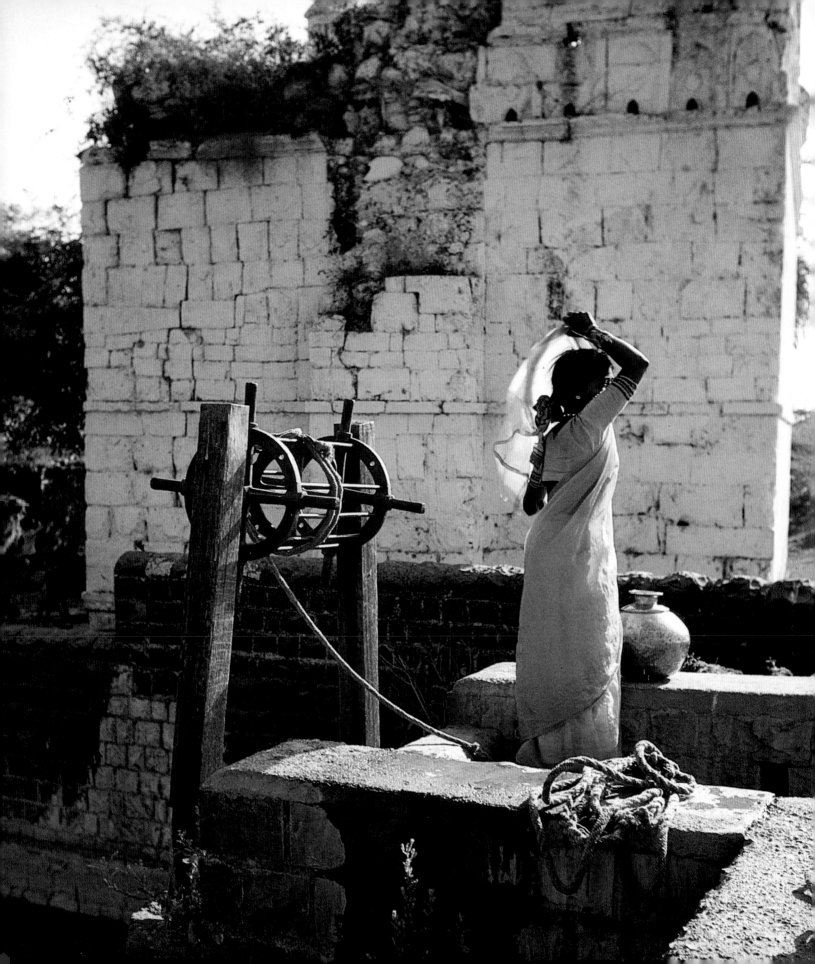

ayurveda

According to Ayurveda, foods have healing properties that are categorised by 'rasa' or taste. The word rasa means both taste and emotion and this aspect of food has a deep effect on our physical and mental health. The six tastes, namely sweet, sour, bitter, astringent, salty and pungent, all have specific effects on each individual constitution and can contribute differently to each person's well-being. Taste is said to have both long term and short term effects. Tastes can be light or heavy, moist or dry. Light tastes include rice, ghee and mung dal, which are easier to digest than heavy tastes, such as black lentils or bananas.

The unique combination of energy present in each individual at birth is that person's constitution or 'prakruti'. Your prakruti is determined by the proportion and balance of the five elements, namely earth, fire, water, air and ether, in your body and therefore no two people are alike. Ayurveda believes that there is no single path to health and each person must be treated individually depending on the prakruti. There are no general rules about which foods to eat because each of us must learn to be aware of the effects that different foods have upon our mind, body and spirit. Indians also believe that peaceful surroundings and a quiet mind at mealtimes help to boost immunity, aid digestion and conserve stamina for future tasks.

The five elements – air, fire, water, earth and ether – exist in nature, in food and even within our bodies. Air promotes health, fire is purification, water signifies movement and fluidity, earth symbolises energy and fecundity and ether or space echoes with vibrations of the Divine. When all the elements are maintained in balance in our bodies, good health follows.

The three basic constitutions are determined by a combination of energies called 'doshas'. The constitutions are Vata (governed by air and ether). Pitta (governed by fire and water) and Kapha (governed by water and earth). Very loosely, if you are a Vata constitution you will find that you suffer from wind, have dry hair and skin and that your hands and feet are often cold. A Pitta constitution means that you will generate a lot of internal heat, you may be moody and angry and you are frequently thirsty. Kapha produces a lot of mucous, is often afflicted by coughs and colds and finds it easy to gain weight. If we understand our own constitution and choose foods as well as a lifestyle accordingly, we provide ourselves with the best chance of good health. Sometimes two doshas form a combination in a single individual and at times, all the doshas are present making it a balanced or 'tridoshic' constitution.

All Indians grow up with this kind of knowledge and understand when to eat what foods for optimum health. We are also taught to respect nature and everywhere in India, great importance is placed on seasonal foods. You would never expect to find mangoes in the winter because they are a summer fruit and this is when they are at their best. An out of season fruit or vegetable will not have adequate healing and nourishing properties. At the centre of Ayurvedic nutrition is the awareness of 'agni' or the digestive fire. In the winter, this demands heavier foods such as grains and proteins or warm foods such as honey and herb teas. In the summer, agni is at a low and we feel like eating fresher, lighter foods such as salads and yoghurt.

Eight rules of an ayurvedic diet

Prakruti – Choose a combination of foods depending on their nature, that is their inherent heaviness or lightness. (Meat is heavy to digest, vegetables are light).

Karana – The processing of foods affects their influence on our bodies. Generally, cooked foods are easier to digest with the exception of fruits and some vegetables. Frying adds heaviness whereas stir–frying helps introduce some lightness. Microwave cooking destroys 'prana' or the life force of foods.

Samyoga – Combine foods healthily and never mix contrary foods. Fish and dairy are not combined as they both need a different rate of acid secretion as well as concentration of acid in the stomach for proper digestion.

Rashi – Control the quantity of food you eat according to your constitution.

Desha – Eat according to your environment. Consider the seasons and factors such as humidity and pollution.

Kala – Be attentive to the time of eating. Eat only when the previous meal has had a chance to be properly digested.

Upayoga Sanstha – Follow the golden rules of eating. Eat food when it is hot. Concentrate on eating rather than on laughing, talking, reading or on distractions. Be calm and unhurried and smoking or drinking too much during a meal is not advisable.

Upabhokta – Every person must decide for herself or himself about what to eat depending on how one feels. Never force yourself or eat against your instinct.

a religious perspective on food

'The purchaser of flesh performs himsa (violence) by his wealth; he who eats flesh does so by enjoying its taste; the killer does himsa by actually tying and killing the animal. Thus, there are three forms of killing: he who brings flesh or sends for it, he who cuts off the limbs of an animal, and he who purchases, sells or cooks flesh and eats it – all of these are to be considered meat-eaters.'
Mahabharata

Most Hindus are vegetarian due to various reasons. Firstly, they consider that Ahimsa, or the law of non-violence, is a Hindu's first duty towards God and all of God's creation must be respected. The love and protection of animals is central to Hinduism and even the ancients associated each deity with an animal with a view to its protection and conservation. Hindu gods and goddesses each have an animal with them as a personal vehicle or companion. Therefore Shiva has the bull, Durga the lion or tiger, Ganesh the mouse and Kartikeya the peacock. Many Hindus feel that killing and eating animals will be disrespectful to the gods who so overtly protect and cherish all beings.

Secondly, they believe that all one's actions, including one's choice of food, have Karmic consequences. The Karma theory is about reaping what you sow, so that each of our actions is rewarded or punished at a later date, sometimes even in following lifetimes. By being a part of the cycle of inflicting pain and death, even indirectly, on other living creatures one brings upon oneself the suffering one has caused to others, in equal measure. Similarly, a good deed will be repaid in equal measure almost like a blessing when one needs it most.

Hindus also believe that food is a source of health and healing and can govern our moods and emotions. By eating the flesh of animals, we eat their innermost being, and introduce into our bodies all their anxieties, fears and instincts. This can bring us into a lower realm of consciousness where spiritual awareness, which is the chief purpose of the Hindu way of life, becomes impossible.

Studies have proved that a vegetarian diet can provide a greater range of nutrients and fewer toxins. Vegetarians are usually less prone to major illnesses and lead longer, healthier lives. Many vegetarians are also non-smokers, have more balanced weights than non vegetarians and consume less alcohol. Also, a vegetarian diet is more ecologically friendly. As Albert Einstein said, 'Nothing will benefit human health and increase chances for survival of life on Earth as much as the evolution to a vegetarian diet.' Animals becoming extinct, air and water pollution all have links to the slaughter of animals. More land is required for the breeding of animals for consumption than for the growing of an equal quantity of protein-rich plant foods. If we are to save our planet, it is important for us all to adopt a vegetarian diet.

Having said this, there is a great variety of beliefs within India. The Christians, Jews and Parsees will eat meat while most Hindus will not. Within the Hindus, some communities such as the Jains are very particular and will not eat even onions or garlic. This is due to the belief that these heat-producing foods can excite the passions and lead the mind away from a constant awareness of spirituality. Most

Hindu temples will only ever serve vegetarian food and in many traditional communities religious celebrations such as weddings will have vegetarian feasts. In some Hindu homes, kitchen utensils for the preparation of meat are kept separately and never mixed with the 'vegetarian' utensils.

It is perhaps true that for some Indians, their being vegetarian is itself their dharma or religious practice. However there are many Hindu communities where meat or fish is very common, especially in the coastal states of Kerala and West Bengal. In Bengal, even religious feasts in honour of the Mother Goddess Kali include several meat and fish dishes. Muslims all over the country eat meat and in north India, the Punjabis are renowned for their chicken fare such as tandoori chicken. Nevertheless, most people around the world see India as being a perfect haven for vegetarians, a land full of rice, wheat, beans and lentils, vegetables and fruit. In many meat-eating Indian families, meat is usually a Sunday afternoon feast and is eaten only on that one day of the week. For some other families, meat – and this most often means chicken or mutton — is eaten a few times a year at weddings or celebrations.

Another practice found in many middle class families in northern, western and central India is that the women of the house will not eat meat whereas the men will. Eating meat is sometimes associated with masculinity, or with the baser instincts to which it is thought that men are more prone, probably going with the belief that to eat an animal is to turn into an animal oneself.

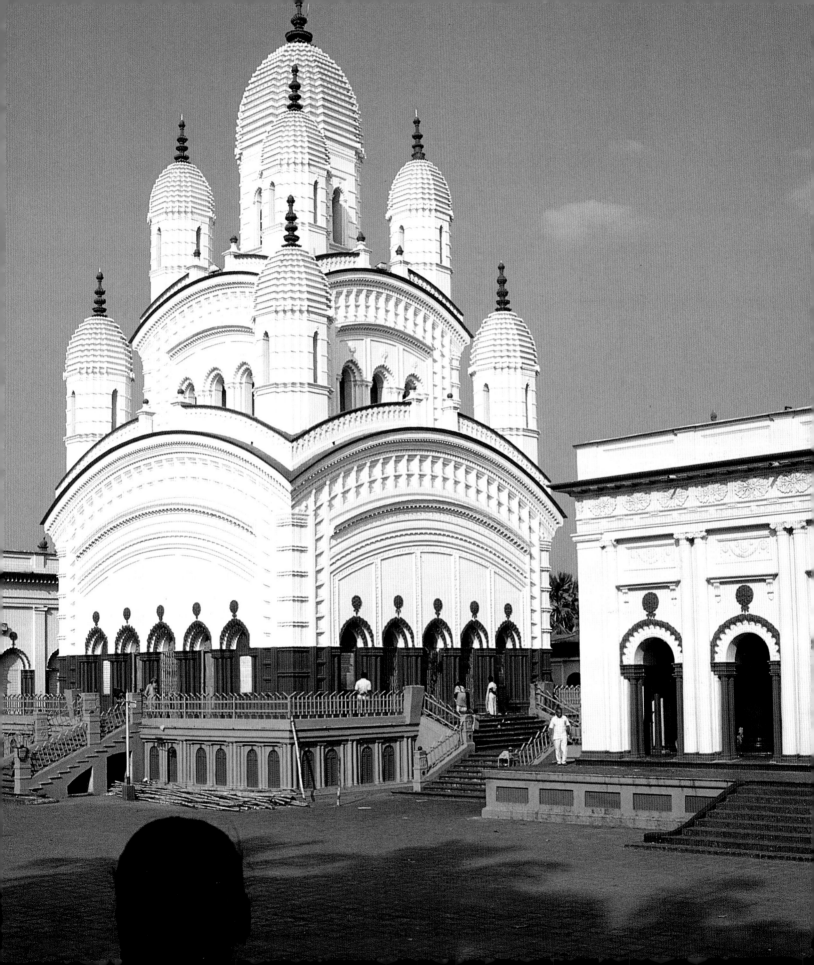

a synergy with the land

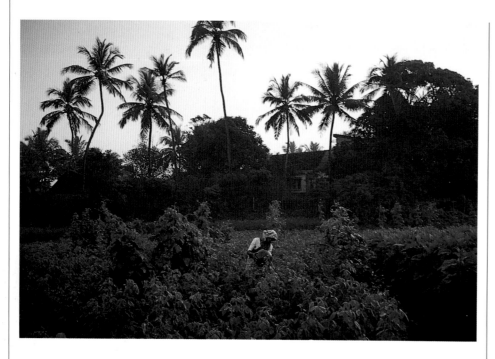

The ancient people who lived in India were nature worshippers. The sun brought warmth and light, the rain fed crops, the earth seemed to mysteriously provide food and the air carried health and comfort. As time went on, the five elements (fire, water, earth, air and ether) became sacred and held a central position in religion and worship. Even today, the five elements are given a special place and they are at the core of many Indian arts, philosophies and sciences.

Thousands of years ago the process of procreation generated awe and respect. People realised that it is the female who conceives and bears both males and females. The similarity between the mother giving birth to a child as a result of intercourse and the earth sprouting plants after the sowing of

seeds glorified both the mother and the earth to a divine status. Worship of fertility was linked with the worship of the mother-goddess. The earth was looked upon as a mother and was symbolically worshipped as such. The terms mother-earth and motherland (Matrubhoomi) are still used today. The ancients had a high regard for the earth and worshipped it as Bhoomi Devi or Earth Goddess, always female because of her fertility and ability to produce plants, trees and crops from deep within herself. Bhoomi Devi had to be kept happy so that she would keep offering her riches. Several stories, rituals and celebrations developed around her and her generosity.

According to later legend, while Siddhartha who later became the Buddha, sat meditating

under the bodhi tree, Mara the Tempter released his mighty armies. But Siddhartha fearlessly continued to meditate. When asked for his account of merit, he touched the fingers of his right hand to the earth and said, 'The very Earth is my witness.' The Earth Goddess materialised at once and agreed that she had witnessed every act of merit that this monk had committed, over several incarnations. Then she wrung out her long hair where the merit had been stored in the form of sparkling water. The water created such a flood that Mara's armies were all drowned in it. In eastern philosophies, the earth is often held as witness, a silent sentinel who observes everything.

In the great epic The Ramayana, Rama's wife Sita was said to be born out of the earth, making her an elemental woman and in the story, when she is asked to prove her chastity, she cannot bear this humiliation and asks to return to her mother. The earth opens up at her feet and accepts her back.

To this day, an Indian dancer will begin a practice session by doing a 'namaskaar' or paying obeisance to the earth. This act is deeply symbolic as the dancer asks for blessings from the primeval Mother as well as for forgiveness for touching her with one's feet, an act considered disrespectful by all Indians.

Harvest festivals all over the world celebrate the fecundity of the earth. In southern India 'Pongal' is celebrated as a happy four-day harvest festival with the cooking of newly harvested rice. Cows and bullocks, who are associated with the land through grass, milk or tilling are beautifully decorated with flowers and fed on 'pongal' which is also a sweet made of rice and jaggery.

The four days of the festival each have their own significance and separate deities are worshipped each day. On the first day the Rain God is worshipped. The day begins with an oil bath and in the evening there is a ceremonial bonfire. The second day is that of the Sun God. The place where the ritual worship is carried out is cleaned and decorated with floor paintings called kolams. Sweet 'pongal' is cooked and offered, on a new banana leaf, to the Sun God in gratitude for showering his blessings on the land and for the bountiful harvest. The third day is that of the cattle worship. On this day, the cattle are decorated and paraded in the village amidst much fanfare and celebration. The final day is when birds are worshipped.

In northern India, the picture is quite different. In Punjab, the granary of India, wheat is the main winter crop, which is sown in October and harvested in March or April. In January, as the fields fill up with the new harvest farmers celebrate the festival of Lohri. This falls in January at a time when the earth is farthest away from the sun. The festival coincides with the point when the earth begins its journey towards the sun and therefore heralds the move towards seasonal warmth and sunshine.

At dusk, huge bonfires are lit in the harvested fields and people gather around the rising flames, circle the bonfire and throw puffed rice or new corn into the fire, sing popular folk songs and dance in joy. This is a ritual to honour Agni, the Fire God, to bless the land with abundance and prosperity. Lohri celebrates fertility and the joy of life.

An ancient belief that is still practised in India today is Vastu Shastra, the science of land, earth and buildings. It takes into account how the five elements will affect the construction of a building and the luck it will bring to its owners. Vastu Shastra depends largely upon astrology and the eight directions. Each direction is ruled by a deity. The North is ruled by Kubera, the god of Wealth and according to the science of Vastu Shastra, this is the direction for the storage of wealth in a home. Money, jewellery and all cupboards that hold valuable possessions should be placed in the northern part of the house near the southern or western wall and facing the east or the north to attract even more wealth.

There are many factors around the building that affect the flow of money and wealth into it. One such factor is the existence of a large open space directly in front of the house. Large empty spaces are governed by the largely malefic planet Rahu (in Hindu astrology), which suppresses growth and prosperity. Another factor is the presence of a road end across the home, that is, if the home is at a T-junction, Rahu will see to it that all the family wealth comes to a dead end and that the inhabitants of the house will face great financial difficulty. If there are such problematic areas in front of the house, they can be corrected by planting beautiful, flowering shrubs or better still, the holy basil (Tulsi) plant that is considered so auspicious all over India and grows well in the summer all over the world.

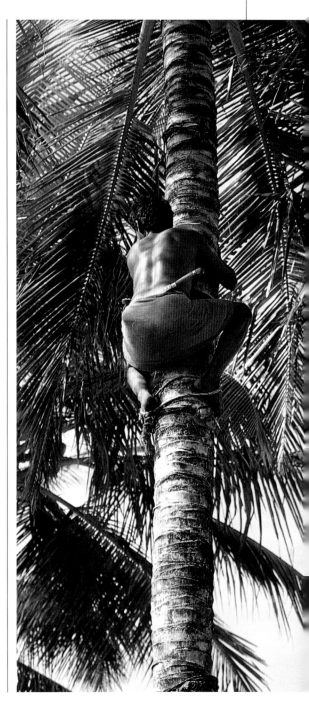

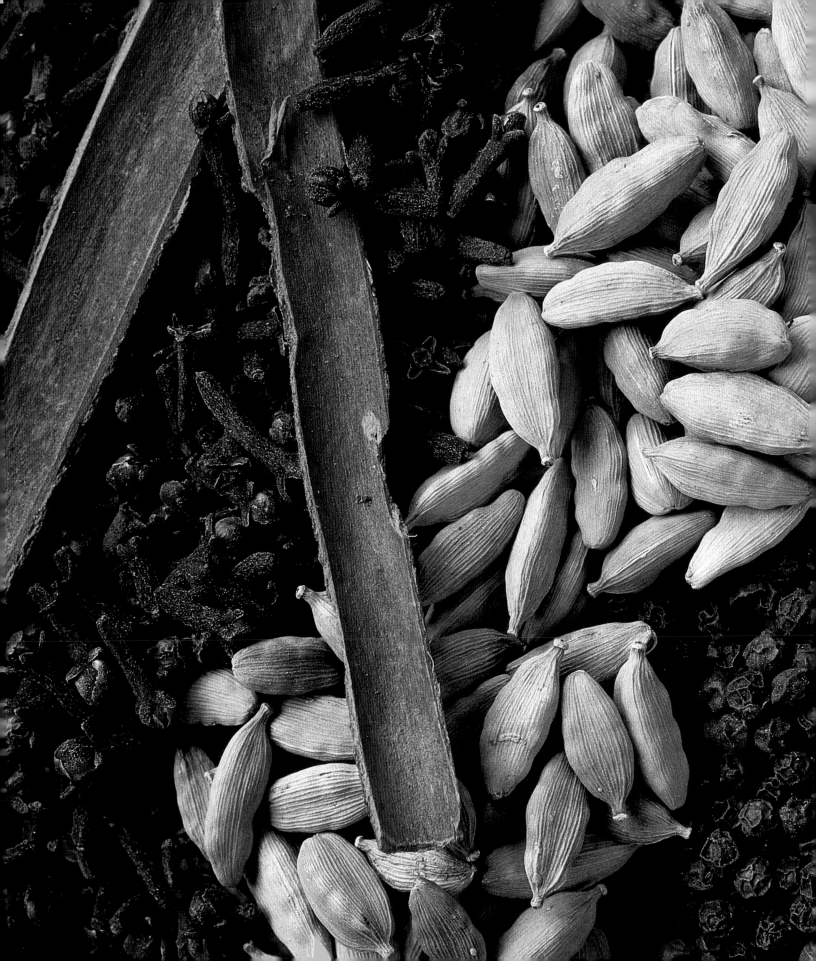

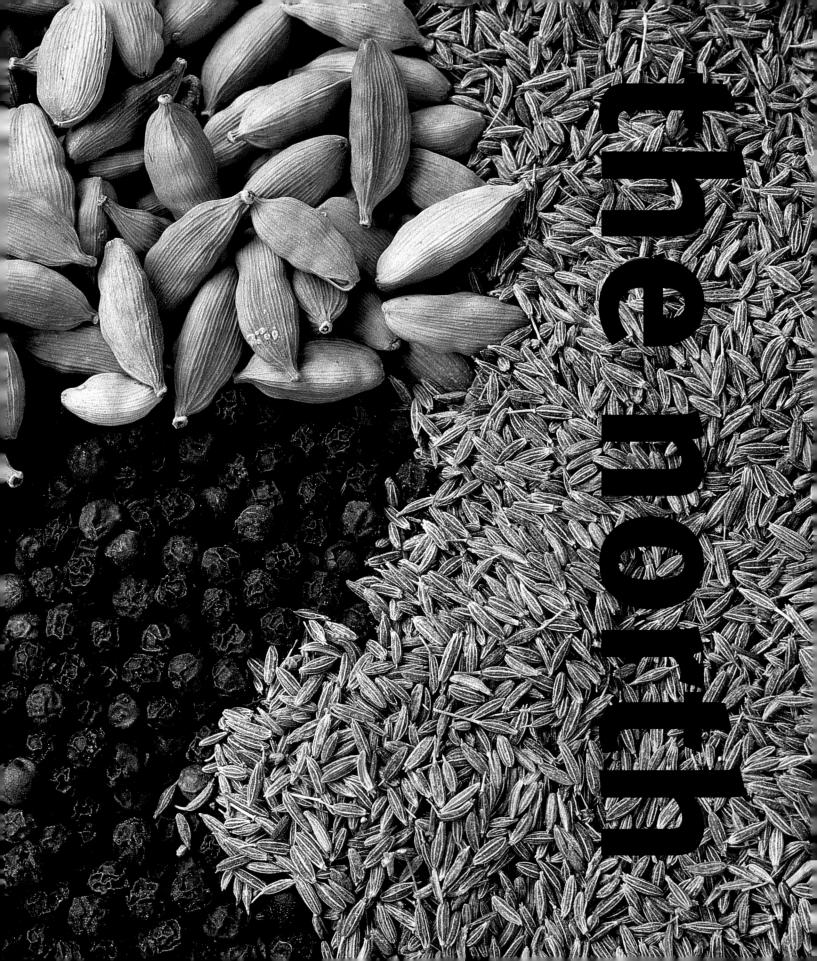

them

My main focus in the north has been on the states of Punjab, Uttar Pradesh, Kashmir and Delhi. The overall style of cooking in the north is fairly similar amongst the states but, perhaps because this area of India has seen the most turbulent phases of history and the most number of invasions, the cuisine is a wonderful blend of many cultures.

punjab

A large number of Indians who live outside of India are Punjabi in origin. In many families, ancestors several generations ago left India in search of better prospects and a new way of life. They carried with them the culture of India so much so that today, in many parts of the world when talking of Indian cooking, it is Punjabi food that is being dissussed. Rich onion- and tomato-flavoured curries or the delicious tandoori foods that are cooked slowly in a clay oven called the tandoor, even the naans and parathas, all originate in Punjab. The Punjabis, both the Hindus and the Sikhs, are possibly the most fun-loving community of India. Ever ready to celebrate with food, drink and dancing, their cuisine is rich and liberally flavoured.

It has sometimes been said that, because much of Punjab is agricultural and rural farming communities abound, the cooking of this state is rather unsophisticated. I would say that, in order to satisfy these hard-working people, the cuisine is hearty and wholesome. In fact, most Indians love Punjabi cooking and restaurants in this style do great business in every Indian town and city. Most non-Punjabis think of this cuisine as being for an occasional treat and look forward to a meal laced with ghee and cream and accompanied by fried treats such as samosas and pakoras. Ingredients that you would commonly find in a Punjabi kitchen are beans such as chickpeas, red kidney beans, and black lentils; vegetables such as cauliflower, potatoes, peas and turnips and wholewheat flour to make many kinds of breads. The Punjab grows a lot of wheat and was known as the granary of India for a long time.

kashmir

This is one of the most beautiful states of India, resplendent with green valleys, flowing waterfalls, pine forests and fruit-filled orchards. Due to its proximity to the Himalayas it was the natural passage to India for many invaders. Its cuisine is therefore a mix of Indian, Persian and Afghani styles. There are two distinct communities who live in Kashmir: the Muslims and the Hindu Brahmins who are known as 'Kashmiri Pundits'. The cuisine of Kashmir makes the most of the local produce such as walnuts, dried apricots and pistachios. As it is a hilly state, not too many vegetables and herbs are grown and the cuisine is largely meat-based. Spices such as dried ginger powder, fennel powder and saffron, which grow in Kashmir, are used. Yoghurt forms the base for many curries. The true cooking of Kashmir can be seen in the Wazawan style which is fragrant with spices including cardamom, cloves and cinnamon. Even today, the master chefs of Kashmir are the descendants of the traditional chefs from Samarkand, the Wazas. The original Wazas came to India with the ruler Timur when he entered India in the 15th century. The royal Wazawan, comprising of 36 courses, is a feast that few can get through.

The meal begins with the ritual of washing the hands, then the 'tramis' or dishes filled with food begin to arrive. The entrées are eaten with a sticky, dense variety of rice which is prized. Much of the Wazawan is meat-based as this is a sign of affluence but vegetarian dishes with lotus root or potatoes are also served. The meal is washed down with Kahwa tea which is flavoured with saffron, cinnamon and almonds.

uttar pradesh

Two of India's most sacred Hindu cities lie in this state. Varanasi and Allahabad are thronged with pilgrims each year and it is not surprising that Uttar Pradesh has a rich and varied vegetarian cuisine. All religious food in India must only include those ingredients which are considered acceptable. An awareness of what is and what is not acceptable is inculcated in each generation by word of mouth. However, Uttar Pradesh does have a non-vegetarian repertoire of food as well. The vegetarian food is light and nutritious and largely free of the heavy spices that dominate much of north Indian cooking. Coriander and cumin are favoured while legumes and pulses form the base of many curries. One of the most famous styles of cooking that originates from this state is the Awadhi style from Lucknow, or Awadh as it was earlier known. Until nearly the middle of the 20th century it was a princely state with Nawab rulers. Their feasts were renowned and even today the 'dum pukht' technique, which literally means 'to choke off the steam', is considered an important skill in any Awadhi chef's repertoire. One story says that 200 years ago Nawab Asaf-ud-Daulah began the construction of a huge edifice, the Bara Imambara (which is the most important site in Lucknow today and is said to have the biggest vaulted hall in the world). He would destroy a part of the day's building work at night so that his workers would be in continuous employment. Food for the workers consisted of rice, meat and vegetables and, as this was required day and night, it was put in a pot and sealed with dough to be slow-cooked all the time. One day, the Nawab tasted this meal, found it truly delicious and had it adopted into the royal kitchens. Awadh's most famous ruler, the artistic Wajid Ali Shah, is said to have refined the technique further. All sorts of fine dishes are made in the dum pukht style and speciality restaurants in many five star hotels around the country specialise in this cuisine.

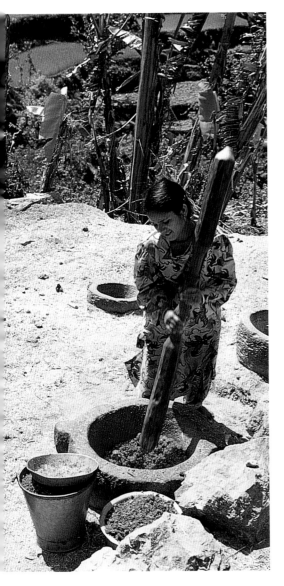

delhi

New Delhi is the capital of India and has a cosmopolitan population of politicians, diplomats and businessmen. The cuisine reflects the diversity of its people and a variety of styles from the rich Punjabi to the vegetarian Bania and the non-vegetarian Kayastha co-exist. The street corners are lined with stalls selling tandoori foods, crisp samosas and syrupy sweets but, as evening turns to dusk and the street lights start to come on, the city's rich and famous dress up in their best silks to attend countless cocktail and dinner parties, often several in one night. At these, the food is a mix of world styles, each tempting the gourmet with newer and fancier creations.

Delhi is famous for its Mughlai cooking, a legacy left by the Mughal rulers who reigned from Delhi, their capital, over a large part of India, before the British took over. This cuisine is Muslim-influenced with several original names such as biryani, kebab and kofta still in use. Mughlai cooking is truly fit for royalty with its buttery sauces, medley of vegetables and rose-flavoured sweets.

cauliflower and potatoes in spices
aloo gobi

This combination of cauliflower and potato is common all over India but, in the Punjab, it is quite a specialty, served with a roti and a lentil dish. I like the cauliflower and the potatoes to turn slightly mushy, but you could cook the vegetables for a little less time and have them hold their shape if you prefer.

Serves: 4
Preparation time: 10 minutes
Cooking time: 25 minutes

3 tablespoons sunflower oil
1 medium onion, sliced
1/2 teaspoon ginger-garlic paste (page 11)
2 fresh green chillies, chopped
150g potatoes, peeled and cubed
100g fresh tomatoes, chopped
150g cauliflower, washed and
 cut into florettes
1/2 teaspoon turmeric powder
1 teaspoon garam masala powder
Salt

1 Heat the oil in a kadhai or heavy-bottomed pan. Add the onion and fry until soft. Add the ginger-garlic paste and fry for a few seconds.

2 Add the chillies and the potatoes. Fry for a couple of minutes, stirring frequently to prevent the mixture from sticking. Add the tomatoes and allow them to soften.

3 Tip in the cauliflower, turmeric, garam masala powder and salt. Mix well. Reduce the heat and cook, adding a few spoonfuls of water if it begins to stick to the pan. When the vegetables are completely done, in about 20 minutes, remove from the heat and serve hot.

spinach with cottage cheese
palak paneer

Indian cottage cheese is known as paneer. It is popular in the Punjab and is made at home by curdling full fat milk and hanging up the milk solids in a piece of muslin to drain off all the whey. The solid cheese is then pressed and cut into cubes. It is quite bland and will not keep very long.

Commercially-available paneer is much denser than the homemade one because it is pressed under heavier weights. This dish can be found on the menu of most north Indian restaurants all over the world.

Serves: 4
Preparation time: 10 minutes
Cooking time: 25 minutes

500g fresh spinach, washed and drained
3 tablespoons sunflower oil
1/2 teaspoon cumin seeds
150g onions, grated
1 tablespoon ginger-garlic paste (page 11) –
 reserve some slivers of ginger for
 the garnish
2 large tomatoes, chopped
1/2 teaspoon chilli powder
1/2 teaspoon garam masala powder
Salt
225g paneer, cubed
2 tablespoons single cream

1 Put the spinach with some water in a heavy pan and cook, uncovered, on high heat until done, for about 5 minutes. Cool slightly and grind along with enough of the cooking water to a thick purée in a blender. Reserve.

2 Heat the oil in a heavy-bottomed pan and fry the cumin seeds until they turn dark. Add the onions and fry until soft.

3 Stir in the ginger-garlic paste and tomatoes and cook on low heat until mushy, for about 5 minutes.

4 Pour in the spinach purée, sprinkle in the spice powders and salt and stir well. Bring to the boil. Reduce the heat and gently add the paneer. Simmer for 1 minute and take off the heat. The paneer will soften in the heat.

5 Serve hot, swirled with the cream and sprinkled with slivers of ginger. This is great with a paratha (page 32) and some slices of fresh tomato, seasoned with salt and pepper.

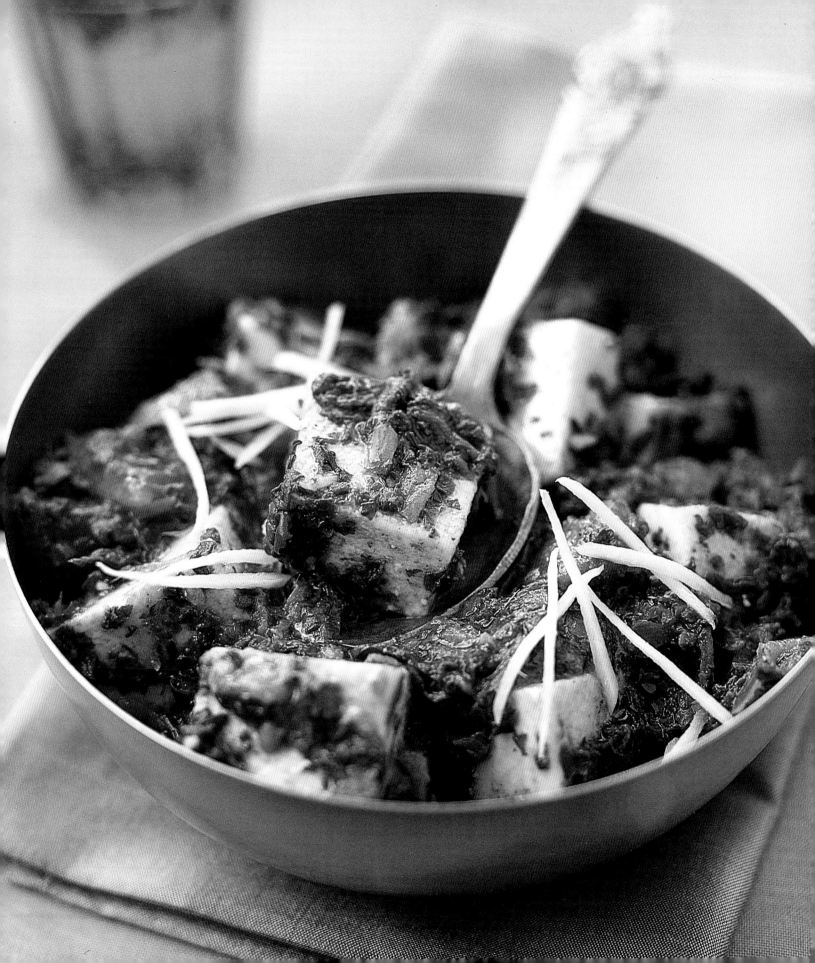

potatoes in sour cream
banarasi aloo

spiced turnips
shalgam masala

Fennel seeds, used a lot in the cooking of Uttar Pradesh, add a sweet richness to curries and desserts, and a special zest to vegetables. They feature powdered or whole with a variety of vegetables and in a popular crisp, golden, fried sweet called 'malpua', which is soaked in fennel-flavoured sugar syrup. Fennel is also used in pickles and chutneys in north India and a fennel infusion makes a delicious base for refreshing drinks. I love adding a few fennel seeds to my tea for a fuller flavour.

Serves: 4
Preparation time: 30 minutes
Cooking time: 15 minutes

3 tablespoons sunflower oil
1 teaspoon fennel seeds
300g potatoes, boiled, peeled and cubed
2 teaspoons tamarind pulp, diluted in a
   little water
4 tablespoons tomato purée
1/2 teaspoon chilli powder
1/2 teaspoon turmeric powder
1/2 teaspoon garam masala powder
Salt
4 tablespoons single cream

1 Heat the oil in a wok or kadhai and toss in the fennel. When the seeds darken, add the potatoes and stir-fry for a couple of minutes.

2 Add the tamarind pulp, tomato purée, spice powders and salt, and stir until well blended. Cook on low heat until the potatoes are done but hold their shape. Gently fold in the cream and heat through. The potatoes should be coated with a thick sauce. Serve hot.

Turnips are commonly used in the north either in stir-fries or in pickles. This pinkish white vegetable adds a crunch to many curries. I like it best when it gets slightly mushy as it seems to take on a creamy texture. Enjoy this with a hot roti (page 32).

Serves: 4
Preparation time: 15 minutes
Cooking time: 35 minutes

2 tablespoons sunflower oil
1 large onion, chopped
1 teaspoon ginger-garlic paste (page 11)
2 fresh green chillies, chopped
2 medium tomatoes, chopped
1 teaspoon cumin powder
1 teaspoon coriander powder
1/2 teaspoon turmeric powder
Salt
300g turnips, peeled and diced
1 teaspoon jaggery or brown sugar
Finely chopped coriander leaves to garnish

1 Heat the oil in a kadhai or heavy-bottomed pan and fry the onion until soft. Add the ginger-garlic paste and the chillies.

2 Add the tomatoes, the spice powders and salt. Stir until well blended.

3 Mix in the turnips. Add about 150ml of hot water and stir well.

4 Cover and bring to the boil, then reduce the heat and cook for about 20 minutes until the turnips are cooked.

5 Stir in the jaggery or sugar, lightly mashing the turnips as you go.

6 Garnish with the coriander leaves and serve the turnips piping hot.

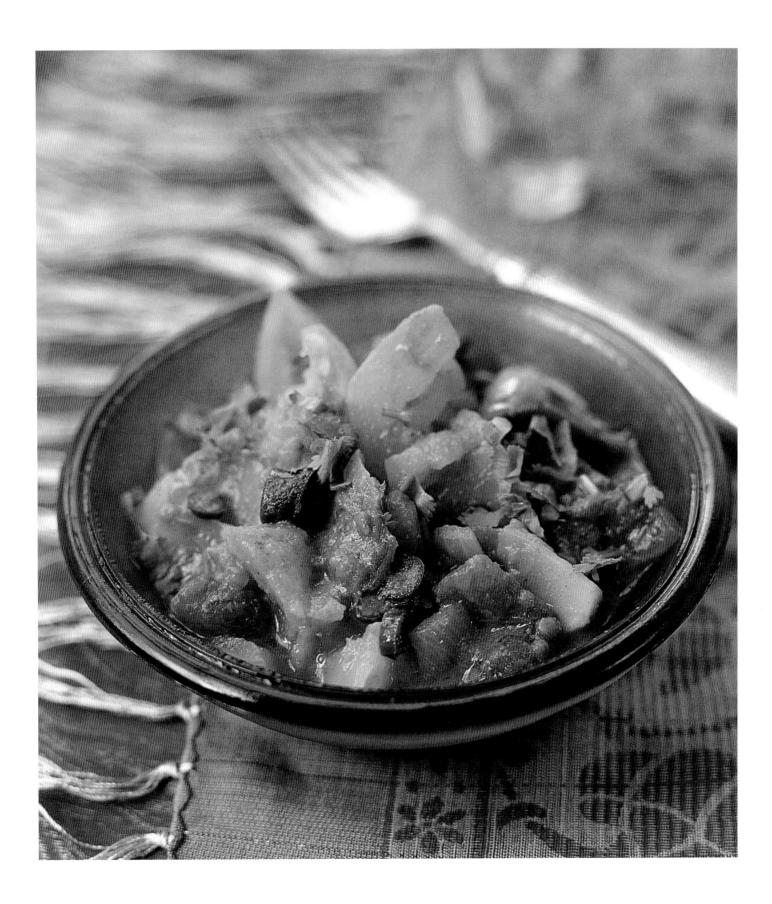

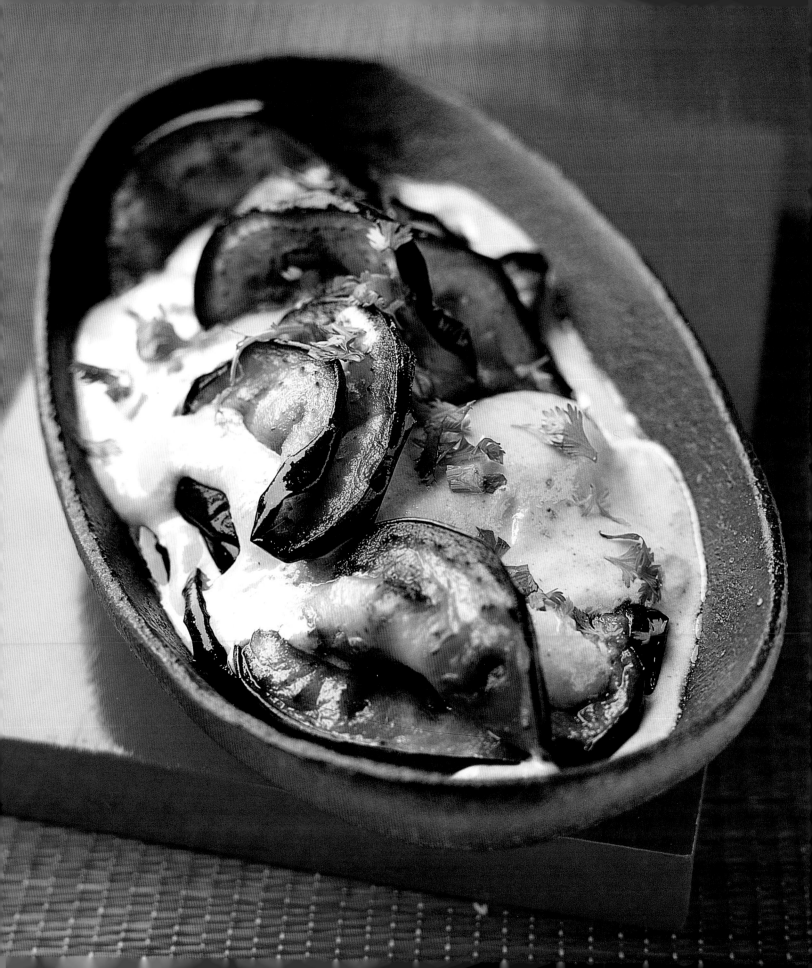

kashmiri-style aubergines in yoghurt
dahi baingan kashmiri

Serves: 4
Preparation time: 10 minutes
Cooking time: (approx.) 30 minutes

Sunflower oil for shallow frying
1 large aubergine, cut into thin discs
4 green cardamoms, bruised
1/2 teaspoon fennel powder
1/2 teaspoon turmeric powder
1/2 teaspoon dried ginger powder
Pinch of asafoetida
300g natural yoghurt
Salt
Finely chopped coriander leaves to garnish

1 Heat the oil in a heavy-bottomed, flat pan and, when very hot, shallow-fry the aubergine discs on both sides, until golden brown in colour. Drain on kitchen paper and reserve. Discard all but 1 tablespoon of the oil from the pan.

2 Drop the green cardamoms, the spice powders and asafoetida into the oil. Add the yoghurt immediately as the spices will burn easily. Season with salt and heat through on low heat, stirring gently.

3 Add the fried aubergine discs and serve at once, garnished with the chopped coriander. This goes well with Aloo Paratha (Page 35).

silky aubergine mash with potatoes
baingan bharta

This most traditional dish is made by cooking the aubergine over an open flame so that it develops a smoky flavour. This process can be done on the hob or in the oven. I have modified the classic version of the recipe slightly to make it faster. This version does not have a smoky flavour but makes the most of the silky texture of the aubergine. The potatoes add a creaminess that goes well with the tomatoes and spices. I sometimes serve this as a topping for canapés or as a dip with cocktail snacks.

Serves: 4
Preparation time: 10 minutes
Cooking time: 40 minutes

1 large aubergine
2 tablespoons sunflower oil
1/2 teaspoon cumin seeds
1 medium onion, finely chopped
1 teaspoon ginger-garlic paste (page 11)
1 fresh green chilli, chopped
2 tablespoons tomato purée
1 teaspoon turmeric powder
1 teaspoon coriander powder
2 medium potatoes, peeled, boiled and cubed
Salt
Chopped coriander leaves to garnish

1 Cut the aubergine into thick slices and place it in a heavy pan with enough water to cover the slices. Cover and cook for 12–15 minutes, reducing the heat when the water begins to boil.

2 Mash the flesh and the skin of the aubergine with a fork. Reserve.

3 Heat the oil in a saucepan or wok and fry the cumin seeds until they change colour, then add the onion and fry it until softened.

4 Add the ginger-garlic paste and the chilli and fry for 1 minute. Then stir in the tomato purée and the spice powders and cook until well blended.

5 Season with salt and stir in the aubergine. Mix well and fold in the potatoes before serving sprinkled with the coriander leaves and a wedge of lemon, if desired.

slow cooked mushrooms
dum ki khumb

Lucknow in the state of Uttar Pradesh is well known for its unique cuisine known as 'Awadhi cooking' (page 21). Rich meat biryanis cooked in this style are very popular but there is also an amazing variety of vegetables such as baby corn, potatoes and yams that are cooked in 'dum'. You will need a saucepan with a tight fitting lid for this dish.

Serves: 4
Preparation time: 10 minutes
Cooking time: 30 minutes

1/2 teaspoon ginger-garlic paste (page 11)
1/4 teaspoon chilli powder
300g closed cap mushrooms, washed and drained
3 tablespoons ghee (you could use sunflower oil as a substitute)
1 large onion, sliced
1 teaspoon coriander powder
1 teaspoon fennel powder
3 tablespoons tomato purée
2 tablespoons ground almonds
Salt
100g natural yoghurt
3 tablespoons condensed milk

1 Mix the ginger-garlic paste, chilli powder and mushrooms and marinate them while you prepare the onion.

2 Heat half the ghee or oil in a heavy-bottomed pan and fry the onion until well browned. Whizz to a paste in a blender and reserve. In the same oil, fry the mushrooms for a few minutes, then drain and reserve.

3 Add the remaining ghee or oil to the pan and add the onion paste, spice powders and the tomato purée. Pour in a few tablespoons of water and blend everything together.

4 Stir in the almonds, salt, yoghurt and condensed milk. Place the mushrooms in this 'masala', stir and cover with a tight-fitting lid.

5 Leave the mushrooms to cook in the steam for about 8 minutes and serve immediately with a roti or rice.

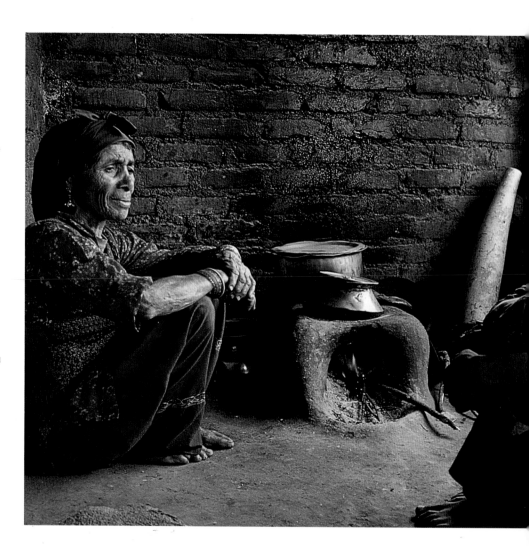

okra with tomatoes and green peppers
kadhai bhindi

Kadhai cooking (India's equivalent of a heavy wok) is a very popular north Indian style. Its close cousin is balti cooking, so popular in the UK. The recipe is cooked and served in the same pan, straight from the fire to the table, so to speak.

When buying okra, make sure that you choose bright green ones. The freshest okra will snap when bent. If they double over, they are too old! Also, when cooking okra, make sure not to add any water to the pan. This makes the okra slimy. To get rid of the natural slime, add something acidic such as lemon juice.

Serves: 4
Preparation time: 10 minutes
Cooking time: 25 minutes

3 tablespoons sunflower oil
1 medium onion, sliced
1 medium green pepper, seeds removed
  and sliced
300g okra, washed, well-dried, tops removed
  and cut in half lengthways
2 ripe tomatoes, chopped
1 teaspoon turmeric powder
1/2 teaspoon chilli powder
1/2 teaspoon garam masala powder
Salt
1 tablespoon lemon juice
Chopped coriander leaves to garnish

1 Heat the oil in a kadhai or heavy saucepan and fry the onion until soft.

2 Add the green pepper and continue to fry for a couple of minutes, then tip in the okra and stir well.

3 Add the tomatoes, spice powders, salt and lemon juice and mix well.

4 Allow to cook on low heat, stirring frequently to keep the mixture from sticking, until the okra is tender. It will change from being slimy to quite firm.

5 Serve hot, sprinkled with the chopped coriander leaves.

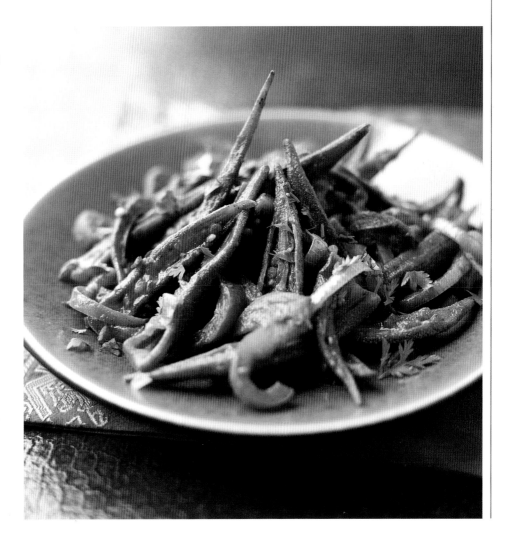

stuffed long chillies
bharwan mirch

There are many kinds of chillies and Kenya (or long) chillies were made for stuffing. These are thick, long and very bright green. They hold their shape well. Some can be very hot while others are quite mild. This dish is for those who like a bit of heat as it is quite a case of Russian Roulette here! For a milder version, try small green peppers instead.

Serves: 4
Preparation time: 10 minutes
Cooking time: 20 minutes

8 long Kenyan chillies
2 tablespoons sunflower oil
Large pinch of asafoetida
2 cloves garlic, minced
4 tablespoons chickpea flour
2 tablespoons cumin powder
2 tablespoons lemon juice
1/2 teaspoon turmeric powder
1/2 teaspoon chilli powder
Salt
1 teaspoon cumin seeds

1 Slit the chillies lengthways and carefully remove and discard all the seeds.

2 Heat 1 tablespoon of the oil in a pan and add the asafoetida and garlic, then add the chickpea flour, cumin powder, lemon juice, turmeric powder, chilli powder and salt, and add a little water to make a thick paste. Cook for a couple of minutes then smear this paste on the inside of each chilli.

3 Heat the remaining oil in a flat, non-stick saucepan until it is hot and add the cumin seeds. When they darken, arrange the chillies in the pan slit-side up.

4 Cover the pan, lower the heat and cook until the chillies are soft and slightly charred on the underside. Serve hot with rotis (page 32).

nine-jewelled curry
navratan korma

I have many good childhood memories associated with this dish. Growing up in Bombay, when going out to a restaurant was not such a commonplace thing as it is today, I would always order this dish. Its delightful combination of fruit and vegetables made all the more exciting with a few cherries and cream was for me a dish made in heaven!

Serves: 4
Preparation time: 15 minutes
Cooking time: 25 minutes

300g mixed vegetables (peas, carrots, beans and potatoes)
2 tablespoons sunflower oil
1 small onion, grated
1 tablespoon ginger-garlic paste (page 11)
3 tablespoons tomato purée
3 fresh green chillies, slit down the middle
1 teaspoon turmeric powder
1 teaspoon garam masala powder
Salt
2 tablespoons cashew nuts
2 tablespoons tinned pineapple chunks, chopped
100ml single cream
Few chopped glacé cherries to garnish
Coriander leaves to garnish
Grated cheddar cheese to garnish

1 Prepare the vegetables by peeling and dicing the carrots and potatoes and chopping the beans finely. Boil all four vegetables in water until just tender, drain and reserve.

2 Heat the oil in a saucepan and fry the onion for a minute or so. Keep stirring to prevent it from sticking and stir in the ginger-garlic paste.

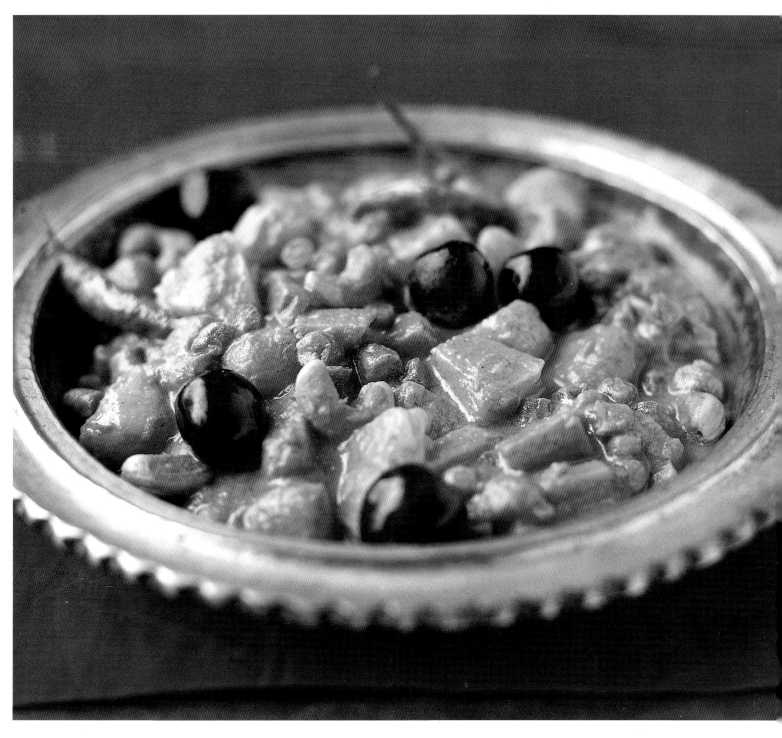

3 Add the tomato purée and chillies and cook until the oil separates, adding a couple of tablespoons of water to hasten the process.

4 Tip in the cooked vegetables, turmeric powder, garam masala and salt. Mix gently and cook for a couple of minutes before folding in the cashew nuts, pineapple and cream. Heat through without allowing to boil.

5 Serve hot, garnished with the cherries, coriander leaves and cheese.

everyday bread
roti/chapati

This is the most commonly made bread all over India. It is flaky and bland and makes a wonderful accompaniment to all the spice and herb flavours of the main dish. The art of making rotis is in getting the dough right and in the rolling out of perfectly round discs that are ready to roast. Many young girls in India, even as little as seven or eight, start out in the kitchen by helping their mothers to make rotis. My own daughter, who is seven, loves to make the balls of dough and has a great time rolling out what she calls 'maps'. We then eat up whole countries!

Serves: 4
Preparation time: 10 minutes
Cooking time: 20 minutes

450g wholewheat flour or atta
2 teaspoons sunflower oil
Warm water as needed
Ghee or sunflower oil for brushing, if desired

1 Combine the flour and oil in a mixing bowl. Using your fingers, mix into a pliable dough with warm water. Knead for 5 minutes (the more you knead the dough, the softer the rotis).

2 Divide the dough into portions the size of a lime. Coat lightly with flour, shape into a ball in your palm and flatten slightly.

3 Roll out into flat discs, 10cm in diameter, flouring the board as necessary.

4 Heat a griddle or shallow pan. Cook the discs on the griddle until the surface appears bubbly. Turn over and press the edges down with a clean cloth to cook evenly. As soon as brown spots appear the roti is done. Make sure that the roti is cooked evenly all over.

5 Remove and smear with ghee or oil, if using. Keep warm, enclosing in tinfoil.

6 Cook all the rotis in the same way. Serve warm or, if serving later on, reheat them for a minute or so in a microwave or re-roast them just enough to heat on a griddle.

garlic bread
lahsun parathas

A meal in a north Indian home will always have some form of fresh bread, and there is an enormous array of different breads including those that are stuffed, layered or flavoured. This bread is strongly flavoured and will go with a mild yoghurt curry such as Kashmiri-style Aubergines in Yoghurt (page 27). You could easily substitute the garlic with half a teaspoonful of cumin seeds for a milder bread.

Serves: 4
Preparation time: 15 minutes
Cooking time: 30 minutes

450g wholewheat flour
Water, as needed
2 tablespoons melted ghee or sunflower oil
1 teaspoon finely crushed garlic
1 teaspoon finely chopped coriander leaves
1/4 teaspoon turmeric powder
Salt

1 Mix all the ingredients, reserving a little flour for dusting and rolling the bread, and knead to form a soft dough.

2 Divide the dough into 8 equal-sized balls. Roll each ball into a flat disc about 8cm in diameter.

3 Smear each one with a little ghee or oil and roll into a hollow cylindrical shape, then flatten with your palm, dust with a little flour and roll out again to the same size.

4 Heat a griddle or frying pan and place one of the parathas on it. As soon as tiny bubbles appear on the surface, turn it over. Press down the edges with a clean cloth to ensure even cooking.

5 When the paratha is done, it should appear slightly puffed with brown patches. Remove it from the pan and keep warm in tinfoil. Cook the remaining parathas in the same way. Serve hot.

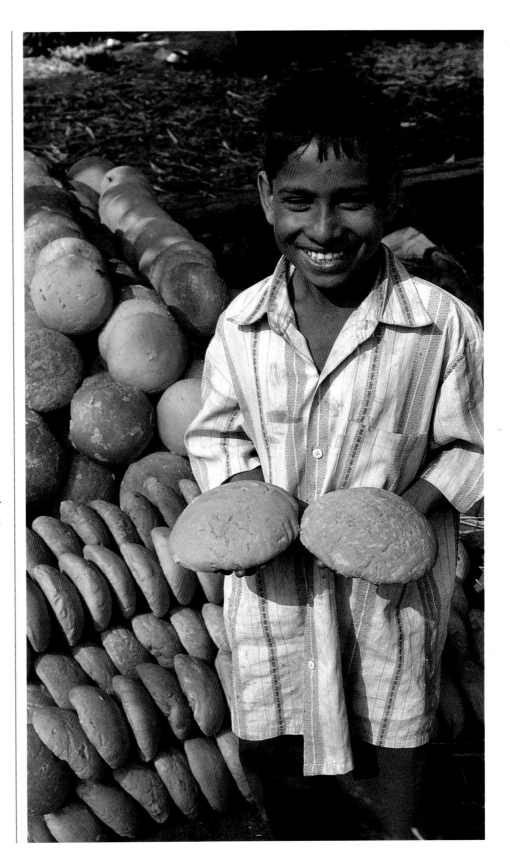

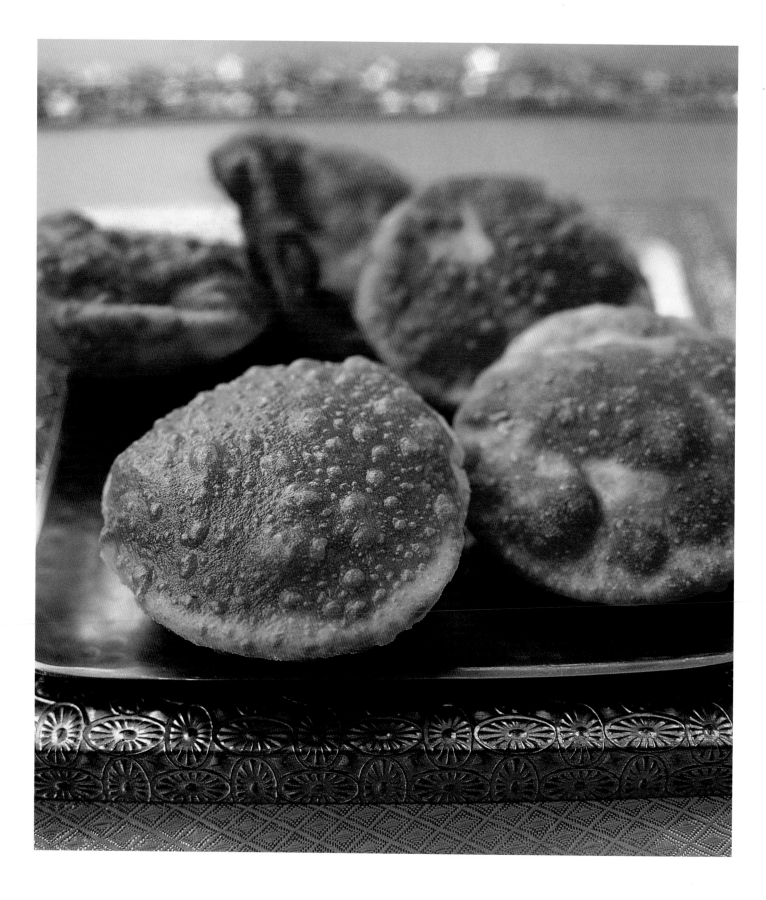

fluffy, soft bread
bhatura

Chole-bhatura is a classic Punjabi combination of chickpeas served with fluffy, fried bread. It is as natural to eat this in a gourmet restaurant as it is to eat it at a roadside stall in any city of India. This combination is served as a complete meal accompanied only by an onion salad and a wedge of lemon.

Serves: 4
Preparation time: 15 minutes
Cooking time: 30 minutes

450g refined white flour
150g natural yoghurt
1/2 teaspoon baking powder
Sunflower oil for deep-frying

1 Reserve a little flour for dusting, and combine the rest with the yoghurt and baking powder and knead together with enough warm water to form a soft dough. Cover with a damp cloth and set aside for 30 minutes.

2 Divide the dough into small balls the size of a lime. Dust a rolling space with flour and roll out each bhatura into a disc 8cm in diameter.

3 Heat enough sunflower oil in a kadhai or deep frying pan. When it is smoking hot, reduce the heat and fry the bhaturas, one at a time, on both sides, until fluffy. Serve hot with Chole (page 43).

potato-stuffed bread
aloo paratha

Breads made with a variety of stuffings are Punjabi specialities. Stuffings can be sweet or savoury but spiced potatoes, cauliflower, turnips and mooli are firm favourites. In many parts of the Punjab, this dish is eaten at any meal in the day. It goes well with a bowl of natural yoghurt and some hot mango pickle.

Serves: 4
Preparation time: 20 minutes
Cooking time: 45 minutes

For the stuffing:
2 medium baking potatoes, peeled and cubed
1 tablespoon sunflower oil
1/2 teaspoon cumin seeds
2 fresh green chillies, finely chopped
1/2 teaspoon turmeric powder
Salt
2 tablespoons finely chopped coriander leaves

For the bread:
450g wholewheat flour
6 tablespoons sunflower oil
Salt
Water, as needed

1 To make the stuffing, boil the potatoes in a large pan of salted water until tender, drain them, then mash and set aside.

2 Heat the sunflower oil and fry the cumin seeds until dark. Add the chillies, turmeric powder and salt to taste.

3 Mix in the mashed potato and coriander leaves. Reserve.

4 To make the bread, combine the flour (reserving some for rolling), 2 tablespoons of the oil, salt and water. Knead the dough until smooth and firm.

5 Divide the dough into 16 equal-sized balls. Roll each one out, dusting with a little flour if sticky, into a flat round about 8cm in diameter.

6 Smear a layer of the potato mixture over one disc then place another rolled out disc of dough over this. Seal the edges to make a potato parcel. Make the other seven parathas.

7 Heat a frying pan and dot with oil. Cook the paratha until tiny, dark spots appear on the underside. Turn over and cook the other side. Keep warm in tinfoil while you cook the rest of the parathas similarly.

fragrant rice with red kidney beans
rajma pulao

Red kidney beans grow plentifully in north India. The area around the Vaishno Devi temple in Kashmir is famous for its rajma or red kidney bean curry and weary travellers who walk long distances to seek the blessings of the Goddess are offered this wholesome meal at every eatery. A combination of rice and beans, it goes well with Navratan Korma (pages 30–31).

Serves: 4
Preparation time: 10 minutes
Cooking time: 30 minutes

3 tablespoons sunflower oil
4 green cardamom pods
6 cloves
8 black peppercorns
2 bay leaves
300g basmati rice, washed and drained
Salt
3 tablespoons tinned red kidney beans, drained
1 large onion, finely sliced

1 Heat 2 tablespoons of the oil in a heavy-bottomed pan and fry the whole spices and the bay leaves for a couple of minutes until you get a wonderful aroma. Add the rice and fry for 2–3 minutes until shiny, stirring all the time to prevent burning.

2 Pour in 600ml of hot water and season lightly with salt. Bring to the boil, reduce the heat, stir the rice once and cover. Simmer for 10 minutes, remove from the heat and leave the pan covered for a further 5 minutes for the rice to finish cooking in the steam.

3 Uncover the pan and gently mix in the red kidney beans.

4 Heat the remaining oil in another pan and fry the onion until golden brown in colour. Drain and toss over the pulao. Serve hot.

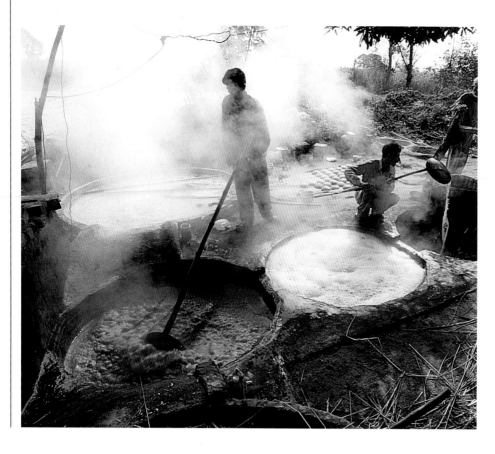

cumin-flavoured rice
jeera pulao

Red kidney beans grow plentifully in north India. The area around the Vaishno Devi temple in Kashmir is famous for its rajma or red kidney bean curry and weary travellers who walk long distances to seek the blessings of the Goddess are offered this wholesome meal at every eatery. This combination of rice and beans goes well with Navratan Korma (pages 30–31).

Serves: 4
Preparation time: 10 minutes
Cooking time: 20 minutes

3 tablespoons sunflower oil
4 green cardamom pods
6 cloves
8 black peppercorns
2 bay leaves
300g basmati rice, washed and drained
Salt
3 tablespoons tinned red kidney beans, drained
1 large onion, finely sliced

1 Heat 2 tablespoons of the oil in a heavy-bottomed pan and fry the whole spices and the bay leaves for a couple of minutes until you get a wonderful aroma. Add the rice and fry for 2–3 minutes until shiny, stirring all the time to prevent burning.

2 Pour in 600ml of hot water and season lightly with salt. Bring to the boil, reduce the heat, stir the rice once and cover. Simmer for 10 minutes, remove from the heat and leave the pan covered for a further 5 minutes for the rice to finish cooking in the steam.

tomato-flavoured rice
tamater pulao

I love to serve this rice at parties because it is so vibrant and delicious! The orange colour complements most dishes and the tang of the tomatoes seems to add to the curry with which it is served. I always blanch the tomatoes because I don't like the skin interfering with the texture. To do this, simply nick the skins of the tomatoes with a sharp knife and immerse them for 1 minute or so in boiling water; the skins will slip off easily.

Serves: 4
Preparation time: 10 minutes
Cooking time: 25 minutes

2 tablespoons sunflower oil
1 teaspoon cumin seeds
10 black peppercorns
300g basmati rice, washed and drained
2 ripe tomatoes, peeled and chopped
2 tablespoons tomato purée
Salt
Fresh coriander sprigs

1 Heat the oil in a heavy pan. Add the cumin seeds and peppercorns. Then add the rice and stir-fry until the rice grains turn shiny, for about 2–3 minutes.

2 Stir in the tomatoes, tomato purée and salt. Mix well and pour in 600ml of hot water. Bring to the boil.

3 Give it a good stir, reduce the heat and cover. Cook for 10 minutes until the rice is fluffy and dry. Turn off the heat and keep the pan covered for a further 5 minutes.

4 Open the pan and run a fork through the rice to loosen it. Serve hot, decorated with the coriander.

rice cooked with garden vegetables, spices and nuts
vegetable dum biryani

The word biryani is derived from the Farsi word 'birian', which means fried before cooking. It is thought to have originated in Persia and could have come into north India via Afghanistan. As the Mughals spread their empire, the biryani travelled to various parts of the country so that today, a south Indian version also exists. A good biryani must have an amazing aroma, should not be too spicy and, above all, the grains of rice must be loose and chewy. It is traditionally made in an earthenware pot and slow cooked to seal in the flavours. Make this as a special treat when you can spend a whole morning in the kitchen. Well worth it!

Serves: 4
Preparation time: 15 minutes
Cooking time: 1¹/₂ hours

Bouquet garni of 10 green cardamoms, 5 black cardamoms, 12 black peppercorns, small stick of cinnamon, 10 cloves, few shavings of nutmeg, 1 teaspoon fennel seeds, 3 bay leaves
4 tablespoons milk
Large pinch of saffron
4 tablespoons rose water
3 tablespoons ghee
3 medium onions, sliced
1 tablespoon ginger-garlic paste (page 11)
2 tablespoons tomato purée
¹/₂ teaspoon turmeric powder
¹/₂ teaspoon garam masala powder
Salt
300g mixed vegetables (carrots, peas, potatoes), peeled, diced and boiled
300g basmati rice
Handful of mint leaves, chopped
Handful of coriander leaves, chopped
3 tablespoons flaked almonds

1 Preheat the oven to 220°C/Gas 6.

2 Put the spices (except 5 of the green cardamoms) for the bouquet garni into a pan with 600ml of hot water and bring to the boil. Turn off the heat, cover the pan and allow to infuse into a savoury aromatic liquid.

3 Crush the reserved green cardamoms finely in a mortar and mix with the milk, saffron and rose water. Set aside. This is the sweet aromatic liquid.

4 Heat 1 tablespoon of the ghee in a pan and fry the onions until brown. Remove half of them and reserve for the garnish. Add the ginger-garlic paste to the remaining onions and stir for a couple of minutes. Whizz the mixture in a blender until smooth.

5 Heat another tablespoon of the ghee in a heavy-bottomed pan and fry the onion mixture over high heat. Add the tomato purée and spice powders. Season with salt.

6 Drain the vegetables and add to the pan. Mix well and simmer for a few minutes until the ghee begins to separate. Remove from the heat and reserve.

7 Heat the remaining 1 tablespoon of ghee in a separate pan and fry the rice over high heat. (Don't wash the rice beforehand.) In a few minutes, when it is shiny, strain half the savoury liquid into the pan. Bring to the boil, reduce the heat, cover and cook for about 6 minutes until the liquid has evaporated.

8 It's time to assemble the dish. The bottom and top layers are always rice. Put a layer of rice at the bottom of an ovenproof dish. Sprinkle over some of the remaining savoury liquid and some of the sweet liquid. Top with a layer of the vegetable curry. Sprinkle over some of the fried onions, mint leaves and coriander leaves. Repeat with another layer of rice. Dot the almonds on top. Keep going until everything is used up and the top layer is rice. Seal the dish with tinfoil.

9 Cook the biryani for 40 minutes in the oven, reducing the heat to 190°C/Gas 5 after 20 minutes. Open the dish just before serving to release a burst of fragrance!

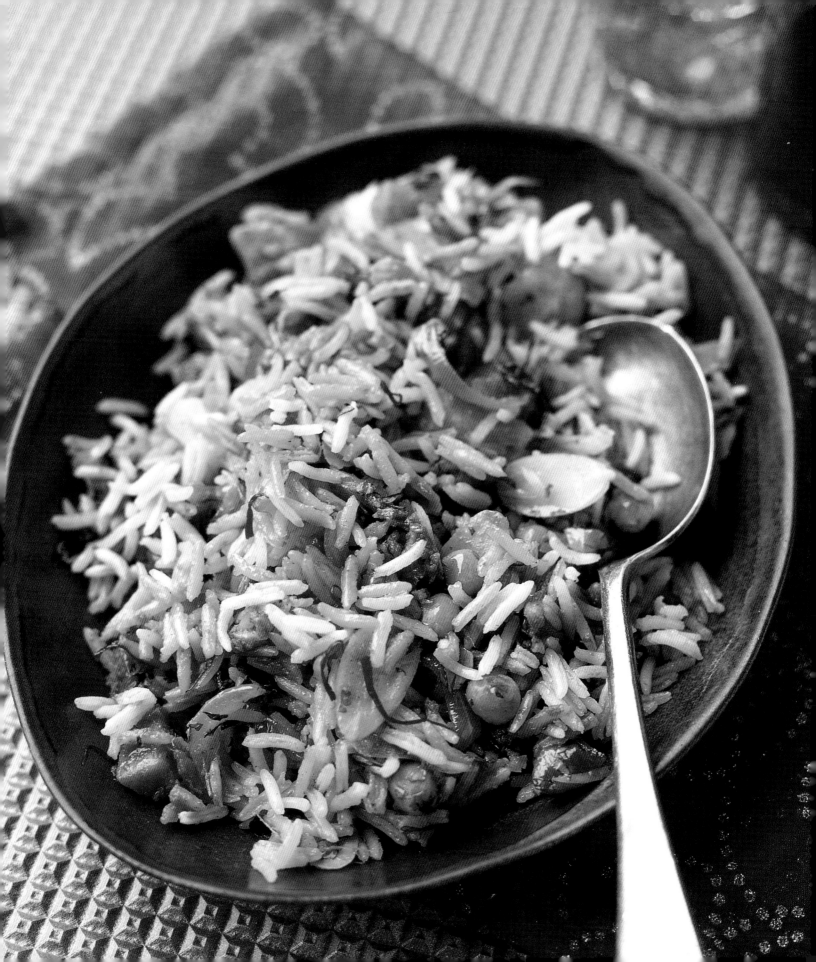

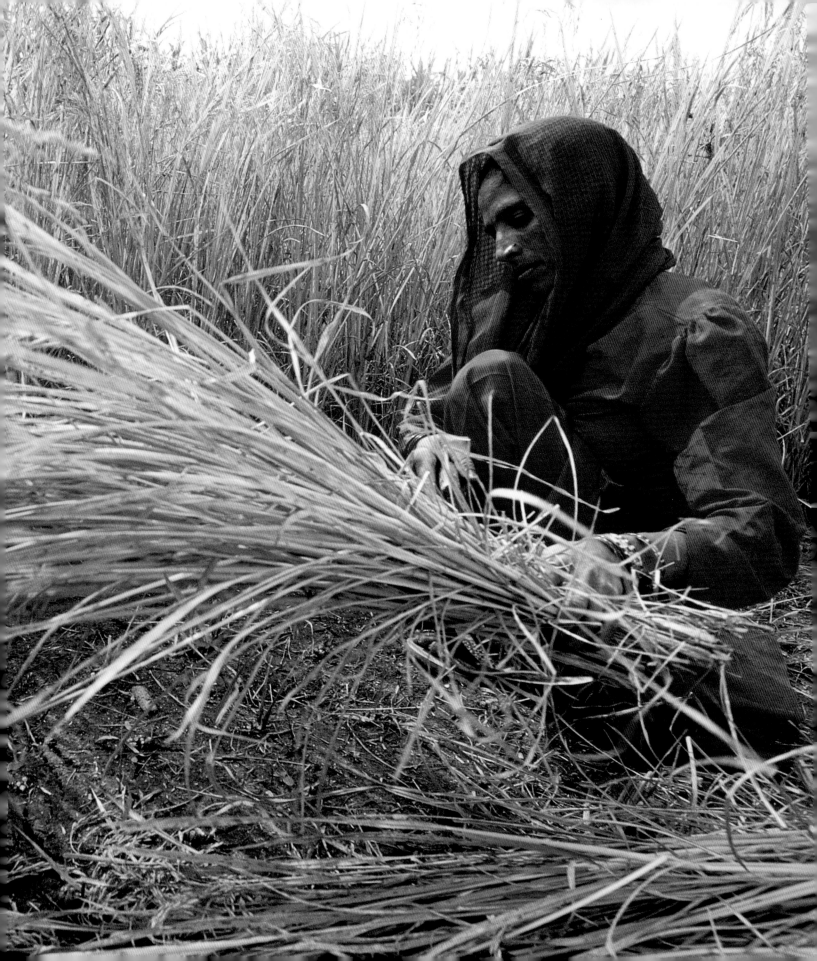

yellow lentils with onion and garlic
tarka dal

This is a very popular dish in north Indian restaurants around the world. The smooth creaminess goes well with rice or rotis, and the flavours of the spices seem to give an extra kick. I make my garam masala just before adding it to the dal as the flavour is strongest when fresh (page 58). Any leftovers can be mixed into wholewheat flour to make some dal roti, a bread that is as tasty as it is nutritious and comforting.

Serves: 4
Preparation time: 15 minutes
Cooking time: 15 minutes

300g yellow lentils (dal)
2 tablespoons sunflower oil
1 teaspoon cumin seeds
1 large onion, sliced
1 tablespoon tomato purée
1 teaspoon ginger-garlic paste (page 11)
2 fresh green chillies, slit
1 teaspoon turmeric powder
Salt
Handful of coriander leaves, chopped
1 teaspoon garam masala powder

1 Pour boiling water over the lentils in a heavy-bottomed pan and set to cook on a medium heat for 30 minutes.

2 Heat the oil in a pan and add the cumin seeds. As they begin to crackle, add the onion and stir until golden and slightly crisp. Remove half the onion with a slotted spoon and drain on absorbent paper.

3 Add the tomato purée, ginger-garlic paste, chillies and salt to the pan and cook until all are well blended.

4 Carefully pour over the cooked lentils and adjust the seasoning. Mix well. Serve hot with the reserved fried onions piled on top and a sprinkling of coriander and garam masala.

black lentils cooked in butter and cream
dal bukhara

This dal is the defining lentil dish of the north, also called 'kali dal'. These are made creamy and delicious with the addition of cream and butter (use sunflower oil for a lighter version), but the dal then becomes quite heavy to digest so it is well spiced. In India, it is cooked overnight on low heat as the lentils get silkier. Serve with plain boiled rice and a fresh green salad.

Serves: 4
Preparation time: 15 minutes + overnight soaking
Cooking time: 1¼ hours

3 tablespoons ghee, butter or sunflower oil
1 large onion, finely chopped
1 tablespoon ginger-garlic paste (page 11)
Large pinch of asafoetida
1 teaspoon turmeric powder
1 teaspoon chilli powder
1 teaspoon garam masala powder
2 large tomatoes, chopped
150g black lentils, soaked overnight
Salt
4 tablespoons double cream
2 tablespoons chopped coriander leaves

1 Heat the butter or oil in a large, heavy-bottomed saucepan and fry the onion until it turns golden. Add ginger-garlic paste and asafoetida. Stir in the spice powders and tomatoes and cook for a few minutes to blend.

2 Drain the lentils and add them to the pan with some salt. Pour in 300ml of hot water and bring to the boil. Reduce the heat and simmer for 1 hour until the lentils are cooked. Take off the heat, stir in the cream and serve, garnished with the coriander leaves.

stir-fried black eyed beans
bhuna lobhia

Black eyed beans are beautifully silky and work very well with tomatoes and onions. They are rich in soluble fibre, which helps to eliminate cholesterol from the body. Most dried beans need overnight soaking but, if you are using cooked beans from a tin, make sure you rinse them well to get rid of the salted water in which they are preserved.

Serves: 4
Preparation time: 15 minutes + overnight soaking
Cooking time: 15 minutes

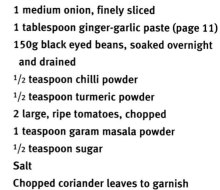

2 tablespoons sunflower oil
1 teaspoon cumin seeds
Large pinch of asafoetida
1 medium onion, finely sliced
1 tablespoon ginger-garlic paste (page 11)
150g black eyed beans, soaked overnight and drained
$^1/_2$ teaspoon chilli powder
$^1/_2$ teaspoon turmeric powder
2 large, ripe tomatoes, chopped
1 teaspoon garam masala powder
$^1/_2$ teaspoon sugar
Salt
Chopped coriander leaves to garnish

1 Heat the oil in a heavy-bottomed saucepan or kadhai. Add the cumin seeds, fry until dark and then add the asafoetida and the onion and stir-fry until golden. Stir in the ginger-garlic paste and mix well.

2 Tip in the beans, sprinkle in the chilli powder and turmeric and fry for 1 minute, before adding the tomatoes, garam masala, sugar and salt. Mix, add a little water, cover and bring to the boil. Reduce the heat and simmer until done. The beans should retain their shape. Mash a few to add thickness to the sauce.

3 Serve hot, garnished with the coriander.

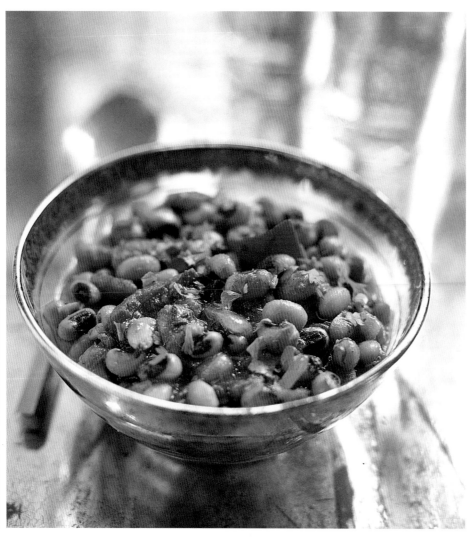

spiced chickpeas
chole

When I was a child, a dish of chole on the table meant that my mum had soaked the peas overnight and then boiled them for a long time to get them to the right texture. Happily today tinned chickpeas are available everywhere making this dish a song. Chole is a classic dish combined with Bhatura (page 35). The pomegranate seeds add a slight tang to the dish. If you can not find them or the mango powder, substitute with 3 tablespoons of lemon juice.

Serves: 4
Preparation time: 15 minutes
Cooking time: 35 minutes

1^1/$_2$ **tablespoon dried pomegranate seeds (anardana), crushed**
1 teaspoon cumin seeds
2 tablespoons ghee or sunflower oil
2 x 400g tins chickpeas, drained
1 teaspoon mango powder (amchoor)
^{1}/$_2$ teaspoon red chilli powder
Salt
2 large onions, chopped
2 fresh green chillies, sliced
3cm piece of ginger, cut in julliennes
2 large tomatoes, chopped
Chopped coriander leaves to garnish

1 Heat a small frying pan and dry-roast the pomegranate and cumin seeds on high heat until the seeds turn dark. Grind to a powder in a mortar and reserve.

2 Heat the ghee or oil in a heavy-bottomed pan. Add the chickpeas and the reserved spice powder. Mix well. Add the mango powder, chilli powder and salt.

3 Add the chopped onions, green chillies and about 150ml of hot water. Bring to the boil, reduce the heat and cook on low heat until the chickpeas are nearly dry.

4 Garnish with the ginger, chopped tomatoes and coriander leaves. Serve hot.

sour lentils flavoured with garlic
khatti dal

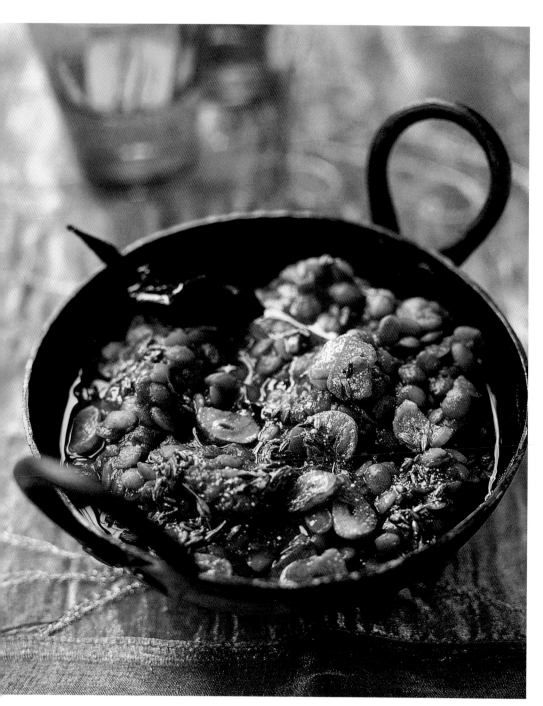

Recipes for sour lentils can be found in every region of India. This recipe is from Lucknow in Uttar Pradesh known for the Awadhi style of cooking. Traditionally, in the days of the nawabs, this was done by highly skilled chefs called 'rakabdars' who would only cook for a few people at a time. This was because presentation was as important as taste. Even today, the 'rakabdars' that remain are considered artists rather than chefs and are very highly respected for their skill.

Serves: 4
Preparation time: 10 minutes
Cooking time: 45 minutes

300g yellow split lentils (toor dal), washed and drained
1/2 teaspoon turmeric powder
1 tablespoon tamarind concentrate
Salt
2 tablespoons ghee or sunflower oil
1 teaspoon cumin seeds
Large pinch of asafoetida
3 dried red chillies, broken in half
3 cloves garlic, chopped
Chopped coriander to garnish

1 Put the lentils and turmeric along with 600ml of hot water in a saucepan and bring to the boil. Reduce the heat and simmer, partially covered, for about 30 minutes until the lentils are soft. If they dry out during the cooking, add a little more water until you get a mushy consistency.

2 Add the tamarind and salt and cook for a couple of minutes. Take off the heat and reserve.

3 Heat the ghee or oil in a small saucepan and add the cumin seeds and asafoetida. When the cumin turns dark, add the red chillies and garlic. Fry on low heat until the garlic is golden brown. Garlic burns easily so quickly pour this mixture over the dal.

4 Serve hot, garnished with the coriander.

soya nuggets in tomato sauce
soya ki subzi

Soya beans grow widely in India and, for a large part of the vegetarian population, provide the protein content in a meal along with the staple dal. Soy protein is available as dried chunks or nuggets which soften on cooking. Their consistency is a bit like that of meat but the taste is blander. This curry goes well with a roti and salad.

Serves: 4
Preparation time: 10 minutes
Cooking time: 30 minutes

300g soya nuggets or chunks
3 tablespoons sunflower oil
2 medium onions, chopped
1 tablespoon ginger-garlic paste (page 11)
2 ripe tomatoes
1 teaspoon cumin seeds
1/2 teaspoon turmeric powder
1/2 teaspoon chilli powder
1/2 teaspoon garam masala powder
Salt
Chopped coriander leaves to garnish

1 Soak the soya nuggets in plenty of water and carry on with the next steps.

2 Heat 2 tablespoons of the sunflower oil in a heavy-bottomed saucepan and fry the onions until soft. Add the ginger-garlic paste and tomatoes and cook till well blended. Take off the heat and whizz in a blender until very smooth.

3 Heat the remaining oil in another saucepan and fry the cumin seeds until they darken. Add the onion and tomato mixture and fry for a couple of minutes.

4 Tip in the spice powders and salt. Squeeze the soya nuggets firmly to remove excess water and add them to the pan. Stir in about 100ml of water. Bring to the boil, reduce the heat and simmer for about 5 minutes to allow the soya to soak up the spices. This dish should be semi-dry and served hot, sprinkled with the coriander.

indian cottage cheese with peas
muttar paneer

In Delhi, no feast is complete without the inclusion of a dish made with paneer. Milk is available in plenty in the north, unlike in some of the drier regions of India, and most households will make this rather bland but wonderfully soft cheese at home. It is often combined with vegetables such as green peppers and mushrooms. The fenugreek in this recipe is available in Indian shops as dried leaves with a wonderful fragrance. If you can't find it, substitute with the same quantity of ginger-garlic paste.

Serves: 4
Preparation time: 5 minutes
Cooking time: 20 minutes

3 tablespoons sunflower oil
1 teaspoon cumin seeds
$1/2$ teaspoon dried fenugreek leaves
1 large fresh green chilli, slit
250g green garden peas
$1/2$ teaspoon turmeric powder
1 teaspoon coriander powder
Salt
Pinch of sugar
100g paneer
Handful of coriander leaves, chopped
Lemon juice

1 Heat the oil and fry the cumin seeds until they darken slightly. Crumble in the fenugreek leaves and stir well.

2 Add the chilli and the peas, together with the spice powders, salt and sugar. Pour in about 100ml of water and cook until the peas are just tender, for about 10 minutes. Add more water if necessary.

3 Fold in the paneer and simmer for a couple of minutes. Serve, hot and sprinkle with the coriander and lemon juice.

indian cottage cheese with green peppers, onions and tomatoes
paneer jalfrezi

Jalfrezi is a dish cooked with peppers and onions and has become one of the most popular Indian recipes in the world. I love the combination of crunchy onions and peppers, creamy paneer and mushy tomatoes that come together with the spices. Serve this with a hot roti and nothing else.

Serves: 4
Preparation time: 15 minutes
Cooking time: 25 minutes

2 tablespoons sunflower oil
1 teaspoon cumin seeds
1 large onion, finely sliced
1 tablespoon ginger-garlic paste (page 11)
$1/2$ teaspoon turmeric powder
$1/2$ teaspoon chilli powder
$1/2$ teaspoon coriander powder
Salt
150g green peppers, sliced
2 ripe tomatoes, sliced
150g paneer, cubed
Chopped coriander leaves to garnish

1 Heat the oil in a heavy-bottomed saucepan and fry the cumin seeds for 1 minute. Add the onion and fry until soft. Add the ginger-garlic paste and fry for a few seconds until well blended.

2 Sprinkle in the spice powders and cook on low heat until the oil begins to separate, in about 3 minutes. Stir frequently to prevent scorching.

3 Add the peppers, stir and simmer gently until they are nearly done but still hold their shape, for about 8 minutes.

4 Add the tomatoes and paneer and cook for a couple of minutes until soft but not mushy; the tomatoes will begin to soften at once because of the salt that has already been added.

5 Take off the heat and serve hot, garnished with the coriander leaves.

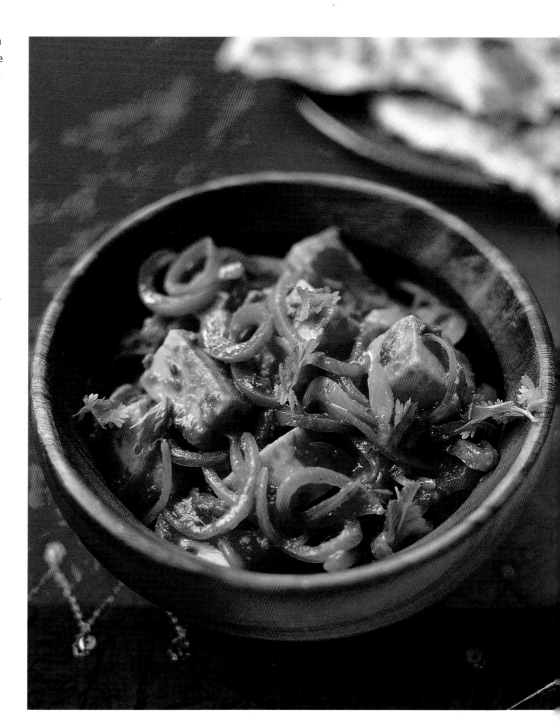

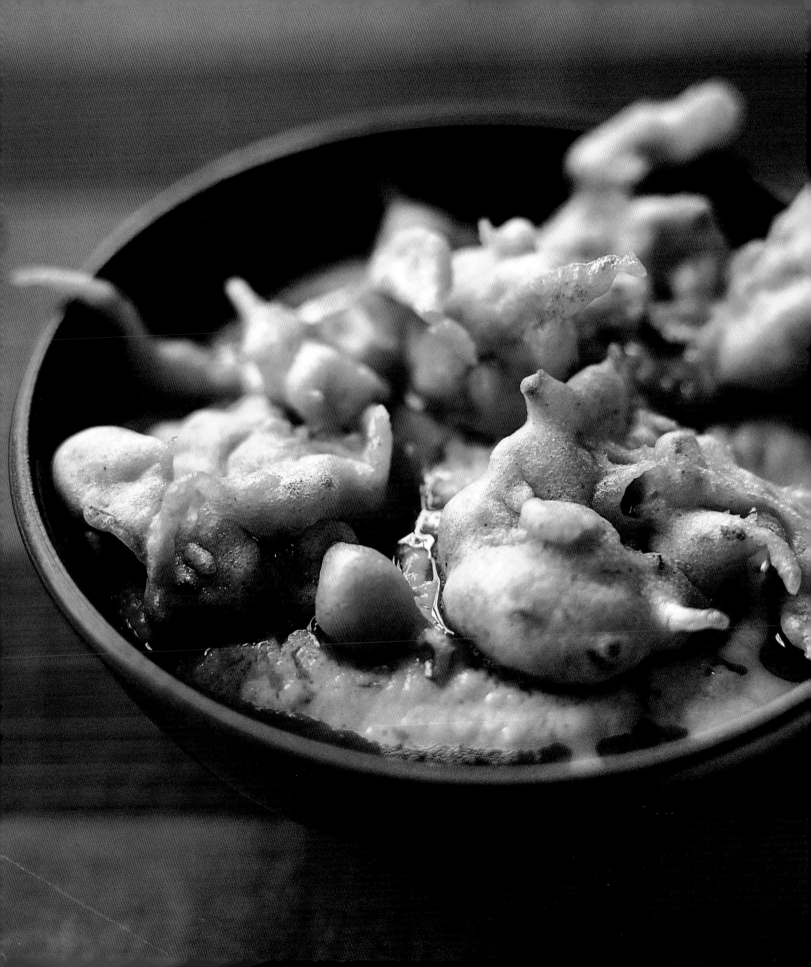

yoghurt curry with fried dumplings
pakodewali kadhi

This is one of the most famous curries from the state of Uttar Pradesh. It is served with rice and hot mango pickle. The pakoras or dumplings that go into the curry can be flavoured with a variety of vegetables such as cooked spinach, grated carrots, fenugreek leaves or florettes of cauliflower.

Serves: 4
Preparation time: 10 minutes
Cooking time: 30 minutes

300g natural yoghurt
150g gram flour (besan)
1 fresh green chilli, finely chopped
$1/2$ teaspoon turmeric powder
2 teaspoons sugar
Salt
2 tablespoons sunflower oil
1 teaspoon cumin seeds
10 black peppercorns
6 cloves
2 tablespoons ghee (optional)
$1/2$ teaspoon chilli powder

For the dumplings:
150g gram flour (besan)
1 medium onion, finely chopped
Pinch of cumin seeds
Sunflower oil for deep-frying

1 Whisk the yoghurt with the gram flour, green chilli, turmeric, sugar, salt and 300ml of cold water.

2 Heat the oil in a heavy pan and add the cumin seeds, peppercorns and cloves.

3 Give the yoghurt mixture a good blend, ensuring that there are no lumps left, and pour into the pan. Bring to the boil. Reduce the heat and cook, stirring frequently, until the consistency resembles that of a thick gravy and the raw flour aroma has gone. Take off the heat.

4 For the dumplings, make a thick batter with the gram flour, onion, cumin seeds and add water as necessary.

5 Heat the oil in a heavy pan. When it starts smoking, lower the heat and drop in 2–3 separate teaspoonfuls of batter at a time. Fry until golden, drain and dip into a bowl of water to soften a bit. Remove immediately, squeeze out the water and add to the yoghurt curry. Make all the dumplings in this manner.

6 Heat the ghee (if using) in a small pan (you could use the hot sunflower oil instead) and add the chilli powder. Pour this mixture over the curry at once and serve without stirring.

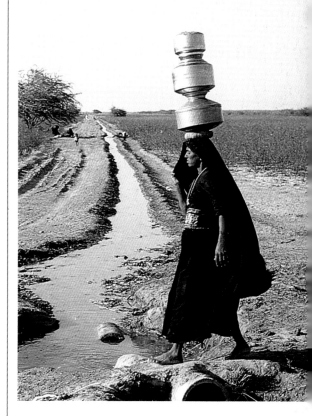

spicy paneer fritters
paneer pakoras

Pakoras, popular snacks or accompaniments not just in India but all over the world, are made with vegetables such as cauliflower, potatoes and aubergine, held together with spiced gram flour. One most relaxing memory is of eating hot pakoras during the Bombay monsoons, a time when it rains in sheets and going out is impossible.

Serves: 4
Preparation time: 15 minutes
Cooking time: 30 minutes

For the batter:
150g gram flour
1 teaspoon chilli powder
1 teaspoon ginger-garlic paste (page 11)
1/2 teaspoon cumin seeds
Handful of coriander leaves, finely chopped
Large pinch of bicarbonate of soda
Salt

Sunflower oil for deep-frying
300g paneer, cut into strips

1 Make a thick mixture of all the batter ingredients with water as needed. Heat the oil in a deep kadhai or frying pan until it smokes.

2 Dip each strip of paneer into the batter and gently add to the hot oil. Reduce the heat to allow the pakora to cook through. Fry until golden, then drain on absorbent paper. Fry 2–3 pakoras at a time, regulating the heat to ensure even cooking.

3 Serve hot with tomato ketchup and a tablespoon of bottled mint sauce stirred into about 5 tablespoons of natural yoghurt.

tiny gram flour balls in yoghurt
boondi raita

This is probably the most popular raita made in north Indian homes. Although ready-made boondi or flour balls are available in many places, it is easy to make your own. The procedure is a little messy but great fun and the kids can have a go if they are supervised by an adult. The semolina helps to make them crunchier. The boondis can be stored in an airtight container for a couple of months. They can also be sprinkled over rice or vegetable stir-fries to add crunch.

Serves: 4
Preparation time: 15 minutes
Cooking time: 25 minutes

For the boondi:
150g gram flour (besan)
1 tablespoon semolina
1/2 teaspoon salt

Sunflower oil for deep-frying
150g natural yoghurt
Salt
Pinch of sugar
1/2 teaspoon cumin seeds

1 To make the boondi, combine the flour, semolina, salt and 100ml of cold water in a mixing bowl. Whisk together to remove any lumps.

2 Heat the oil in a kadhai or deep frying pan.

3 When it comes to smoking point, reduce the heat. Hold a perforated spoon (one with large enough holes) about 10cm above the pan and pour some batter onto it. It should drip in droplets into the oil.

4 The drops of batter float up to the surface of the oil quite quickly. Fry for 1 minute or so, drain and remove with a slotted spoon on to absorbent paper. Fry the rest of the batter similarly.

5 Make the raita by combining the yoghurt, salt and sugar in a serving bowl. Reserve.

6 Heat a small saucepan and dry-roast the cumin seeds until they turn dark. Then crush them to a fine powder in a mortar. Stir into the yoghurt.

7 Just before serving, stir in some of the boondis to make a semi-liquid raita. The next time you make this dish, it will be a lot easier if you have some boondis left over!

onion and mint raita
dahi kuchumber

sweet star fruit preserve
karambal ka murabba

A raita is usually a yoghurt-based salad and is almost always served with a north Indian meal. The name of this dish literally means yoghurt salad. Mughlai food, with its rich sauces and creamy curries, is served with this fresh onion raita. I use Greek yoghurt for a fuller flavour but do use low-fat natural yoghurt if you prefer.

Serves: 4
Preparation time: 15 minutes
Cooking time: nil

150g natural Greek yoghurt
Salt
1 fresh green chilli, very finely chopped
1 medium onion, finely chopped
Handful of mint leaves, washed and
  finely chopped

1 Beat the yoghurt with the salt for 1 minute. Add the rest of the ingredients and serve.

2 If preparing in advance, add the salt at the last minute.

Preserve- and pickle-making are traditional skills passed down from mother to daughter. I remember my grandmother making a variety of mango preserves every summer – hot, sweet and salty. I especially loved her raw mangoes in brine which would keep for a whole year. This star fruit preserve can be stored for about a month in the fridge.

Serves: 4
Preparation time: 5 minutes
Cooking time: 30 minutes

2 large juicy star fruits (carambola), sliced
100g sugar
Juice of 1 lemon
Pinch of saffron strands

1 Put the star fruit with half the sugar in a heavy-bottomed pan. Pour in 150ml of water and bring to the boil. Reduce the heat and simmer for 5 minutes until the fruit is tender but holds its shape. Strain the fruit out of the syrup and reserve.

2 Add the remaining sugar to the cooking liquor in the pan and cook until it becomes a syrup of single thread consistency. Test this by putting a drop of syrup on a plate and dabbing it with your finger – it should feel sticky and thick.

3 Add the lemon juice, saffron and cooked fruit to the syrup and simmer for 1 minute. Remove from the heat, cool completely and store in a clean, airtight glass jar in the fridge.

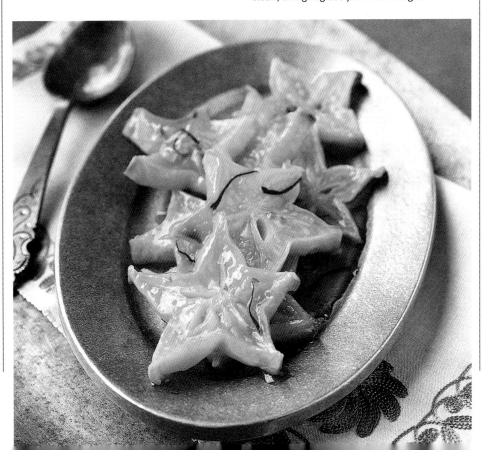

sweet potato kebabs
shakarkand ke kebab

I remember as a teenager in Bombay going to a friend's farm for a sleepover and having the most delicious farm meal. Her dad cooked us some meat on a barbeque and then he had a hole dug in the ground, put the live coals from the barbeque into it and placed some sweet potatoes and onions in their skin on top. He covered this with some stones and in a while we had charred vegetables that we peeled and ate with the meat. Fabulous and fun! Commercially bought paneer has been pressed to make it hard and therefore easy to grate.

Serves: 4
Preparation time: 15 minutes
Cooking time: 40 minutes

4 tablespoons cashew nuts
100g gram flour
300g sweet potatoes, boiled, peeled
 and grated
100g paneer, grated
1 tablespoon peeled and grated fresh ginger
Small handful of mint leaves, chopped
Few shavings of nutmeg
Salt and pepper
Lemon juice to drizzle on top

Wooden skewers

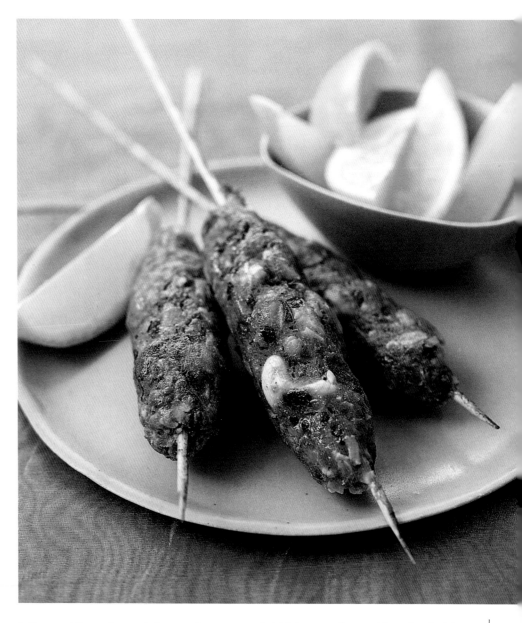

1 Dry-roast the cashew nuts in a small pan. When they turn golden, remove and reserve. In the same pan, dry-roast the gram flour. Keep stirring to prevent it from sticking. When the raw aroma has transformed into a cooked aroma, in about 6–7 minutes, remove and reserve.

2 Preheat the oven to 220°C/Gas 6. Combine the sweet potatoes, paneer, ginger, mint leaves, nutmeg, cashew nuts and the seasoning.

3 Add the gram flour and knead well with your fingers until a dough is formed.

4 Divide the dough into 8 portions and shape around wooden skewers.

5 Reduce the oven temperature to 180°C/ Gas 4. Place the skewers on a lined baking tray and bake for 20 minutes until golden. Serve hot, drizzled with the lemon juice.

potatoes and green pea samosas
mutter ke samose

Samosas are very popular all over the world and can be served as a snack, a main meal or a picnic treat. In India, they are served with tomato ketchup, sweet and sour tamarind chutney or a spicy mint relish. The potatoes in this recipe need to be cut up finely, almost the size of a fingernail. They should retain their shape but melt in the mouth. Although they are traditionally deep-fried, I bake my samosas as a healthier option.

Serves: 4 (makes 12 samosas)
Preparation time: 15 minutes
Cooking time: 1 hour

2 tablespoons sunflower oil
1/2 teaspoon cumin seeds
1/2 teaspoon turmeric powder
1/4 teaspoon chilli powder
1 teaspoon coriander powder
300g potatoes, peeled, cut into small cubes, boiled and drained
150g frozen green peas, cooked and drained
Salt
500g frozen ready-to-use filo pastry

1 Heat the oil in a heavy saucepan and fry the cumin seeds until they turn dark, for a few seconds. Reduce the heat.

2 Add the spice powders and stir in the potatoes at once as the spice powders will scorch easily. Add the peas and salt and cook until well blended, for a couple of minutes.

3 Line a baking tray with tinfoil and preheat the oven to 220°C/Gas 6.

4 Lay a sheet of pastry on a flat surface. Fill with a bit of the potatos and peas mixture. Fold the pastry to make a triangle and continue similarly for the rest of the filling. (Folding technique: lift the top left corner and fold over the filling to be in line with the bottom edge, making a triangle shape. Now lift the right bottom corner over to the top and then the top left down again. Carry on until you have a triangular parcel.)

5 Bake in the oven for 25–30 minutes, turning over once to cook both sides. Serve hot.

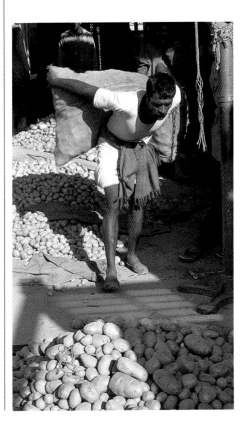

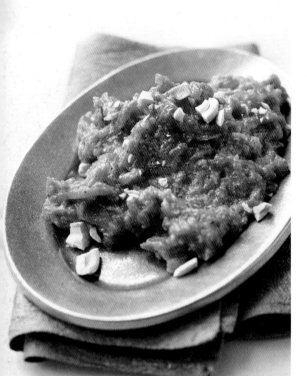

carrot halwa
gajar ka halwa

crisp toast in nutty saffron milk
shahi tukre

This is a winter favourite in north India as its carotene content helps to protect against the harmful pollution that lingers in the cold, heavy air. Winter carrots grown in India are bright red giving this dish its unique jewelled colour. Serve it all through the year; in the summer, serve it warm with vanilla ice cream and in the winter with a dash of cream.

Serves: 4
Preparation time: 15 minutes
Cooking time: 40 minutes

100g sugar
2 tablespoons ghee
300g carrots, grated
300ml full fat milk
1/2 teaspoon powdered cardamom
1 tablespoon finely chopped cashew nuts

1 Mix the sugar with double its volume of water in a heavy saucepan and bring to the boil. Reduce the heat and cook until the syrup has thickened slightly. Take off the heat and reserve.

2 In the meantime, heat the ghee in a heavy-bottomed pan and fry the carrots, stirring occasionally to prevent them from sticking. When they turn translucent, add the sugar syrup and stir until blended.

3 Pour in the milk, reduce the heat and cook until the carrots are mushy and the milk has been soaked up. The ghee should begin to separate at this point.

4 Take off the heat, mix in the cardamom and serve warm, decorated with the nuts.

This classic pudding was created for the Mughal rulers a few centuries ago and is still served at feasts and banquets. As a child, I remember my mother making it for Sunday lunch and it was always a firm favourite! Although the toast needs to be crisp, I quite like it soft and chewy, full of the sweet saffron milk that envelops it.

Serves: 4
Preparation time: 10 minutes
Cooking time: 30 minutes

Sunflower oil for deep-frying
4 slices of white bread, each cut into
 4 squares
150ml full fat milk
150ml evaporated milk
120ml sweetened condensed milk
Sugar to taste
Generous pinch of saffron
2 tablespoons crushed pistachios

1 Heat the oil and fry the squares of bread on both sides until golden. Lift from the pan and drain on absorbent paper.

2 Mix all the milks, sugar and saffron and bring to the boil. Simmer for 10 minutes or so until the mixture thickens. Remove from the heat and allow it to cool.

3 To serve, put the fried bread toasts on a platter and sprinkle half the pistachios over them. Pour the saffron milk on top and decorate with the rest of the pistachios.

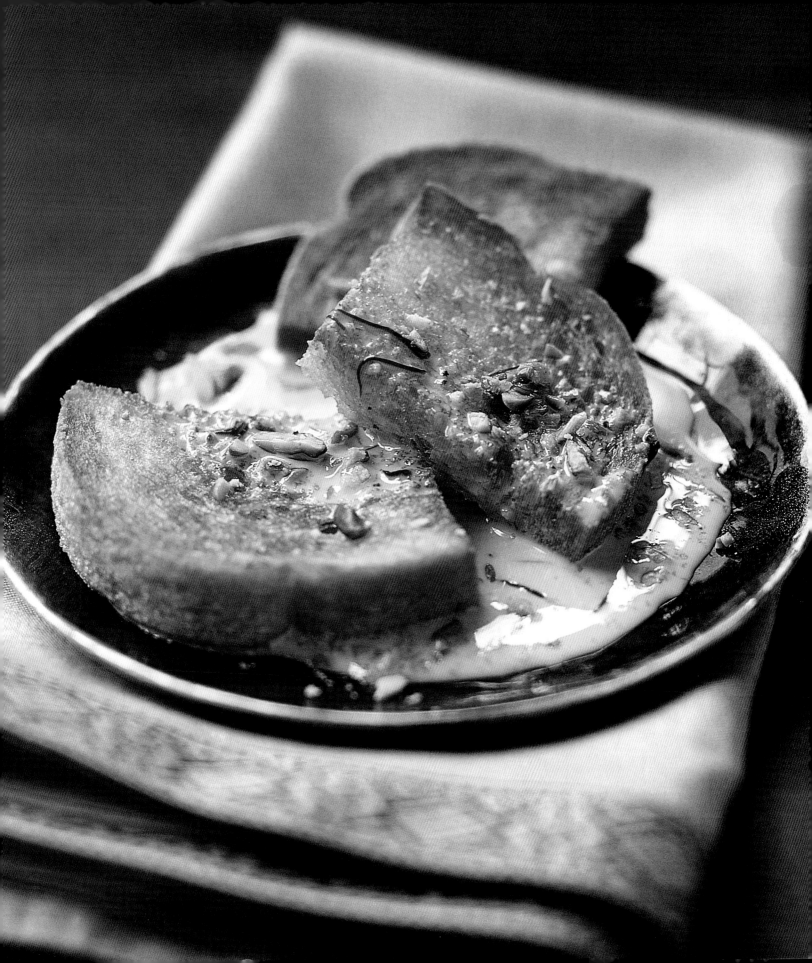

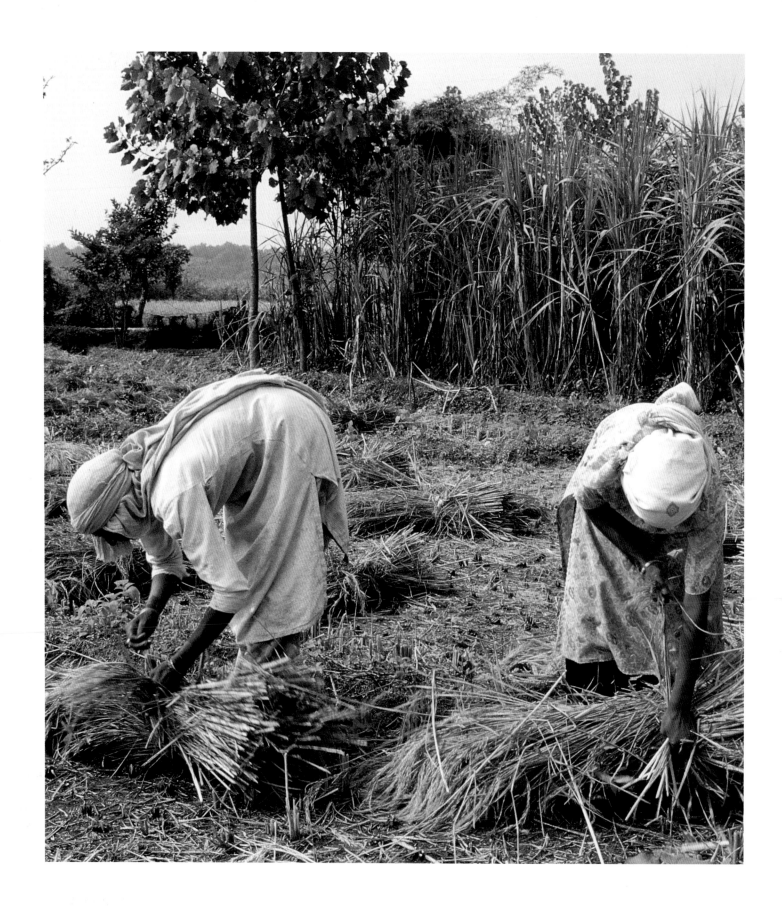

mangoes with semolina
shakaramba

A summer speciality in Lucknow and surrounding areas, this Awadhi dish makes the most of the seasonal fruit. The beauty of Awadhi sweets lies in their charming combination of Hindu and Muslim cultures so that there is a place for wonderful Eid sweets such as sevaiyan and for traditional Diwali sweets such as jalebis and laddoos. I have sometimes made this with other fruit such as strawberries and nectarines.

Serves: 4
Preparation time: 10 minutes
Cooking time: 25 minutes

2 tablespoons ghee or butter
300g mangoes, peeled, stoned and cut into small chunks
3 tablespoons sugar
4 cloves
4 green cardamom pods, bruised
4 tablespoons semolina
150ml warm milk

1 Heat half the ghee or butter in a pan and sauté the mango for a couple of minutes until slightly mashed. Reserve.

2 Combine the sugar and double its volume of water in a small pan and bring to the boil. Reduce the heat and simmer for a couple of minutes until slightly thickened. Add the mango and cook for 1 minute and reserve.

3 Heat the rest of the ghee in a heavy saucepan and fry the spices for 1 minute.

4 Add the semolina and fry, stirring constantly to prevent it from sticking. In about 5 minutes, add the milk and stir continuously to prevent lumps from forming, until the milk has been absorbed and the semolina is soft.

5 Pour in the mango mixture and serve warm.

indian rice pudding
chaaval ki kheer

Kheer is a generic term given to puddings that resemble creams. They can be made with nuts or fruit and always have a milk component. They are considered food for the gods: in fact the god Rama was thought to have been conceived after his mother ate some magical kheer. Rice kheer is made all over India and this is the northern version. In the south, cooks add slivers of coconut or flavour the dish with edible camphor. Broken basmati rice is available commercially.

Serves: 4
Preparation time: 30 minutes
Cooking time: 1 hour

150g broken basmati rice (this gives a better, sticky texture to the pudding)
600ml full fat milk
4 tablespoons ground almonds
150ml evaporated milk
Sugar to taste
2 tablespoons chopped pistachio nuts
1/2 teaspoon powdered cardamom

1 Bring the rice to the boil with the milk in a heavy pan, then allow to simmer for 1 hour or until mushy. Mash the rice roughly with a whisk while still on the heat.

2 Blend the ground almonds into the evaporated milk and add to the rice. Stir until thick and creamy.

3 Add the sugar and pistachios. Sprinkle over the cardamom powder and stir well. Serve chilled or warm, depending on the weather; delicious warm on a winter's evening.

salted lassi with ginger
adrak ki lassi

This is a wonderful drink in the summer. Ayurveda, the Indian system of holistic health, suggests that ginger is good for stimulating the appetite, a much needed thing in the summer! It is also called 'maha aushadhi' or great medicine because it has so many health properties. It is best to peel ginger lightly: the essential oil to which it owes its efficacy lies just beneath the skin.

Serves: 4
Preparation time: 10 minutes
Cooking time: nil

1 teaspoon cumin seeds, dry toasted and
 crushed in a mortar
300ml cold water
200g natural yoghurt
1 teaspoon finely grated fresh ginger
Salt

Combine all the ingredients, whisk well and serve chilled.

raw mango cooler
panha

Serves: 4
Preparation time: 10 minutes
Cooking time: 30 minutes

1 raw green mango
100g sugar
Pinch of salt
Few strands of saffron
Couple of twists of the peppermill
Seeds from 3 green cardamom pods, crushed

1 Peel the mango and chop roughly, taking care to cut around the stone. Place the flesh in a pan with 300ml of water and bring to the boil. I always boil the mango stone for its flavour. Reduce the heat and simmer for 15 minutes until the mango is pulpy.

2 Take off the heat, cool and whizz in a blender until smooth. If the pulp is stringy or thick, strain it through a fine strainer.

3 Add the rest of the ingredients and return to the heat. Cook for a few minutes until the sugar has dissolved completely.

4 Cool and store in the fridge. To make a glassful, add 2–3 tablespoons of this concentrate and top with chilled water.

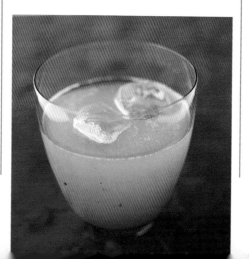

garam masala

In the north, where the winters are bitterly cold, a blend called garam masala, meaning hot spice, is preferred to chillies to add heat to many dishes. Chillies cool the body by promoting perspiration whereas garam masala creates heat within the body, keeping it warm. Some of the most expensive spices go into the making of garam masala and there are as many recipes for it as there are households in India. Depending on individual taste, the proportions of the various ingredients can be adjusted but every blend of garam masala has a rich, warm fragrance and tastes hot and aromatic.

Commercially produced garam masala is often sold in large quantities that cannot be used up quickly enough by most of us so I always make my own blend at home just when I need to use it. It takes a few minutes and the flavours are astounding. Here is my simplest recipe and it will make enough for one curry for four people.

10 black peppercorns
1 teaspoon cumin seeds
Small stick of cinnamon
Seeds from 2–3 green cardamom pods
3 cloves

Dry-roast all the spices in a small saucepan for a couple of minutes until a delicious fragrance wafts up. Put the spices in a mortar and bash to a fine powder or blitz in a coffee mill. Use at once.

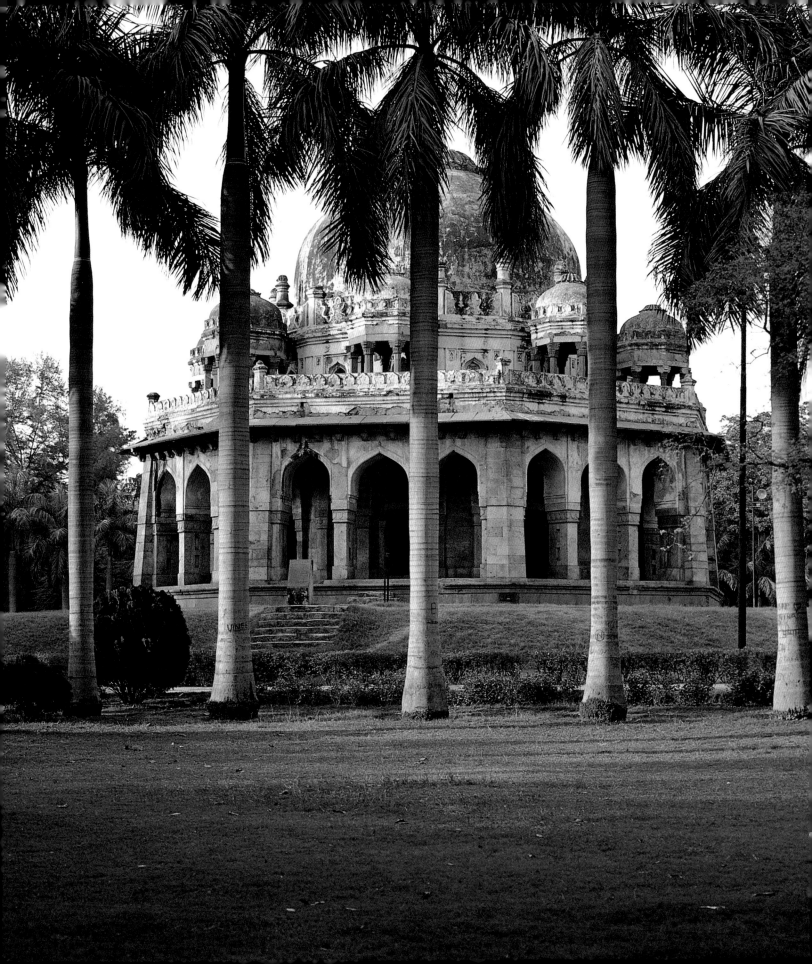

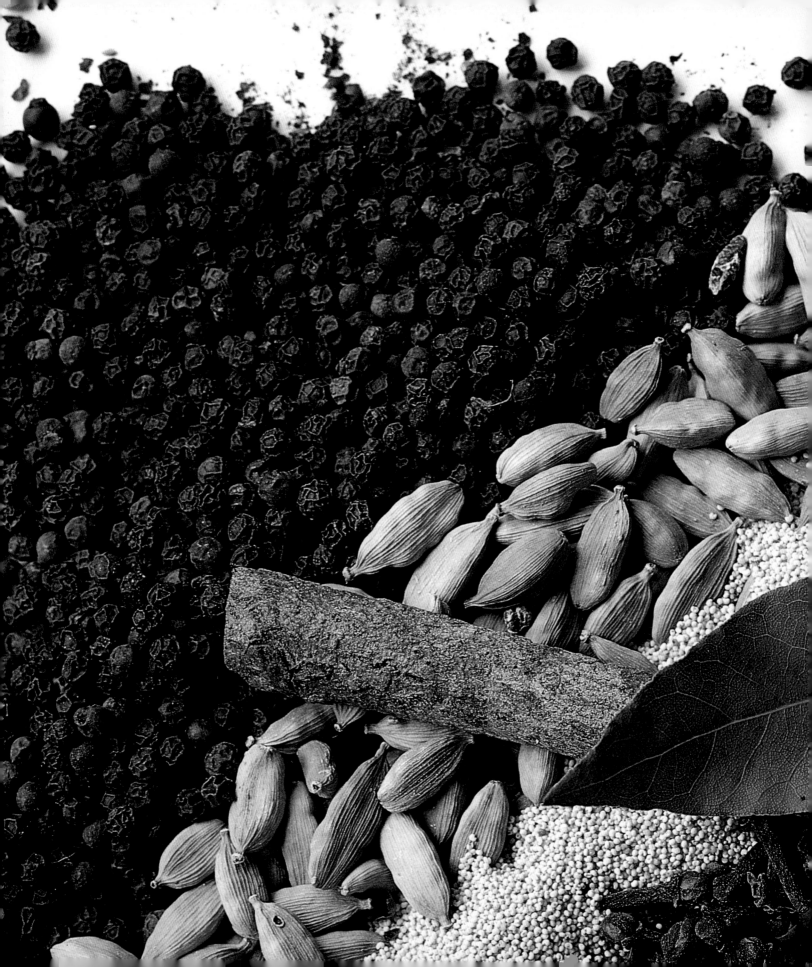

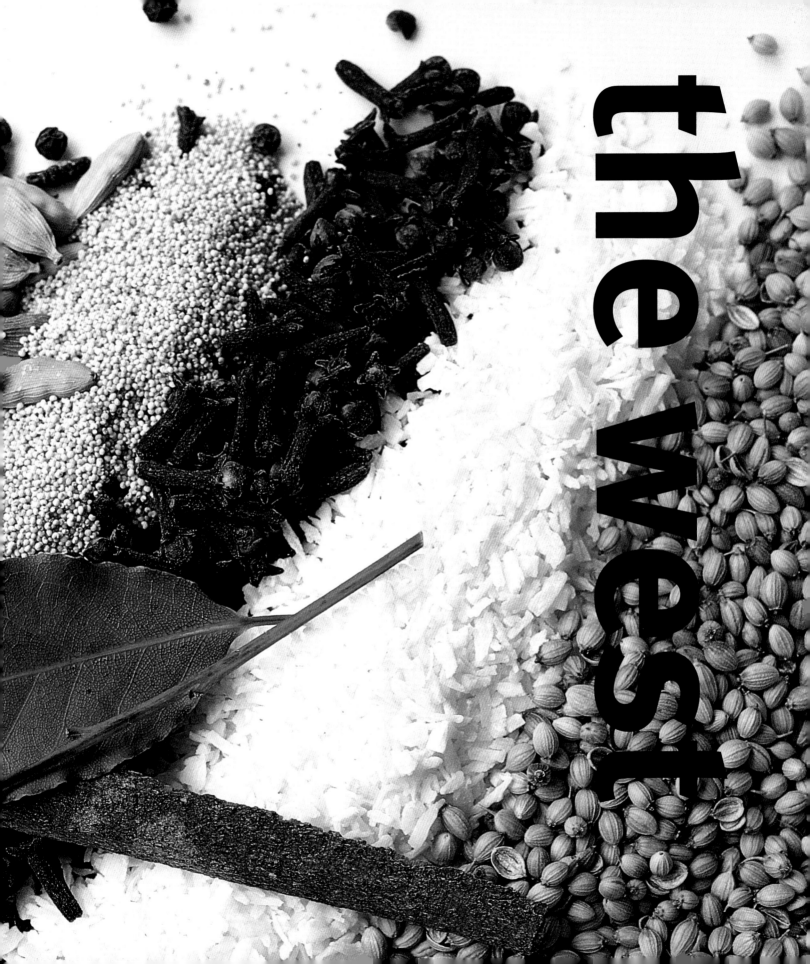

the west

the states

rajasthan

The west includes the states of Rajasthan, Gujarat, Maharashtra and Madhya Pradesh. Within these states exist many communities such as the Bohri Muslims of Gujarat, the Parsees who live predominantly in Mumbai and Gujarat and the Sindhis who have made Mumbai and Pune their home. Mumbai, the capital of the state of Maharashtra and the largest commercial city, has its own unique cuisine because it is home to every community of India. Mumbai street food is famous and it is common to see groups of people eating at little roadside carts all through the day.

Rajasthan, which lies in the Thar desert is also called the Land of Princes because of the many princely kingdoms that existed here before Independence in 1947. In all the royal kitchens of Rajasthan, the preparation of food was raised to the levels of an art form. The Khansamas or royal cooks were artists who guarded their recipes with pride and passed them down only to a known successor. I have spoken to several who, when asked about a recipe, would smile and say something like, 'Master liked my cooking'.

Everyday Rajasthani cooking was designed for the war-like lifestyle of medieval Rajasthan when war lords spent many days away from home, in battle. Also being an arid desert the availability of ingredients of the region was relatively limited. Food that could remain unspoilt for several days and could be eaten without heating was preferred, more out of necessity than choice. The scarcity of water, fresh vegetables and delicate spices has had its effect on the cooking of this state. Most foods are still cooked in ghee.

In the desert belt of Jaisalmer, Barmer and Bikaner, chefs use less water and more milk, buttermilk and ghee. A special feature of Marwari cooking is the use of amchoor or mango powder, making up for the scarcity of tomatoes in the desert, and asafoetida, to flavour curries that do not have the luxury of onions and garlic. Generally, most bright red Rajasthani curries look spicier than they actually are and, if you travel through Rajasthan, you will see heaps of brilliant red chillies drying in the strong sunshine for use later on.

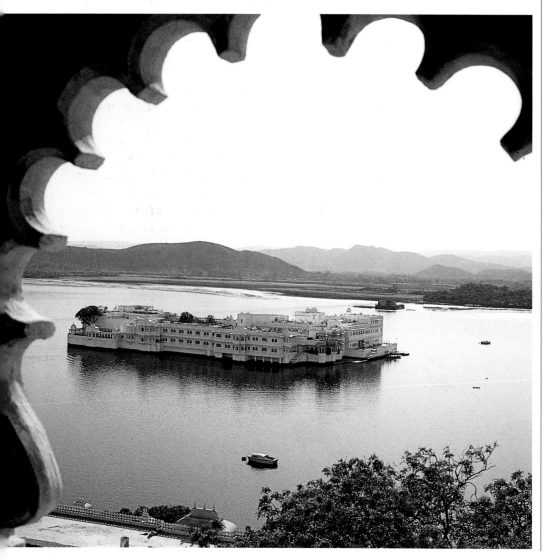

gujarat

Gujarat is the mango shaped state to the west of India. Its northern region is famous for a delicate, vegetarian cuisine and most especially for the thali, a metal plate with several small bowls filled with an array of tempting dishes. The thali has rice, breads, fried accompaniments called farsans, vegetables, lentils and sweets all served at the same time.

Although Gujarat has had many foreign influences over the years, the basic cuisine has remained the same. Even within Gujarat, the cuisine is varied within the different areas. Some areas are drier than others. Kathiawari and Kachchi food both use red chilli powder to create heat. In the southern part of the state, green chillies are used for the same purpose, most often in conjunction with fresh ginger. In Surat, sugar is added to many dishes, even lentils and vegetables and much of the cuisine has a sweet, tangy flavour. The food of Surat is renowned all over India. Oondhiyoon, which is a delicious combination of winter vegetables, contains sweet, sharp and herby flavours. The delicate balance of flavours – sweet, tangy and sharp – is what makes the food of Surat unique.

Gujarat was also home to the Bohri Muslim community which migrated to Mumbai in large numbers. Their cooking is a mix of the local Gujarati with Islamic overtones and some of the delicacies such as lamba pau, a bread that is smoky from being baked in a wood oven, is found only in exclusive eateries today.

maharashtra

Maharashtra lies to the west of India and has a long coastline along the Arabian Sea. Many communities live here – different sects of Maharashtrians and the settlers who came from other states.

Native Maharashtrian cooking has many styles, the Pune Brahmin style with its sweet, simple flavourings and use of peanuts, the fiery curries of the Deccan Plateau and the coconut and tamarind flavourings of the coastal areas. The state grows a large variety of crops such as peanuts, coconuts, rice and mangoes. The most sought after mango in India, the Alphonso, is grown here in Ratnagiri.

The biggest city in the state is Mumbai. This cosmopolitan city is dotted with innumerable restaurants serving up every type of regional cuisine. The Parsees who came from Persia and settled in Gujarat later moved to Mumbai. Their cooking is a mix of Iranian and Hindu and, out of respect to the local community, they do not eat beef. Their cooking is exemplified by the sweet and sour dhansak, stews and dessert custards.

The Sindhi community migrated from Pakistan and many of them set up homes in Mumbai. They are known for their love of food and their cooking is fresh and flavourful. Leafy vegetables imbued with cumin, fried breads and spiced lentils with garlic are specialities. Their love of various poppadoms is legendary and they make them using anything from lentils to lotus root.

madhya pradesh

This state lies at the centre of India and is often called her 'heart'. The cooking is influenced by all the surrounding states, most importantly by Gujarat and Maharashtra. MP, as it is known, has a great culture of hospitality and I have never been to any other place in the world where the people eat and offer others so much food. There seem to be six meals a day – breakfast, elevenses, lunch, tea, dinner and supper with many 'munchings' in between!

Much of MP has Hindu cooking. Indore is famous for its pickle shops that sell preserved fruit and vegetables. I was once taken to a pickle shop that was heaven for a foodie like me, every imaginable pickle made in the region filled rows and rows of clean glass jars. As I pointed out my choices, the vendor weighed and filled tiny plastic bags with flaming scarlet, golden yellow or rich terracotta coloured pickles. There were whole lemons with cloves and ginger, stuffed red chillies (surprisingly mild) and sliced green mango with fennel and mustard seeds at home for many months afterwards. In Indore, the local high street turns into a food lane called the sarafa after the shops close and every night people stroll along this road to eat fresh samosas, hot sweet jalebis and to drink warm nut-flavoured milk.

Bhopal, the capital, is an exception. Ruled for many years by a Muslim ruler, the cuisine is a mix of Islamic and Hindu styles. Kebabs and biryanis sit next to simple stir-fries and fresh breads. Sweets are much loved and tiny milk burfies and halwas are served at each meal.

gujarati-style cabbage and peas stir-fry
kobi vatana

Gujarati cooking is very delicate and this recipe works well if the cabbage is finely shredded. It should look translucent and shiny when served and is best cooked with the pan uncovered as this helps get rid of the rather unpleasant smell. This slightly sweet stir-fry goes well with roti (page 32).

Serves: 4
Preparation time: 10 minutes
Cooking time: 25 minutes

2 fresh green chillies, finely chopped
1 teaspoon grated, fresh ginger
2 tablespoons sunflower oil
1 teaspoon black mustard seeds
1/2 teaspoon cumin seeds
Pinch of asafoetida
1 teaspoon turmeric powder
300g cabbage, finely shredded
150g fresh or frozen peas
Salt
2 tablespoons freshly grated coconut

1 Crush the chillies and ginger to a paste in a mortar or coffee mill (wash it well after use!).

2 Heat the oil in a wok or a heavy saucepan until almost smoking. Add the mustard seeds and let them pop. Add the cumin seeds, asafoetida and chilli-ginger paste and stir for a few seconds. Sprinkle in the turmeric powder and add the cabbage and peas at once. Season with salt and stir until the vegetables start to turn translucent. Pour in a few tablespoons of water. Reduce the heat and cook, adding a little more water as necessary, until the vegetables are al dente. Serve hot sprinkled with the coconut.

aubergines and potatoes in peanut sauce
vengan bataka

I first tasted this in a friend's house in Mumbai and have always made it for special occasions since then. The ingredient list may seem a bit daunting, but the final dish is well worth it. Also, most of the ingredients are not too difficult to get hold of. Fenugreek leaves add a curry-like flavour and, if you are using them, pinch off the leaves and discard the stalks. Serve this with a roti or with poories (page 74).

Serves: 4
Preparation time: 15 minutes
Cooking time: 45 minutes

1 teaspoon white sesame seeds, toasted
2 teaspoons peanuts, toasted
2 tablespoons gram flour (besan)
400g tin chopped tomatoes
1 tablespoon ginger-garlic paste (page 11)
Handful of fenugreek leaves, chopped (optional)
Handful of coriander leaves, chopped
1/2 teaspoon turmeric powder
1/2 teaspoon chilli powder
Salt
1 teaspoon brown sugar
300g small aubergines, slit down the middle but stalks left on
2 tablespoons sunflower oil
1/2 teaspoon black mustard seeds
100g potatoes, peeled and quartered

1 Whizz the sesame seeds and peanuts in a coffee mill or crush them finely in a mortar and reserve.

2 Heat a pan and dry roast the gram flour, stirring constantly for 2–3 minutes, and then mix well into the chopped tomatoes in a small bowl and reserve.

3 In a mixing bowl, combine the peanut mixture, tomato mixture, ginger-garlic paste and the chopped leaves. Add the spice powders and season with salt, then the sugar.

4 Stuff the aubergines with this mixture saving any that is left over to add to the pan later.

5 Heat the oil in a heavy-bottomed saucepan or kadhai. Add the mustard seeds and allow them to pop.

6 Gently place the aubergines and potatoes in the pan and pour in any leftover spice mixture. Pour in a few tablespoons of water and cover the pan.

7 Bring to the boil, reduce the heat and simmer until the vegetables are cooked, for about 25 minutes. Serve hot. The sauce should be quite thick.

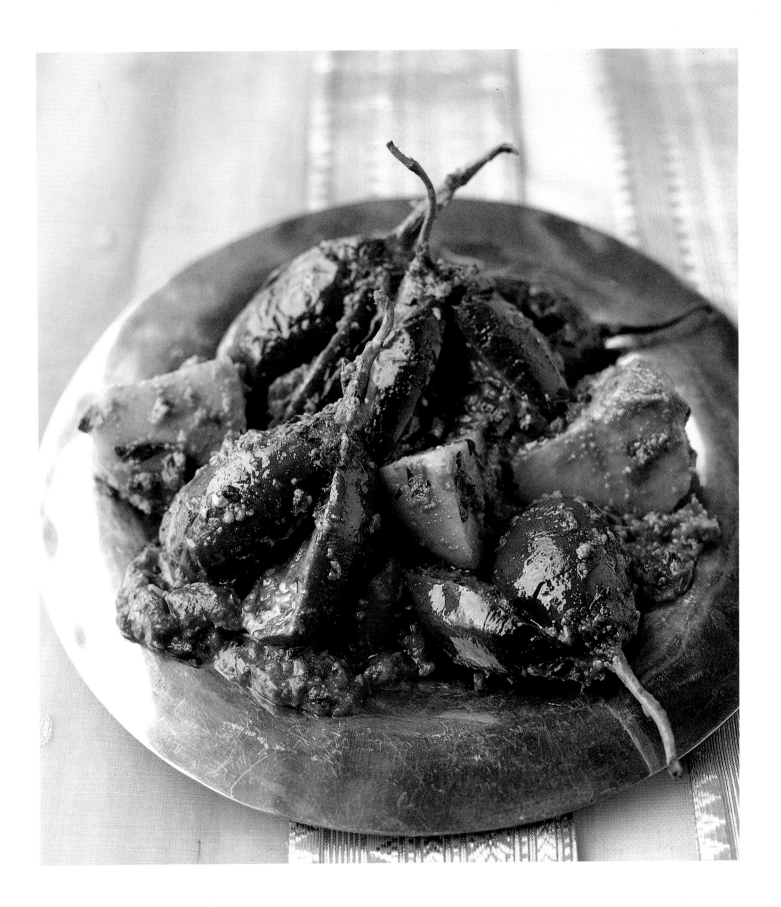

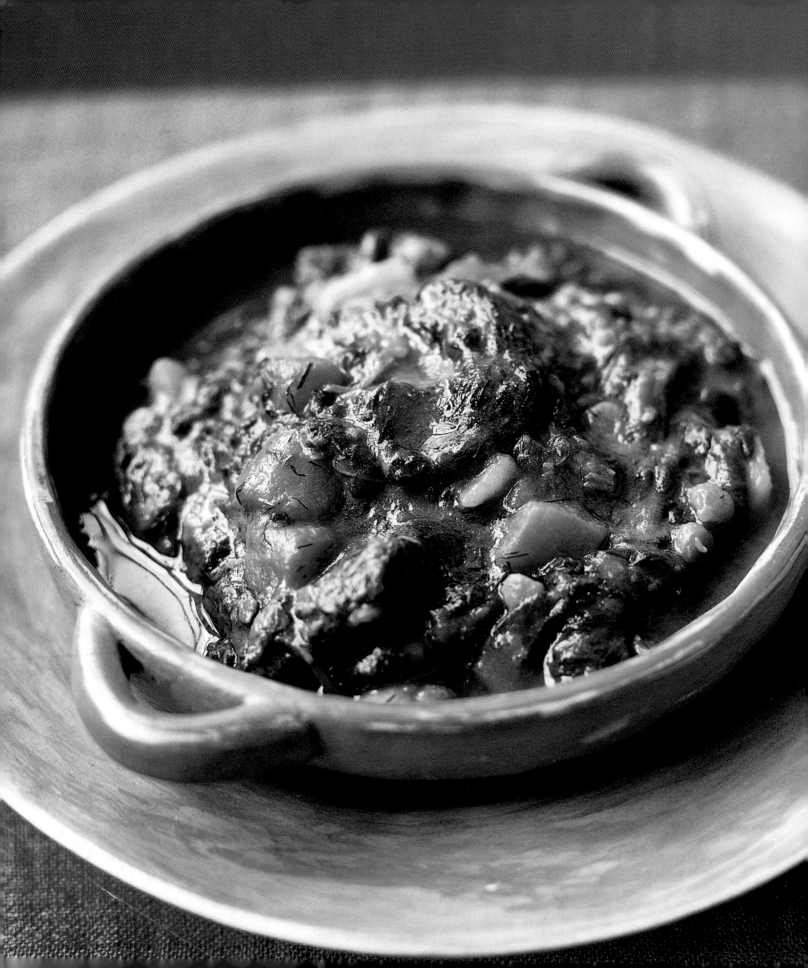

dilled vegetables
saibhaji

This is a Sindhi favourite of mine. The dish is creamy and nutritious and goes well with rotis. Dill leaves are popular amongst certain communities of India – the Sindhis and the Gujaratis to name two. Dill combines well with lentils and garlic to make a herby dal that is delicious with rice. Dill leaves are wispy and delicate and they cook fast. Their strong flavour is unpopular with some people but, in this dish, it seems to complement the spinach rather than overwhelm it.

Serves: 4
Preparation time: 20 minutes
Cooking time: 45 minutes

2 tablespoons sunflower oil
1/2 teaspoon cumin seeds
2 teaspoons ginger-garlic paste (page 11)
4 teaspoons split gram lentils (channa dal), washed and drained
600g spinach, washed and chopped
Handful of dill leaves, chopped
2 medium tomatoes, chopped
1 small potato, peeled and chopped
2 small aubergines, chopped (or half a large one)
2 carrots, peeled and chopped
1/2 teaspoon chilli powder
1/2 teaspoon turmeric powder
Salt

1 Heat the oil in a pan. Add the cumin seeds and as they begin to darken, in a minute or so, add the ginger-garlic paste.

2 Stir and add the lentils, spinach, dill, tomatoes and vegetables. Mix in the chilli and turmeric powders and salt. Pour in about 150ml of water and simmer gently until the lentils are cooked, for about 35 minutes. The vegetables will be mushy by now.

3 Remove from the heat and whisk gently to blend into a smooth but thick consistency. Serve very hot.

french beans with mustard
farasbeechi bhaji

This stir-fry from Maharashtra is one my mum made quite often when I was a child. The beans must be chopped quite finely to get the best flavour – you could use runner beans equally well. I find that the zing of mustard seeds and the bitter taste of cumin seeds complement this vegetable beautifully. Cooking without a lid on the pan keeps the beans green and fresh looking. I sometimes add a few tablespoons of tinned black peas for a bit of variety.

Serves: 4
Preparation time: 5 minutes
Cooking time: 15 minutes

2 tablespoons sunflower oil
1 teaspoon black mustard seeds
1/2 teaspoon cumin seeds
1 medium onion, finely chopped
300g French beans, finely chopped
Salt
1 tablespoon lemon juice
3 tablespoons desiccated coconut

1 Heat the oil and add in the mustard seeds. As they pop, add the cumin and onion. Stir and fry until the onion is soft.

2 Add the French beans and salt. Pour in a few tablespoons of water and cook uncovered until the beans are tender.

3 Take off the heat, stir in the lemon juice and serve hot, sprinkled with the coconut.

corn on the cob in coconut curry
bhajani makka

This recipe is from the coasts of Maharashtra, a region rich in coconut and native fruits such as mango and jackfruit. The basic curry paste in this recipe is very versatile and tastes better the next day. In its place of origin, it is used with a variety of vegetables such as cauliflower, potatoes and peas. It has always proved a great hit at my parties.

Serves: 4
Preparation time: 15 minutes
Cooking time: 40 minutes

600g corn on the cob, cut into 2cm chunks
3 tablespoons sunflower oil
10 black peppercorns
2cm stick of cinnamon
6 cloves
2 teaspoons coriander seeds
1 large onion, finely sliced
150g freshly grated or desiccated coconut
1 teaspoon cumin seeds
150g tomatoes, chopped
1 teaspoon chilli powder
1 teaspoon turmeric powder
Salt

1 Put the corn into a pan with enough water to cover it and bring to the boil. Reduce the heat and cook until tender. Drain (save the water for the curry) and reserve.

2 Meanwhile, make the curry paste. Heat half the oil in a kadhai or heavy-bottomed saucepan. Add the whole spices and fry for 1 minute. Then add the onion and stir-fry until brown.

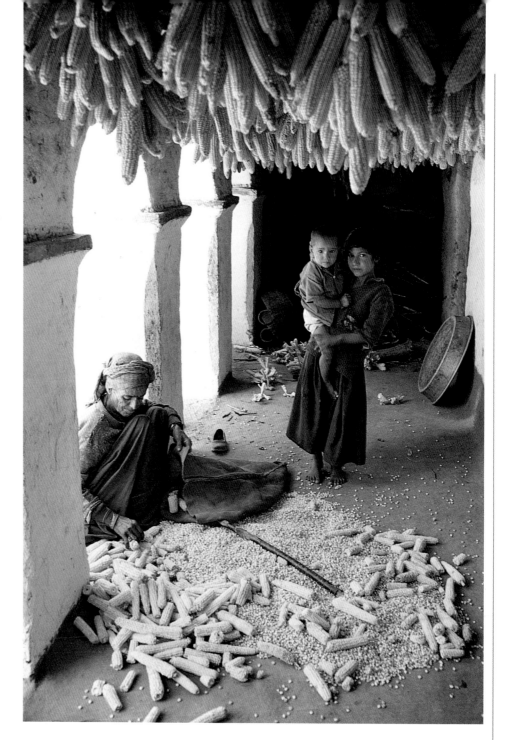

3 Add the coconut and continue stirring until the whole mixture is a rich brown. Take off the heat and allow it to cool. Add a little water and grind to a fine paste in a blender. Reserve.

4 In another saucepan heat the remaining oil and add the cumin seeds. When they darken, add the corn and mix well.

5 Mix in the tomatoes, spice powders and salt. Add a few tablespoons of the reserved corn water.

6 Gently stir in the curry paste and simmer for 3 minutes to blend well. Add more water if necessary to make a thick sauce.

crushed yam with chilli and garlic
suranacha thecha

Yam is popular in the west of India where it is known as suran. Be careful while peeling certain varieties of suran as the sap can cause a mild itching of the hands. The trick is to oil them lightly before handling all varieties of yam. On cooking, yam develops a creamy, mild potato-like taste, without being floury.

Serves: 4
Preparation time: 15 minutes
Cooking time: 30 minutes

300g yam, peeled, washed and cut into
  1cm cubes
1 tablespoon sunflower oil
1/2 teaspoon black mustard seeds
Pinch of asafoetida
2 fresh green chillies, minced
1 teaspoon ginger-garlic paste (page 11)
1 teaspoon turmeric powder
Salt
2 teaspoons crushed peanuts
Handful of coriander leaves, chopped
Large pinch of sugar

1 Put the yam into a heavy-bottomed saucepan, cover with water and set to boil. Reduce the heat and simmer until it is just tender, each cube being cooked through but still holding its shape. Drain and reserve.

2 Heat the oil and fry the mustard seeds for 1 minute until they pop. Add the asafoetida, green chillies and the ginger-garlic paste. Reduce the heat and fry for a couple of minutes, stirring.

3 Stir in the turmeric powder and add the cooked yam. Turn up the heat, season with salt and stir to blend. Don't worry if the yam disintegrates a bit – it is meant to!

4 Add the peanuts, coriander and sugar, mix lightly and take off the heat. Serve hot with rotis (page 32) or poories (page 74).

green peas with cumin and ginger
vatana bhaaji

This is a fresh looking and great tasting stir-fry. I sometimes fill it into wraps, add a few sliced tomatoes and offer it to the kids for a weekend lunch. You can sprinkle a bit of coconut on top for variety and also stir in a few spoonfuls of Greek yoghurt for an instant summer salad. This goes well with poories (page 74).

Serves: 4
Preparation time: nil
Cooking time: 15 minutes

2 tablespoons sunflower oil
1/2 teaspoon cumin seeds
300g green peas
1/2 teaspoon turmeric powder
2 fresh green chillies, slit down the middle
  but kept whole with the stalk
Pinch of sugar
Salt
2cm piece of fresh ginger, peeled

1 Heat the oil in a kadhai or saucepan and add the cumin seeds.

2 As they sizzle, add the green peas and stir. Sprinkle in the turmeric and add the green chillies. Stir for 1 minute.

3 Pour in a couple of tablespoons of water, add the sugar and salt and bring to the boil. Reduce the heat and cook without a lid until the peas are soft and done.

4 Remove from the heat, grate the ginger on top and gently fold it in with a wooden spoon. Serve warm.

puffy fried bread
poories

Poories are fried and therefore rich in taste (and calories!). They form a part of a wedding feast or banquet and are sometimes flavoured or stuffed with spices and herbs. They are often served with fresh mango purée or a yoghurt-based pudding called shrikhand and this is quite usual in India – in a traditional meal, the sweet is always served as a part of the main meal.

Serves: 4
Preparation time: 15 minutes
Cooking time: 20 minutes

300g wholewheat flour, plus extra for flouring
Sunflower oil for deep-frying
150ml warm water

1 Blend the flour, 1 tablespoon of oil and warm water to make a stiff dough. You may need a little less or more water than the quantity given, depending on the quality of the flour. Divide the dough into equal balls, the size of a large cherry. Smear your palms with oil and smooth each ball.

2 Heat the oil in a deep frying pan or kadhai. Roll each ball out into a flat disc 2cm in diameter, flouring the board as necessary.

3 Gently place the disc into the hot oil, pressing it down with the back of a slotted spoon until puffy and golden. Turn over and fry for 1 minute. It will puff up only if the oil is hot enough and the disc has been submerged. Lift out with a slotted spoon and drain on absorbent paper. Proceed similarly for all the poories, adjusting the heat so that the poories do not brown excessively.

fenugreek leaf bread
thepla

This is the ideal bread to take on picnics or long journeys. It keeps well because of its yoghurt content and stays soft for a couple of days. It is eaten with a spicy mango chutney. Fenugreek leaves can be bought in Indian shops in bundles. You need to pinch the leaves off and discard the stalks. The leaves are often dried to make kasuri methi, and used to give many curries a distinctive curry smell.

Serves: 4
Preparation time: 20 minutes
Cooking time: 30 minutes

300g wholewheat flour, plus extra for flouring
150g gram flour (besan)
2 handfuls of fenugreek leaves, washed and finely chopped
1/2 teaspoon chilli powder
1/2 teaspoon cumin seeds
1 tablespoon sunflower oil plus extra for brushing
150g natural yoghurt
Salt

1 Combine the two flours, fenugreek, chilli powder and cumin seeds in a mixing bowl and mix well with your fingers.

2 Drizzle in the oil and mix again. Pour in enough yoghurt to make a firm dough and season with salt, before kneading well to bring everything together.

3 Divide the dough into portions the size of a lime. Coat them lightly with flour, shape into a ball in your palm and flatten slightly. Roll out into flat discs, 10cm in diameter, flouring the board as necessary.

4 Heat a griddle or shallow pan. Cook the discs on the griddle until the surface appears bubbly. Turn over and press the edges down with a clean cloth to cook evenly. As soon as brown spots appear the thepla is done. Make sure that the thepla is cooked evenly all over. You can do this by cooking them on medium heat and raising the temperature if the pan cools down.

5 Remove, brush with oil and keep warm by enclosing in tinfoil. Cook all the theplas in the same way.

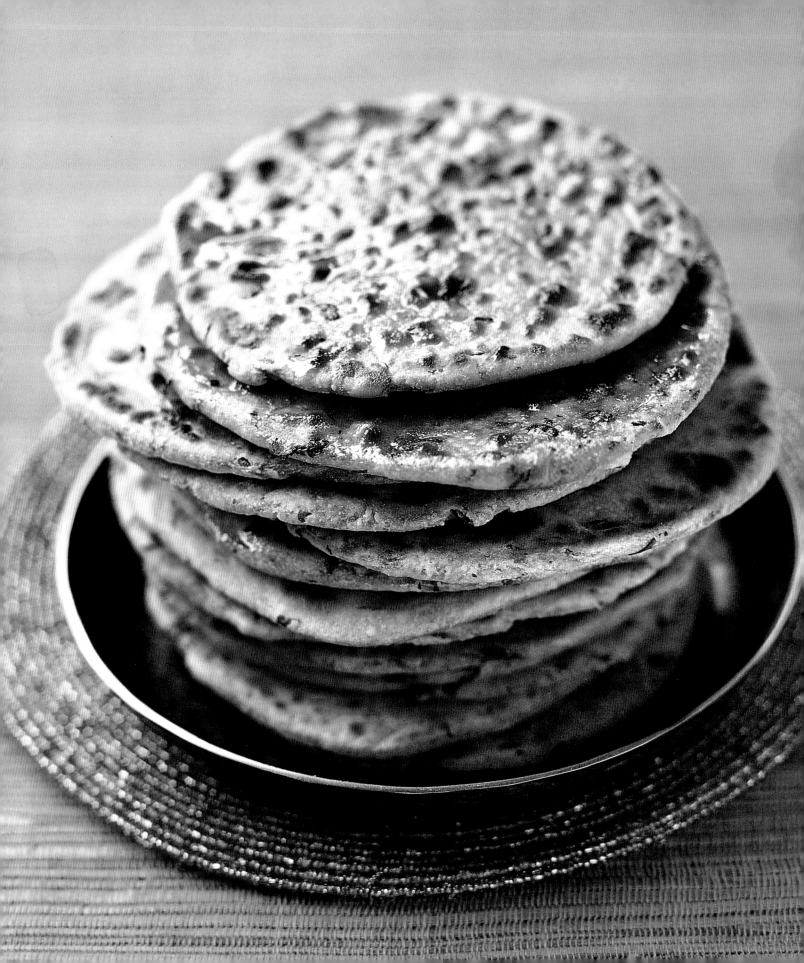

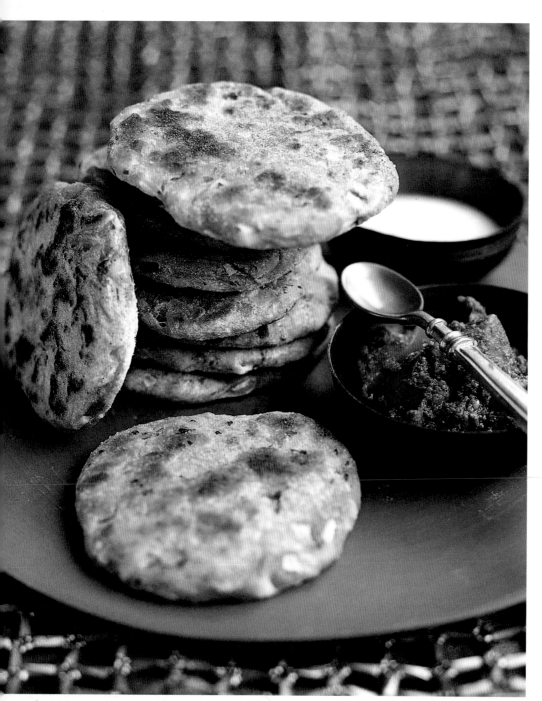

sindhi-style rotis
koki

This is a favourite of the Sindhi community. They are fond of spicy, rich food but I have used far less oil than a traditional Sindhi cook would!

Serves: 4
Preparation time: 15 minutes
Cooking time: 40 minutes

300g wholewheat flour, plus extra for flouring
1 medium onion, finely chopped
2 fresh green chillies, minced
Handful of coriander leaves, chopped
Salt
2 tablespoons sunflower oil plus extra
** for brushing**

1 Combine the flour, onion, green chillies and coriander leaves in a large mixing bowl. Season with salt and add the oil to the mixture.

2 Blend all the ingredients with your fingers and add enough warm water to form a firm dough. Knead for 5 minutes or so but make sure that the dough is not too soft. Leave it to rest for about 5 minutes.

3 Divide the dough into 8 lime-sized balls. Flour the board and roll out each ball into a thick disc about 8cm in diameter.

4 Heat a flat saucepan and place a koki in it. When the underside begins to brown, brush the top with oil and turn over to cook the other side. Make sure that both sides are cooked by keeping the flame at medium. Brush with oil and remove. Make the rest of the kokis similarly. Serve hot with a hot mango pickle and natural yoghurt.

plain boiled rice
bhaat

This is the simplest form of cooked rice and is the one most commonly eaten all over India. Its neutral, unflavoured taste goes well with the spices in the accompanying curries and stir-fries. In Maharashtra and Gujarat, people use many local varieties of rice such as ambemohar or surti kolam. These are quite fragrant and delicious. However, I have used basmati rice in this recipe as it is quite easily found outside India, almost anywhere in the world. Also, I never add salt to plain rice – it simply isn't needed.

Serves: 4
Preparation time: 5 minutes
Cooking time: 20 minutes

300g basmati rice, washed and drained
600ml hot water

1 Put the ingredients in a heavy saucepan and bring to the boil. Reduce the heat, cover and simmer for 10 minutes until the rice is fluffy and cooked. This may take a bit more or less time depending on the age and quality of the rice. In the West it is difficult to find out the age of the rice but in India people will ask the grocer for old rice that cooks better without becoming sticky.

2 Gently run a fork through the rice to loosen the individual grains and serve hot with a lentil or vegetable curry.

spiced vegetable rice
pulao

This wonderfully glamorous dish can also be made with brown rice, but this takes a bit longer to cook. Brown rice has more fibre than basmati and is also high in Vitamin B. I like its rough taste combined with the smoothness of the vegetables and raisins. You could jazz up this pulao with mushrooms, mixed peppers or diced, fried potatoes.

Serves: 4
Preparation time: 15 minutes
Cooking time: 30 minutes

6 tablespoons sunflower oil
2 tablespoons cashew nuts
1 tablespoon cumin seeds
150g carrots, peeled and finely diced
150g fresh or frozen green peas
90g fresh or frozen sweetcorn
Salt
1 teaspoon garam masala powder
300g basmati rice, washed and drained
2 tablespoons raisins

1 Heat the oil in a heavy pan and fry the cashew nuts until golden. Drain and reserve.

2 Add the cumin seeds to the pan. When they pop, add the vegetables and salt, then stir in the garam masala powder.

3 Add the rice and fry until translucent, before pouring in 600ml of hot water; mix gently and bring to the boil. Lower the heat, cover and simmer for about 10–15 minutes until the vegetables are soft but still crisp.

4 Serve hot garnished with the raisins and reserved cashew nuts.

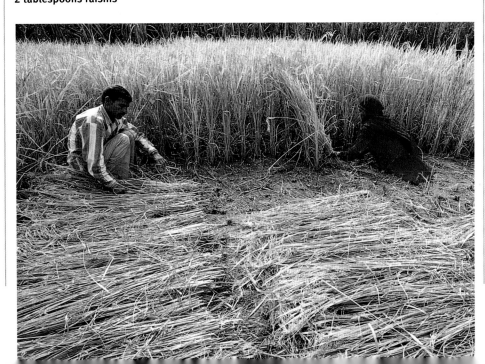

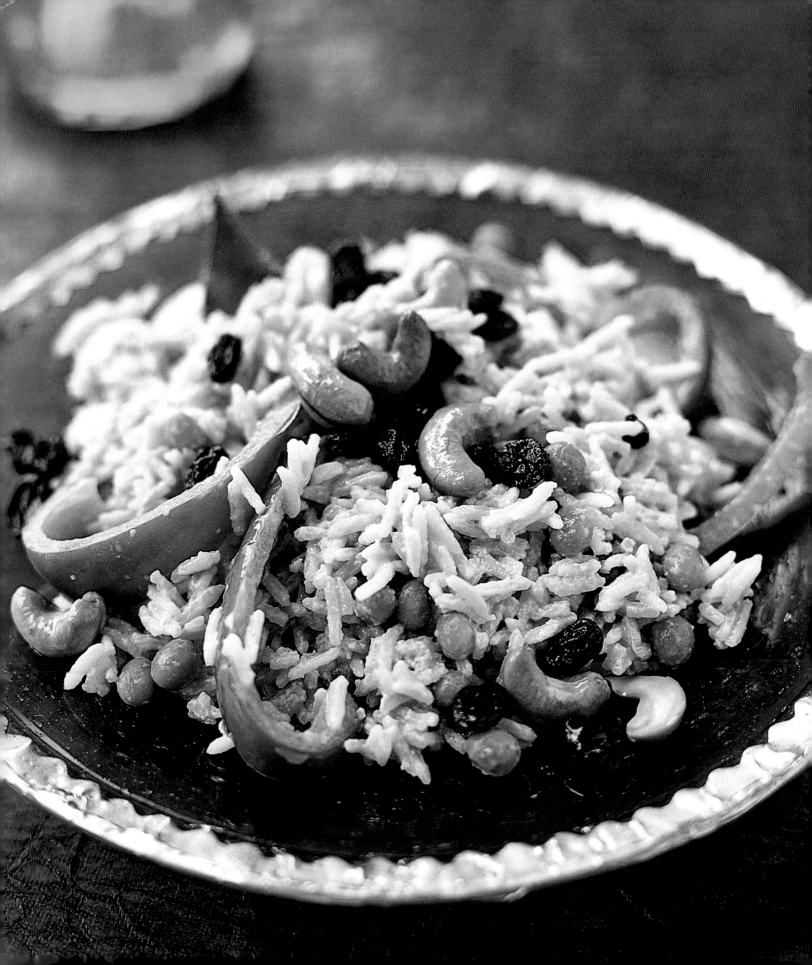

parsee-style coconut and cashew nut rice
kaju saathe khichdi pulao

A khichdi is a rice dish made with either vegetables or nuts or lentils. The texture of a khichdi can vary from firm to almost risotto-like and many khichdis are almost soupy. They are considered very healthy and nutritious and often someone who is convalescing will be offered khichdi to boost their energy levels! This one is quite festive and warming on a cold evening.

Serves: 4
Preparation time: 10 minutes
Cooking time: 35 minutes

3 tablespoons sunflower oil or ghee
1 medium onion, sliced
10 black peppercorns
3 cloves
3 green cardamom pods, bruised
2 bay leaves
300g basmati rice, washed and drained
300ml tinned coconut milk
Salt
1 green pepper, deseeded and sliced
3 tablespoons frozen green peas
2 tablespoons raisins
2 tablespoons cashew nuts

1 Heat 2 tablespoons of the oil or ghee in a heavy-bottomed saucepan and fry the onion until golden brown. Add the whole spices and bay leaves and swirl around for 1 minute. Add about 300ml of water and bring to the boil.

2 Add the rice to the pan together with half the coconut milk and salt. Bring back to the boil, then reduce the heat and add the green pepper and peas.

3 As soon as the liquid has been absorbed add the rest of the coconut milk. Cover the pan and simmer until the rice is cooked through.

4 Heat the remaining oil or ghee in a small saucepan and fry the raisins and cashew nuts for 1 minute. Pour over the rice to garnish and serve hot with Laganshala (page 70).

rice and mung stew
mung khichdi

Khichdis are at the heart of Pancha Karma or Ayurvedic cleansing therapy, because they are easy to digest and they promote lubrication. Various spices are added for specific functions. This khichdi is a meal in itself with good amounts of protein, carbohydrate and fat, and combined with a vegetable stir-fry and a fresh salad, can be one of the healthiest Indian meals.

Serves: 4
Preparation time: 10 minutes
Cooking time: 35 minutes

1 tablespoon ghee (or sunflower oil if you prefer)
5 cloves
10 black peppercorns
1 bay leaf
1/2 teaspoon cumin seeds
1/2 teaspoon turmeric powder
250g basmati rice, washed and drained
4 tablespoons split mung beans, washed and drained
Salt

1 Heat the ghee in a large heavy-bottomed saucepan and fry the cloves, peppercorns, bay leaf and cumin seeds for about 1 minute until the aroma fills the kitchen.

2 Add the turmeric, rice, mung beans, salt and 600ml of hot water and bring to the boil. Reduce the heat and simmer, covered, until the rice is creamy and soft, for about 30 minutes, adding more hot water as necessary. This dish will be quite moist which only increases its digestibility. Serve with natural yoghurt on the side.

stir-fried mung sprouts
mugachi usal

The process of sprouting induces a riot of bio-chemical changes in which complex components break down into simpler substances that are easy to digest. Sprouted legumes have higher amounts of vitamin C, iron and calcium than those that are not sprouted. Sprouted beans are a common addition to a Maharashtrian or Gujarati meal and are a must in a thali from this region.

Serves: 4
Preparation time: 10 minutes + 5 hours
 soaking time + overnight sprouting time
Cooking time: 25 minutes

150g dried mung beans
1 tablespoon sunflower oil
1/2 teaspoon black mustard seeds
1/2 teaspoon cumin seeds
8 curry leaves
1 small fresh green chilli, cut in half
 and deseeded
1 medium onion, finely chopped
1/4 teaspoon turmeric powder
Salt
2 tablespoons desiccated coconut
1 tablespoon chopped coriander leaves
1 tablespoon lemon juice

1 Soak the mung beans in cold water for 5 hours, then drain them and tie them in a cheese cloth or muslin and put in a warm place, such as an airing cupboard, to sprout overnight. Refresh the sprouted beans in cold water and reserve.

2 Heat the oil and add the mustard seeds. When they pop, add the cumin seeds, curry leaves and the green chilli. Swirl around and add the onion, frying it until soft.

3 Tip in the sprouted beans, turmeric and salt. Add about 3 tablespoons of water and bring to the boil. Reduce the heat, cover the pan and cook until the beans are soft but firm, for about 20 minutes, adding more water if necessary.

4 Finish off by sprinkling the coconut, coriander and lemon juice on top. Serve warm.

maharashtrian sweet and sour lentils
aamti

I have often been asked during my cookery demonstrations about the cooking of lentils. My advice is to wash them well and cook them in plenty of water. They should mash up in the cooking process and if you have to use a whisk or beater, it often means that they need more cooking time. This recipe uses jaggery which is manufactured commercially in Maharashtra. Soft brown sugar makes an acceptable substitute.

Serves: 4
Preparation time: 10 minutes
Cooking time: 35 minutes

150g yellow lentils (toor dal)
2 tablespoons sunflower oil
1/2 teaspoon black mustard seeds
Large pinch asafoetida
1/2 teaspoon cumin seeds
10 curry leaves
2 fresh green chillies, sliced
1/2 teaspoon turmeric
2 tomatoes, chopped
1 tablespoon jaggery or soft brown sugar
Salt
Juice of 1/2 lemon
Small handful of coriander leaves, chopped

lentil fritters
moong dal bhajia

1 Bring the lentils to the boil in a quantity of hot water double their volume and simmer until soft and mushy, adding more water as necessary. This should take about 30 minutes. I usually cover the pan partially when the simmering starts, to hasten the process. Reserve the cooked lentils which should have a thick, custard-like consistency.

2 Heat the oil in a saucepan and add the mustard seeds. When they pop, add the asafoetida, cumin, curry leaves and chillies, and fry for 1 minute.

3 Tip in the turmeric and add the cooked lentils at once.

4 Bring to the boil. Add the tomatoes, jaggery or sugar and salt and turn off the heat. The tomatoes should turn mushy in the pot. Stir in the lemon juice and top with the coriander.

5 Serve hot with plain, boiled rice (page 77).

Every Indian meal is served with accompaniments and in the western region of Rajasthan and Gujarat these are usually fried. Bhajias are common all over India and can be also be added to yoghurt to make another traditional accompaniment, Dahi Vada. Bhajias can be served as cocktail snacks or for tea when the kids come home from school. They make a great alternative to chips!

Serves: 4
Preparation time: 15 minutes
Cooking time: 30 minutes

150g split mung beans, washed and
   soaked for 1 hour
2 fresh green chillies
Small handful of coriander leaves,
   finely chopped
1/2 teaspoon coriander seeds, coarsely
   crushed
1/2 teaspoon cumin seeds, coarsely crushed
1/2 teaspoon ajowan seeds (optional,
   although they taste great!)
Salt
Sunflower oil for deep-frying

1 Drain the soaked mung beans and put them into a blender with about 80ml water. Whizz until coarsely ground. The batter should be quite thick.

2 Mix in all other ingredients, except the oil.

3 Heat the oil in a kadhai or deep frying pan. When it is quite hot, spoon out 3 tablespoons of the oil and add it to the lentil batter. Mix well, as this will make the bhajias crisp.

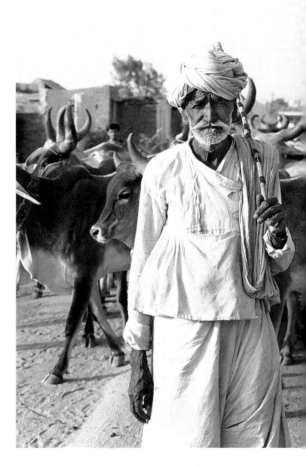

4 Using a tablespoon, drop spoonfuls of the lentil batter into the hot oil, 2–3 at a time depending on the size of the pan. Lower the heat to medium and fry the bhajias until golden brown.

5 Make sure that they are cooked through and keep going with the rest of the batter.

6 Serve hot with tomato ketchup and papaya chutney (page 83).

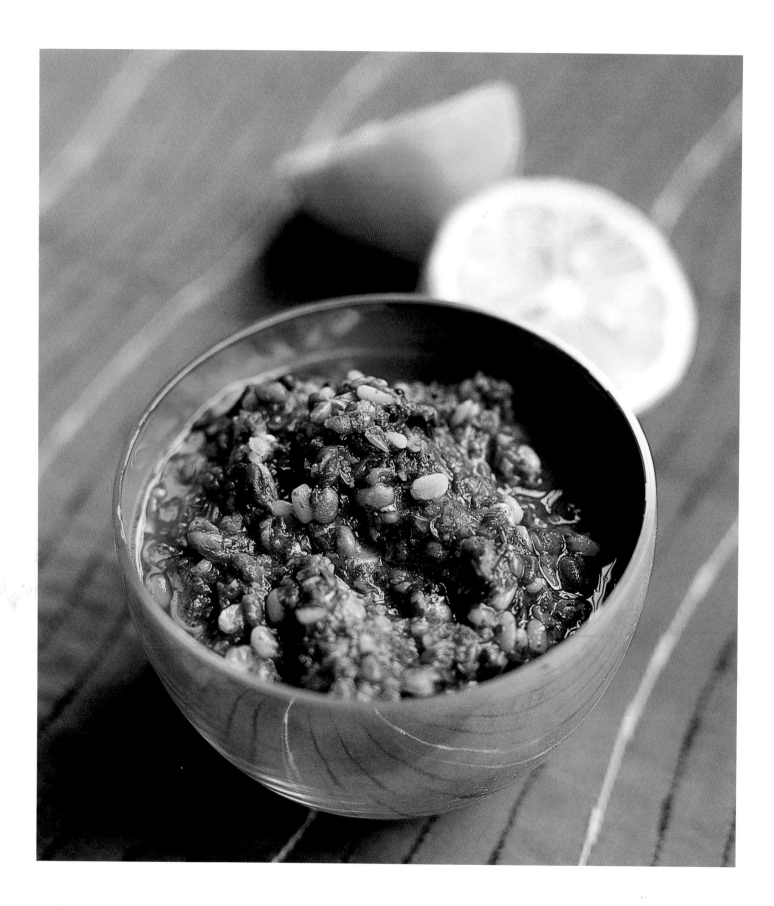

gujarati-style spinach with lentils
palak dal

Many regions in India combine lentils with vegetables to add flavour, nutrition and variety to a meal. I sometimes use fresh fenugreek leaves or even greens in this recipe. I like the vegetables to be really finely chopped so that they almost melt into the lentils. That is why I have suggested that you whizz the spinach in a blender.

Serves: 4
Preparation time: 10 minutes
Cooking time: 40 minutes

150g split mung beans, washed
  and drained
150g fresh spinach, washed, drained
  and chopped
2 tablespoons sunflower oil or ghee
1/2 teaspoon black mustard seeds
1/2 teaspoon cumin seeds
1 teaspoon grated fresh ginger
1/2 teaspoon garlic, minced
2 fresh green chillies, finely chopped
Juice of 1/2 lemon
Salt

1 Put the lentils into a heavy-bottomed saucepan and pour in double their volume of hot water. Bring to the boil, reduce the heat and simmer, covered, until the lentils are mushy, for about 25 minutes.

2 In the meantime, put the spinach in a blender and pulse 4–5 times, until it is quite fine but not mushy. Add the spinach to the lentils and allow to cook for 3–4 minutes.

3 Heat the oil or ghee in a small saucepan and add the mustard seeds. When they pop, add the cumin, then the ginger, garlic and green chillies almost at once. Pour this into the cooked lentils and simmer for 1 minute more. Remove from the heat.

4 Squeeze in the lemon juice and season with salt. Serve hot with plain rice and a good vegetable stir-fry.

curried black chickpeas
kala channa masala

This has to be one of the simplest recipes ever. You can substitute the black chickpeas with white ones. Black ones are coarser in taste and often associated with feasts cooked in honour of the Mother Goddess. Asafoetida is always added to beans and lentils to make them more digestible and to aid flatulence.

Serves: 4
Preparation time: 10 minutes
Cooking time: 10 minutes

1/2 teaspoon turmeric powder
1 teaspoon cumin powder
1 teaspoon coriander powder
1/2 teaspoon chilli powder
2 tablespoons sunflower oil
Pinch of asafoetida
Salt
400g tin black chickpeas, drained
1 tablespoon lemon juice
Few coriander leaves, chopped

1 Mix all the spice powders with about 4 tablespoons of water and reserve.

2 Heat the oil in a heavy-bottomed saucepan and add the asafoetida. Reduce the heat, stand back and pour in the spice liquid. Let it sizzle for 1 minute or so and add the salt and the chickpeas.

3 Pour in about 150ml of hot water and bring to the boil. Simmer for a couple of minutes, crushing a few of the peas with the back of the spoon to thicken the sauce. This should be fairly liquid but have some consistency. Take off the heat and serve hot, sprinkled with the lemon juice and coriander.

tangy lentils with crisp bread
dal pakwan

This is a popular Sindhi breakfast but I could eat it at any time of the day. The lentils must be cooked until soft but should still hold their shape. I soak them for at least 5–6 hours but, if you forget to do that (and I sometimes do), be prepared for a slightly longer cooking time. Also, this dish tastes so much more delicious when made with ghee rather than with oil. Serve with some sliced onions and a wedge of lemon and enjoy with friends!

Serves: 4
Preparation time: 15 minutes + soaking time
Cooking time: 1 hour

For the dal:
150g channa dal (split gram lentils), washed and soaked for 5–6 hours
1/4 teaspoon turmeric powder
1 tablespoon tamarind concentrate
Salt
1 tablespoon ghee
1/2 teaspoon garam masala powder
1/2 teaspoon red chilli powder
1/2 teaspoon cumin powder
1/2 teaspoon amchoor (dried mango) powder

For the pakwan:
300g plain flour, plus extra for flouring
1 tablespoon ghee
Pinch of salt
Sunflower oil for deep-frying

To make the dal:
1 Put the lentils in a heavy-bottomed saucepan with double their volume of water and set to boil. Add the turmeric and, when boiling, reduce the heat and simmer until the lentils are cooked, for about 30 minutes. The dal should not be mushy. I like to see the shape of the lentils rather than a sludge!

2 Stir in the tamarind concentrate and season with salt.

3 Heat the ghee in a small pan. When nearly smoking hot, take off the heat and add all the spice powders. Pour over the cooked dal at once or else the spices will burn. Serve hot with the crisp bread or pakwan.

To make the pakwan:
1 Mix the flour, ghee and salt and add enough warm water to make a soft dough.

2 Knead well, then divide the dough into cherry-sized balls and roll out into thin discs 8cm in diameter. Flour the board as necessary to prevent sticking.

3 Prick the discs all over with a fork.

4 Heat the oil in a deep saucepan or kadhai. When nearly smoking, reduce the heat and gently slide the pakwans in one at a time. Fry them until golden and crisp.

5 Drain and keep warm in tinfoil while you make the rest of the pakwans similarly.

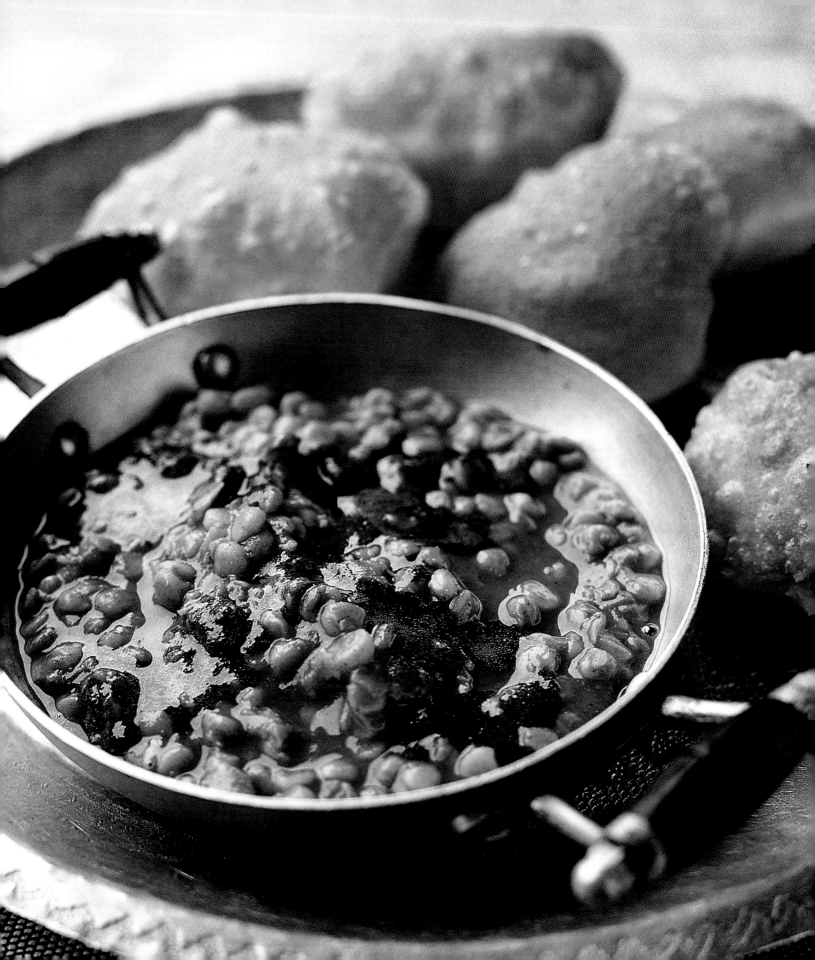

silky pumpkin in yoghurt
bhoplyache bharit

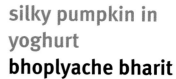

I love this dish for the sweet and silky feel that the pumpkin takes on when added to the yoghurt. Choose a very bright orange pumpkin for good flavour. Peel as thinly as possible, and take care to get rid of the seeds and membranes. I chop the chilli very finely or even bash it in a mortar as I think that there are few things worse than biting into a piece of chilli unintentionally!

Serves: 4
Preparation time: 15 minutes
Cooking time: 10 minutes

300g red pumpkin, peeled and diced
4 tablespoons natural yoghurt
Few coriander leaves, chopped
1 fresh green chilli, minced
Salt
3/4 teaspoon sugar
2 teaspoons sunflower oil
1 teaspoon black mustard seeds
1/2 teaspoon asafoetida

1 Put the pumpkin with enough hot water to cover it in a saucepan and bring to the boil. Reduce the heat and simmer for 3–4 minutes until soft. Drain and mash the pumpkin with a fork. (You can use the cooking liquid in a lentil dish or even for boiling rice.)

2 Add the yoghurt, coriander leaves, chilli, salt and sugar to the pumpkin.

3 Heat the oil in a small pan and add the mustard seeds. As they start popping, add the asafoetida. Pour this tempering over the pumpkin at once. Serve cool.

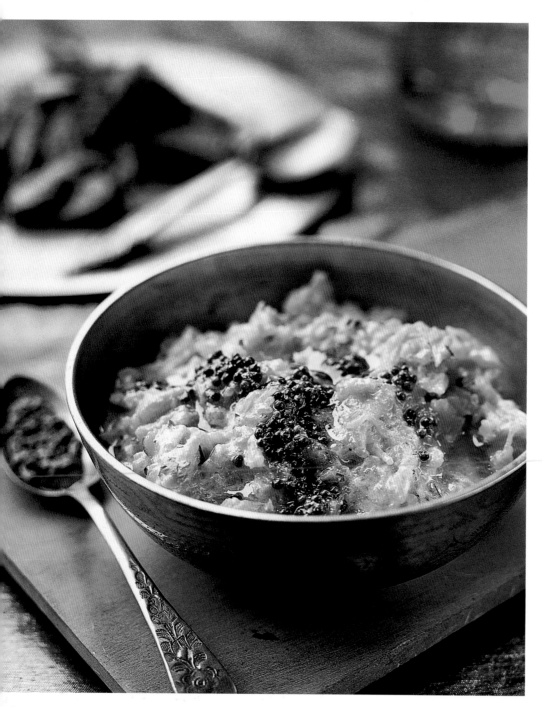

gujarati-style yoghurt yoghurt curry
gujarati kadhi

The real flavour of this curry is in the tempering, where spice seeds are fried in hot oil and then poured over it. I love the fenugreek seeds that smell rather sweet but have a bitter taste. The dish can be tricky sometimes as the yoghurt can split on cooking; to avoid this, use low heat and stir frequently. Kadhi is served with Mung Khichdi (page 79) and hot pickle.

Serves: 4
Preparation time: 15 minutes
Cooking time: 25 minutes

300g natural yoghurt
6 tablespoons gram flour
750ml water
Salt
3 teaspoons sugar
1 tablespoon sunflower oil
1/2 teaspoon black mustard seeds
1/2 teaspoon cumin seeds
Few curry leaves
1/4 teaspoon fenugreek seeds
10 black peppercorns
6 cloves
4 dried red chillies, deseeded and broken up

1 Whisk the yoghurt, flour, water, salt and sugar to a smooth mixture. Pour it into a heavy-bottomed saucepan and cook on high heat for 3–4 minutes. Reduce the heat and continue cooking, stirring frequently, until the curry is creamy. This should take about 15 minutes. The test is in the aroma that should not be of raw flour. Take off the heat and pour into a warmed dish.

2 Heat the oil in a small pan and add the mustard seeds. When they crackle add all the other ingredients. Swirl the pan for 1 minute and pour the oil and the spices over the yoghurt curry.

3 Serve hot. Gujarati kadhi can be made ahead, in which case heat gently, taking care not to boil the curry.

gram flour dumplings in spices
gatte ki subzi

A typical Rajasthani dish, this has quite a bit of oil and chilli powder and makes an occasional, indulgent treat, not for the faint hearted, with a roti or poories. The yoghurt must not be overheated as it will curdle.

Serves: 4
Preparation time: 10 minutes
Cooking time: 25 minutes

150g gram flour (besan)
1 teaspoon coriander powder
1 1/2 teaspoons red chilli powder
1 teaspoon turmeric powder
Salt
4 tablespoons ghee or sunflower oil
150g natural yoghurt
1/2 teaspoon cumin seeds

1 Mix the gram flour with half the coriander powder, a third of the chilli powder and half the turmeric. Season with salt. Pour in half the ghee or oil and enough water to make a stiff dough. Knead well. Make 4 thin, long rolls of the dough. Boil a pan of water and put the rolls in to simmer for 5–7 minutes. Drain and cool slightly. Cut these strips into small pieces called gatte.

2 Combine the remaining spice powders (reserving 1/2 teaspoon of the chilli powder) and the yoghurt in a heavy saucepan. Add the gatte and heat well without actually allowing them to boil. Simmer for 5 minutes and remove from the heat.

3 Warm the remaining oil in a small saucepan. Add the cumin seeds and, as they turn dark, add the remaining chilli powder. Pour this into the yoghurt mixture and serve hot.

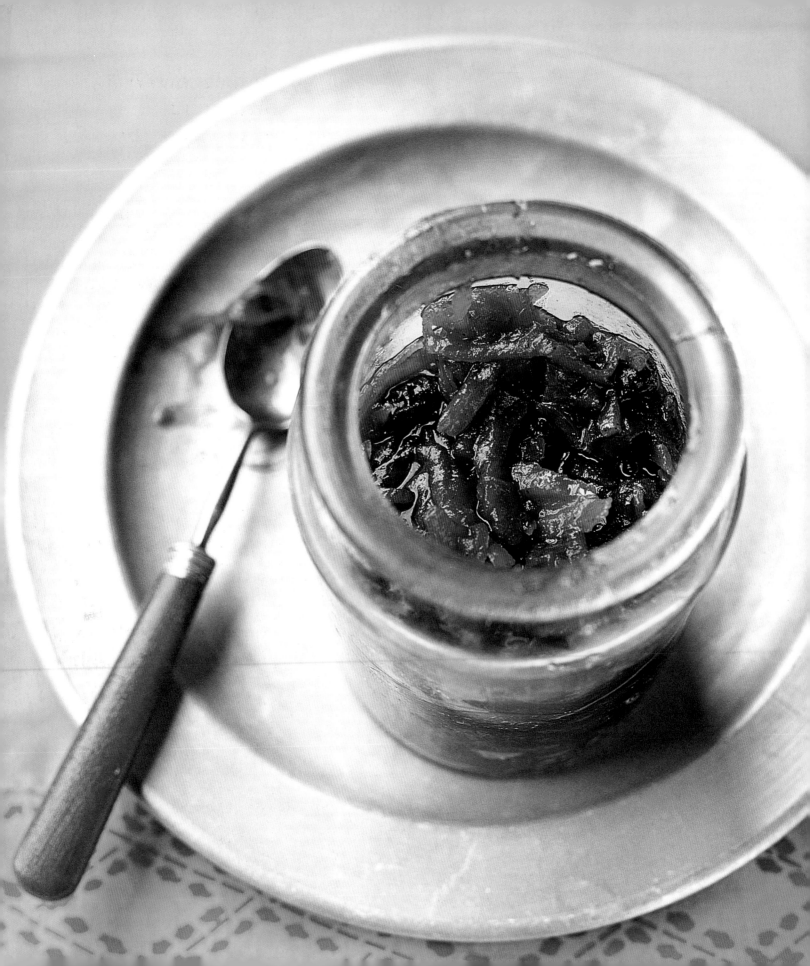

carrot and dried fruit pickle
gajar meva nu achaar

Whenever my Parsee friends invite me to a traditional wedding feast, I make sure to eat a good portion of lagan nu achaar which is the special wedding pickle with many kinds of dried fruit and berries. This is a simpler version of that sweet and sour relish and one that goes well with hot dal and rice.

Serves: 4
Preparation time: 15 minutes + overnight
 soaking
Cooking time: 40 minutes

2 tablespoons raisins
8 dried apricots, thinly sliced
6 dates, thinly sliced
150ml malt vinegar
150g carrots, peeled and grated
150g sugar
1/2 teaspoon garlic powder
1/2 teaspoon garam masala powder
1/2 teaspoon turmeric powder
1/2 teaspoon chilli powder
Salt

1 Soak the dried fruit overnight in 3 tablespoons of the vinegar.

2 To make the pickle, place the carrots with the sugar and the remaining vinegar in a heavy saucepan and cook on high heat until the sugar begins to melt but take care not to let it burn.

3 Add the garlic powder, reduce the heat and continue cooking until the carrots are soft.

4 Add the soaked, dried fruit and cook for about 5 minutes to blend.

5 Sprinkle in the spice powders and season with salt. Cook until thick and syrupy. Take off the heat, cool thoroughly and store in a clean, dry glass jar. This will keep for a couple of months in the fridge.

papaya chutney with mustard seeds
papaya chutney

There are countless papaya farms in Maharashtra therefore the fruit is inexpensive and sold very fresh. Indian papayas can be large and vary between the size of a honeydew melon and a watermelon! In fact, the little papayas we see in the West are known as disco papaya and are a novelty. Preparing a papaya means removing all the seeds and pith around the centre and, because it is so soft when ripe, this fruit hardly needs any cooking at all.

Serves: 4
Preparation time: 10 minutes
Cooking time: 10 minutes

80ml malt vinegar
80g sugar
4 tablespoons water
150g ripe papaya, peeled, seeds discarded
 and flesh diced
1/2 teaspoon garam masala powder
Salt
1 teaspoon sunflower oil
1 teaspoon black mustard seeds

1 Put the vinegar, sugar and water in a heavy-bottomed saucepan and bring to the boil. Reduce the heat and simmer until syrupy. Add in the papaya and garam masala powder and cook for a couple of minutes, stirring constantly. Season with salt and remove from the heat. Reserve.

2 Heat the oil in a small saucepan and add the mustard seeds. When they pop, pour over the chutney and mix well. Serve with rice and Kadhi (page 81). This chutney will keep for 1–2 days in the fridge.

potato and garlic balls encased in batter
batata vada

A classic dish from Maharashtra and one that is sold on every street corner in Mumbai. It is often eaten as a mid-morning snack or served at teatime with a cup of sweet tea. I prefer to use baking potatoes for this to get a really buttery texture but you can choose any variety you like. Eat them fresh as keeping them for any length of time makes the outer shell of batter go limp.

Serves: 4
Preparation time: 30 minutes
Cooking time: 15 minutes

300g potatoes, peeled, boiled and mashed
Salt
1/2 teaspoon turmeric powder
2 tablespoons chopped coriander leaves
2 fresh green chillies, finely chopped
2 cloves garlic, finely chopped
2 tablespoons sunflower oil
1 teaspoon black mustard seeds
Large pinch of asafoetida
1 teaspoon cumin seeds

For the batter:
150g gram flour
Large pinch of bicarbonate of soda
1/2 teaspoon turmeric powder
Salt
Sunflower oil for deep-frying

1 Combine the potatoes, salt, turmeric, coriander leaves, green chillies and garlic in a mixing bowl.

2 Heat the oil in a small pan and add the mustard seeds. When they crackle add the asafoetida and cumin seeds. Pour this into the potato mixture and mix well.

3 Divide the potato mixture into 8 small balls and reserve.

4 Make a batter of pouring consistency with the gram flour, bicarbonate of soda, turmeric and salt and as much water as is needed.

5 Heat the oil in a deep frying pan or kadhai.

6 When it is nearly smoking, dip each potato ball in the batter and deep-fry it until golden. Reduce the heat to prevent the balls from browning too quickly. Serve hot with tomato ketchup as a snack or with a main meal as an accompaniment.

bananas stuffed with coriander chutney
bharela kela

If you have ever wondered what to do with slightly overripe bananas that have not gone mushy, here is the perfect recipe. Traditionally these are made with ripe plantains which are firm and sweet but dessert bananas also work well too. My mother makes these for me even now as a special treat and, unusual as they may sound, they taste delicious with everything. I like them a little over-fried with a few burnt bits.

Serves: 4
Preparation time: 15 minutes
Cooking time: 15 minutes

2 good handfuls of coriander leaves
3 cloves garlic, peeled
3cm piece of ginger, peeled and chopped
2 fresh green chillies, roughly chopped
4 tablespoons desiccated coconut
Salt
1/2 teaspoon sugar
4 ripe but firm bananas
Sunflower oil for shallow frying

black eyed beans with coconut and raisins
lobhia ka salad

1 Put the coriander into a blender with the garlic, ginger, chillies and coconut.

2 Whizz to a fine paste with a few tablespoons of water. Season with salt and add the sugar. Mix well and reserve.

3 Peel the bananas and make a shallow slit along the top of each one, keeping them whole. Stuff a little of the coriander chutney into each banana. Any extra chutney can be served on the side or frozen for later use. (This makes an excellent accompaniment to a meal and freezes very well.)

4 Heat some oil in a wide saucepan and shallow-fry the bananas, turning them occasionally until they are golden brown and slightly caramelised. Serve warm.

This is a great all-rounder, good for lunch, brunch or to accompany a more substantial meal. Also, what could be simpler? I love the creaminess of black eyed beans and what a great way to add protein and fibre to a meal! I sometimes stir some natural yoghurt into this salad to turn it into an exceptionally delicious raita. Toss a few finely chopped green chillies on top if you like a bit of heat.

Serves: 4
Preparation time: 10 minutes
Cooking time: nil

400g tin black eyed beans, drained
Salt
1/2 teaspoon sugar
4 tablespoons freshly grated or
   desiccated coconut
2 teaspoons raisins
1 teaspoon lemon juice
Few chopped coriander leaves

Mix all the ingredients together and serve at once.

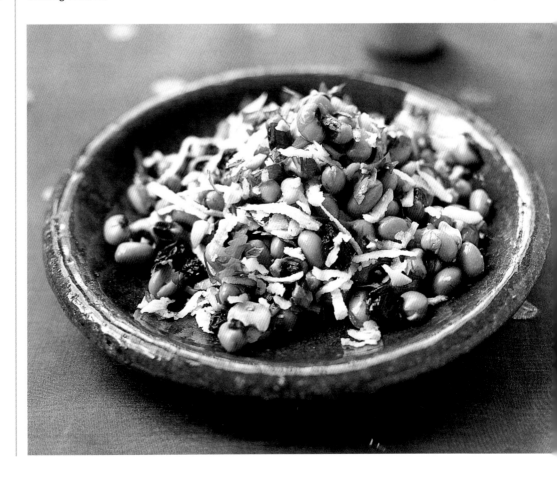

quick no-fuss mango ice cream
keri nu ice cream

Both Gujarat and Maharashtra are famous for their delicious seasonal mangoes. Kesar from the former and Alphonso from the latter being the most popular. During the mango season in the summer, most households make all sorts of wonderful recipes from this fruit. Ice cream is very quick to make but be sure you use soft, non-fibrous mangoes. You might want to move the ice cream from the freezer to the fridge half an hour before serving it to soften it slightly.

Serves: 4
Preparation time: 30 minutes + 7–8 hours
  freezing time
Cooking time: nil

300ml double cream
200ml cold milk
200ml sweetened condensed milk
300ml fresh mango pulp (or tinned pulp if
  using out of season)

1 Pour the cream into a mixing bowl and beat it until it is thick and fluffy, for about 3–4 minutes. Take care not to overdo this or else you will end up with butter!

2 Beat the milk and condensed milk together in a separate bowl until well blended.

3 Fold the milk and condensed milk mixture into the cream, then the mango pulp as well. Tip into an ice cream tray and freeze for about 7-8 hours until firm.

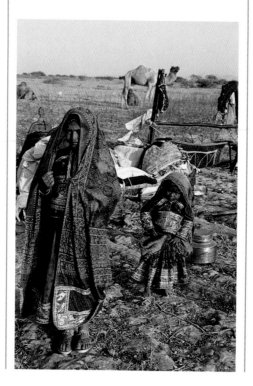

mango and yoghurt medley
amrakhand

This is the traditional method of making Amrakhand which tastes rich and delicious. I have a lighter version made with Greek yoghurt that cuts out the hanging up of the set yoghurt. Amrakhand is very popular in Maharashtra and its close cousin Shrikhand, made in exactly the same way but without the mango, is popular in Gujarat as well.

Serves: 4
Preparation time: 15 minutes + 5 hours
  draining time
Cooking time: nil

900g full fat set bio yoghurt
About 6 tablespoons caster sugar, or to taste
150ml mango pulp (tinned or fresh)
Pinch of cardamom powder
2 tablespoons crushed pistachio nuts

1 Tie the yoghurt in a clean piece of muslin and hang up to drain off the whey. I usually do this over the kitchen sink.

2 When the yoghurt is quite dry, scoop it out of the cloth and place it in a bowl. Beat well with a wooden spoon or whisk, adding the caster sugar a little at a time.

3 When the yoghurt is light and fluffy in texture, stir in the mango pulp and cardamom, and spoon into decorative glasses and chill. Serve sprinkled with the pistachio nuts.

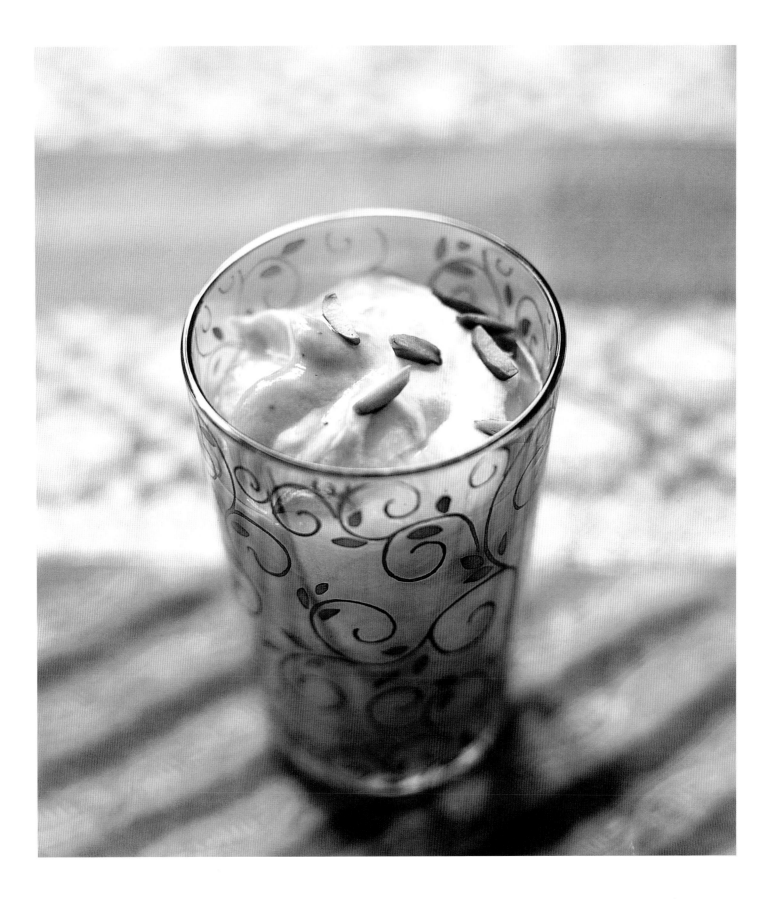

sweet sparkly diamonds
bombay ice halwa

This is a popular sweet in Mumbai, earlier known as Bombay, as is its cousin, the sticky Bombay chewy halwa. That is made with wheat flour and, to eat some versions of it, one needs fangs instead of teeth. This one is fine and glassy and quite delicate in taste. It keeps well in the fridge for up to a week.

Serves: 4
Preparation time: 10 minutes
Cooking time: 45 minutes

150g very fine semolina
150g ghee
600ml milk
300g sugar
1 tablespoon rose water
1 tablespoon flaked almonds
1/2 teaspoon powdered cardamom seeds
Large pinch of saffron

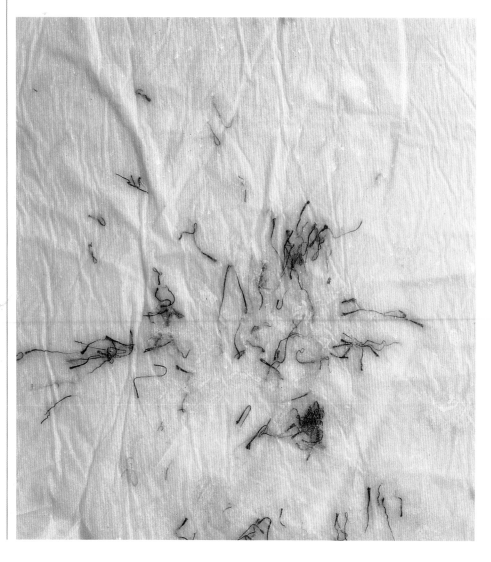

1 Put the semolina, ghee, milk and sugar in a large, heavy saucepan and cook on high heat until the mixture begins to bubble. Reduce the heat and continue cooking, stirring all the while, until the mixture thickens into a very soft ball. Take off the heat.

2 Add the rose water and mix well with a wooden spoon. The mixing should be almost like kneading because this brings a shine to the finished product.

3 Take a sheet of greaseproof paper and place a large spoonful of the semolina dough on it. Cover with another sheet and roll out the dough as quickly as possible into a thick, flat cake.

4 Remove the top sheet of paper and sprinkle some of the almonds, powdered cardamom and saffron strands onto the semolina cake. Replace the greaseproof paper on top of the cake and roll again very quickly until the dough is very thin, almost like a sheet of ice. Repeat with the rest of the dough.

5 Cut into roughly 16 diamond shapes and allow to cool. Serve cold. Store between sheets of greaseproof paper to prevent the diamonds from sticking.

sweet saffron rice
keshar bhaat

This is quite a festive dish from Maharashtra although versions of it are made all over the country. I like to cook the rice until slightly soft and serve it warm especially in the winter. The amount of ghee may seem excessive but this is quite an indulgent sweet and can be a great treat on a cold winter's evening!

Serves: 4
Preparation time: 10 minutes
Cooking time: 30 minutes

150g basmati rice, washed and drained
4 tablespoons ghee
80g sugar
Large pinch of saffron strands, soaked in
** 1 tablespoon milk**
50g raisins
50g cashew nuts, roughly crushed
Large pinch of powdered cardamom

1 Put the rice in a heavy-bottomed saucepan with double its volume of hot water and bring to the boil. Reduce the heat, stir the rice, cover the pan and simmer until cooked, for about 10 minutes.

2 Add the ghee and sugar and continue cooking on low heat, stirring constantly.

3 Add the saffron along with the milk, raisins and cashew nuts. Stir gently until well blended and the rice has turned a yellowy-orange colour. Take off the heat, stir in the cardamom powder and serve warm.

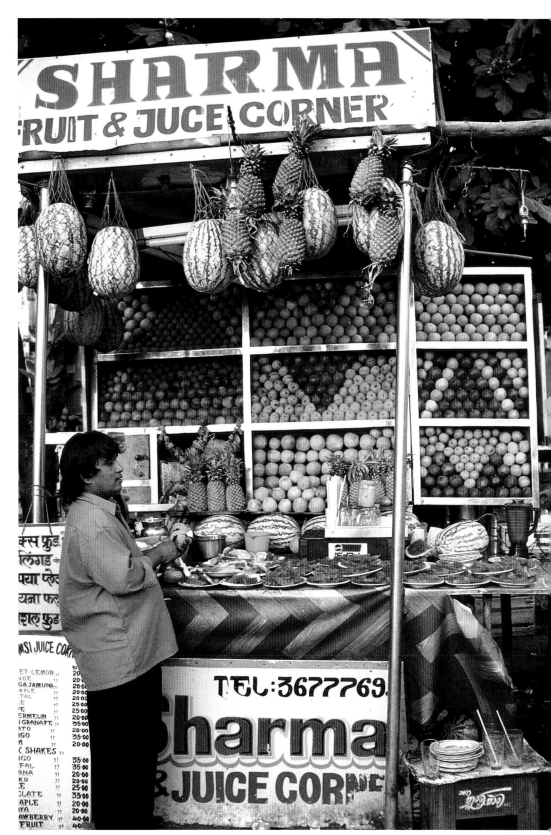

coconut and poppy seed pastry
karanji

A favourite childhood memory of mine was eating these during Diwali, the Hindu festival of lights. My grandmother would make batches days before the festival with a strict warning that we were not to touch them until the day arrived. The temptation almost always proved too great and my cousin and I would sneak a few to eat under the table, my favourite hiding place at the time!

Serves: 4
Preparation time: 40 minutes
Cooking time: 30 minutes

300g plain flour, plus extra for flouring
2 teaspoons sunflower oil
Large pinch of salt

For the filling:
150g soft brown sugar
300g freshly grated or desiccated coconut
2 teaspoons white poppy seeds, dry-roasted
2 teaspoons raisins
1/2 teaspoon powdered cardamom seeds
Sunflower oil for deep-frying

1 Make a stiff dough with the flour, oil, salt and water as needed. Reserve.

2 Combine the sugar, coconut, poppy seeds, raisins and cardamom powder in a heavy saucepan and set on high heat. As the sugar melts, reduce the heat and cook for a few minutes to blend everything, taking care not to let the mixture burn. Take off the heat and allow the mixture to cool.

3 Divide the dough into 12 equal-sized balls. Roll each one out to a thin disc about 5cm in diameter, dusting it with a little flour if necessary.

4 Place a little of the coconut mixture in the centre of the disc. If the mixture is slightly runny, strain it and use the liquid as a dipping sauce. Fold the disc in half to make a half-moon shape and seal the edges properly or the filling will come out during the frying.

5 Heat the oil in a deep frying pan and fry each pastry individually until golden. Remove with a slotted spoon and drain on absorbent paper. Serve at room temperature.

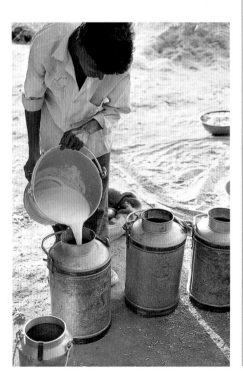

spiced tea
masala chai

If you travel through Gujarat, you will find that you are offered this version of tea everywhere. People here love sweet, spicy tea that leaves a zing on the tongue. It is especially great as an after-dinner digestive and helps to wash down the grease and spice of a meal. Fennel is known to promote good digestion and it is often boiled in water, strained out and the water fed to even very tiny babies.

Serves: 4
Preparation time: 5 minutes
Cooking time: 15 minutes

1 teaspoon fennel seeds
5 black peppercorns
3 green cardamom pods, bruised
600ml hot water
3 teabags
Sugar to taste
Dash of milk

1 Crush the fennel seeds, peppercorns and cardamoms in a mortar. Put the spices in a heavy-bottomed saucepan and pour in the water. Bring to the boil.

2 Reduce the heat and simmer for 3–4 minutes. The water will have turned golden.

3 Add the teabags and simmer for 1 minute or so. Take off the heat, strain through a fine strainer and discard the spices and teabags.

4 Serve sweetened with sugar if desired and add a dash of milk.

rose-flavoured ice cream float
bombay falooda

Small shops that are run by the Iranians or Muslims who settled in Bombay many years ago sell this delicacy. It also has tiny subja seeds that are cooked and put at the bottom of each glass but I have omitted them in this recipe as they are so hard to find outside of India. Rose syrup is sweet, red and fragrant and, in India, it is also mixed with water and served as rose sherbet.

Serves: 4
Preparation time: 15 minutes
Cooking time: nil

6 tablespoons rice noodles, broken into
    short lengths
600ml milk
Sugar
4 teaspoons rose syrup (available in
    Indian shops)
4 scoops of vanilla ice cream

1 Put the noodles in a pan with enough water to cover them and bring to the boil. Stir, reduce the heat and simmer until soft. Drain and rinse under cold running water so that they do not get sticky.

2 Mix the milk, sugar to taste and rose syrup.

3 Divide the noodles between 4 tall glasses and pour the rose milk over them. Chill well. Just before serving, float a scoop of vanilla ice cream on top of each glass.

cumin seed cooler
jaljeera

This is a popular drink in Rajasthan and Gujarat where the summers are dry and fierce. The cumin acts as a digestive and this drink is served with main meals. Indian rock salt is mined from stone quarries and has a strong aroma that goes well with tamarind or yoghurt dishes. If you cannot find rock salt, sea salt can be used instead.

Serves: 4
Preparation time: 45 minutes
Cooking time: nil

2 teaspoons cumin seeds
1 tablespoon tamarind concentrate
600ml hot water
6 tablespoons soft brown sugar
1/2 teaspoon chilli powder
1 teaspoon rock salt
Few coriander leaves, finely chopped
Few mint leaves, finely chopped

1 Dry-roast the cumin seeds in a small pan. When they turn dark, pour into a mortar and bash them until fine and powdery; reserve.

2 Dilute the tamarind in the water. Stir in the sugar, chilli powder, rock salt and reserved cumin powder and mix well. Allow the mixture to cool.

3 Stir in the coriander and mint leaves and chill the jaljeera in the fridge. Serve cold.

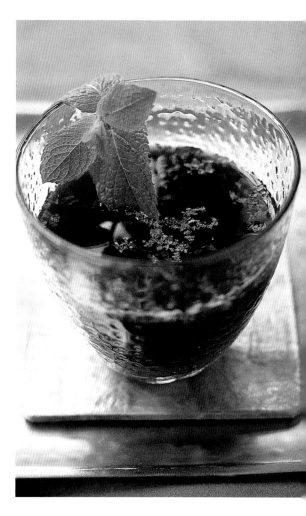

goda masala

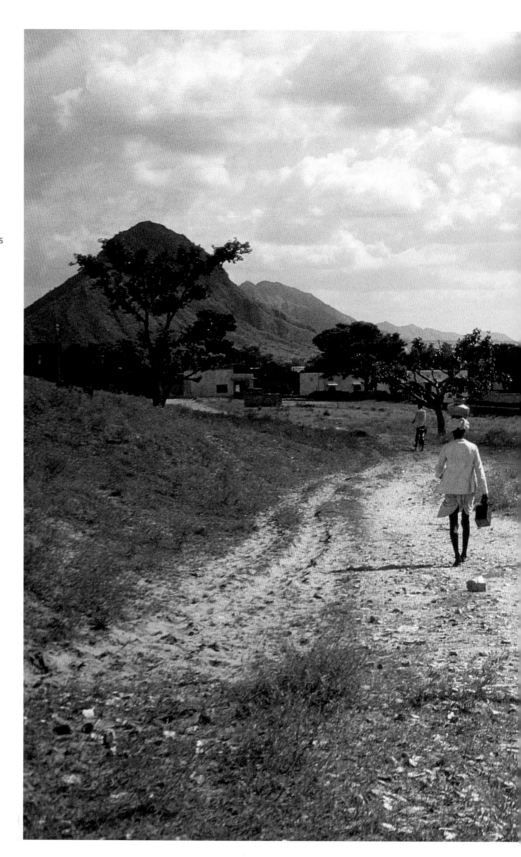

Goda Masala which literally means sweet spice is used in certain parts of Maharashtra, such as the city of Pune, to enhance the flavour of vegetarian cooking. The masala is a black aromatic powder with a burnt sweetness which comes from the coconut in the mixture. It can be added before or after the main ingredient to vary the taste from strong to subtle. Make enough for one-time use. It can be sprinkled onto the Aamti (page 80) or the Farasbeechi Bhaji (page 67) or into a variety of lentil or vegetable dishes.

1 teaspoon sunflower oil
Seeds from 2 green cardamom pods
Small stick of cinnamon
2 cloves
1 bay leaf
5 black peppercorns
$^1/_2$ teaspoon coriander seeds
2 tablespoons desiccated coconut
1 teaspoon white poppy seeds

1 Heat the oil in a small saucepan and fry the cardamom seeds, cinnamon, cloves, bay leaf, peppercorns and coriander seeds for a couple of minutes until the cloves swell.

2 Add the coconut and poppy seeds and continue cooking, stirring constantly, until the coconut is well browned.

3 Take off the heat, cool slightly and grind to a fine powder in a coffee mill (or a pestle and mortar). Store in an airtight container.

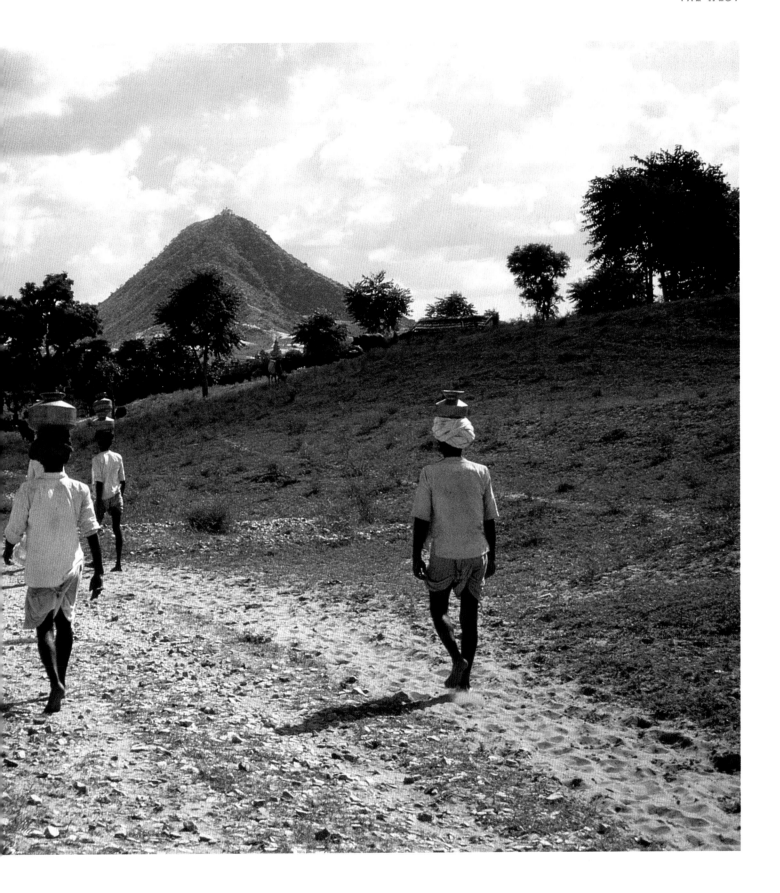

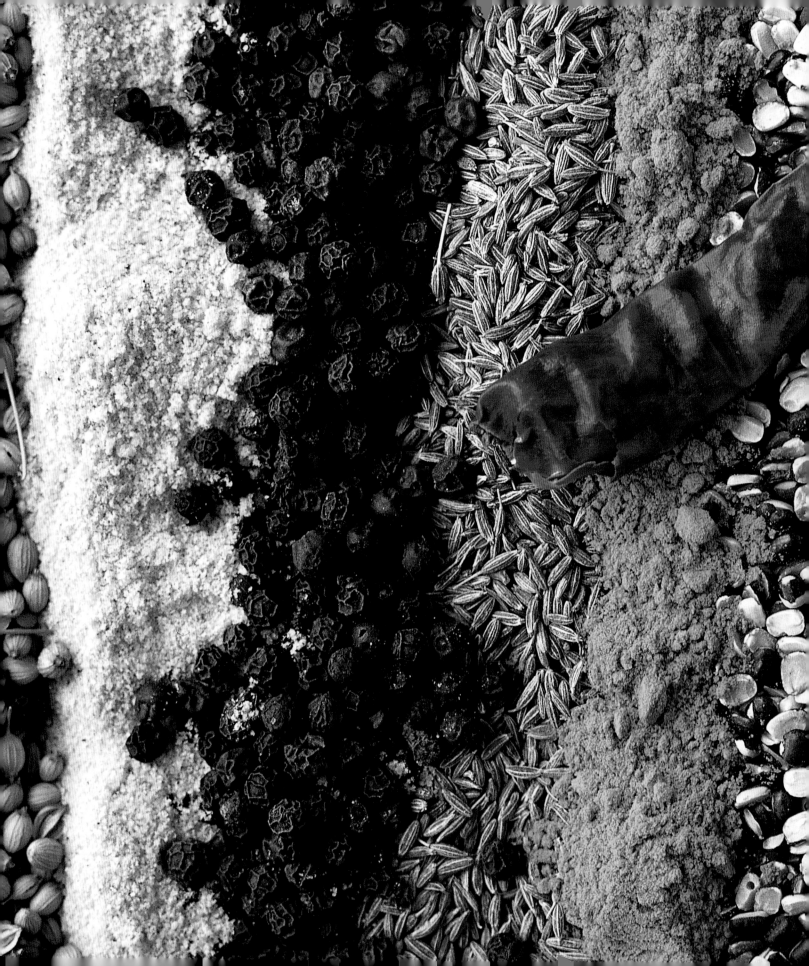

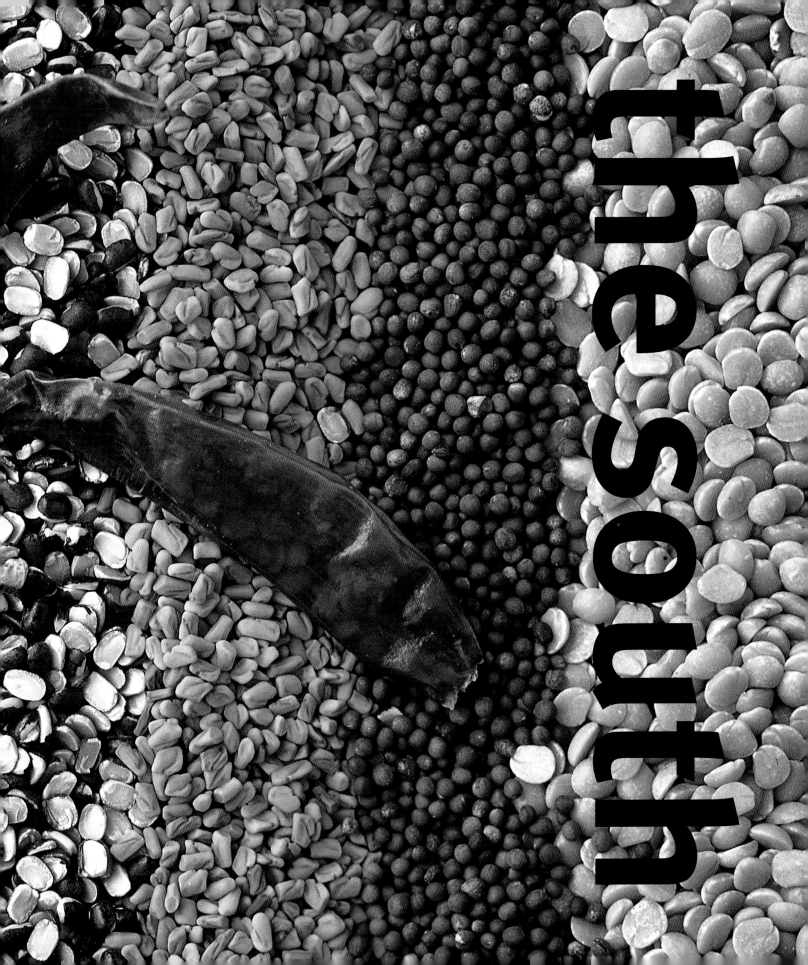

the south

This section deals with the cooking of Tamil Nadu, Andhra Pradesh, Karnataka, Kerala and Goa. The south was less affected by invasions (although many foreign powers did make forays) than the north and many south Indians feel that their style of cooking is the original style of India.

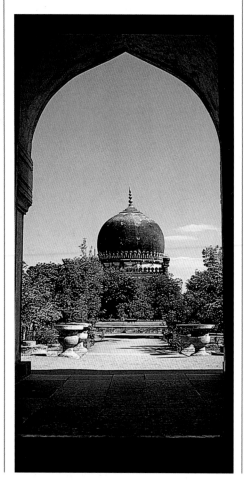

tamil nadu

Tamil Nadu is situated on the south-eastern coast of India by the Bay of Bengal. Some of the oldest and most famous of all Hindu temples are here, such as the Nataraja temple in Chidambaram and the Brihadeeshwara temple at Tanjore. Tamil culture is resplendent with classical literature and dance, fascinating bronze sculptures and awe inspiring architecture. One sees the best of the Dravidian way of life here. Chennai is the capital and home to some of the finest artists and artisans in the country. Fine, shimmering silks come from Kanjeevaram, beautiful stone-studded temple jewellery is crafted in the jewellery quarter of each town. The people of Tamil Nadu are disciplined and adhere greatly to tradition. Worship, education, the arts and food are all treated with great respect and the social order is maintained through a strict hierarchy and the passing down of knowledge about how things should be from one generation to the next. For religious reasons, most Tamilian food is vegetarian, very fresh and fragrant. A meal here is made mainly of rice served in three different courses. First with sambhar, a thick lentil dish flavoured with fresh vegetables. Then comes rasam, a thinner version of the sambhar and one that is slurped up along with the rice (a great experience!) and, finally, yoghurt and rice to cool one in the strong southern heat. Other rice preparations include coconut rice, tamarind rice, lemon rice and countless other flavourings that provide variety and taste. Black pepper, red chillies, cumin, turmeric, coriander, fenugreek and mustard seeds are used in the cooking of vegetables such as plantains, yams, gourds and greens.

andhra pradesh

Situated in the central south, Andhra Pradesh is a combination of Hindu vegetarianism and Muslim meat cookery. Before Partition, the beautiful city of Hyderabad was ruled by the Nizam, a man reputed to be the wealthiest in the world at the time. His kitchens produced some of the richest and tastiest fare and many of his favourite recipes have become trademarks of the region. Hyderabadi cookery is characterised by slow cooking methods. Many dishes are tempered, that is the spices are fried in hot oil and poured over at the last minute.

An Andhra meal is also served in courses. In Hyderabad, it is the Mughlai set of courses, replete with kebabs and biryanis. In other parts of the state, the food is mainly vegetarian and again with rice forming a staple part of it.

Andhra Pradesh is most famous for its many pickles and chutneys. The hot, spicy food is set off by chutneys made of just about anything – from mangoes, aubergines and tomatoes to ginger and gongura, an aromatic reddish-green leafy vegetable not seen in any other state. The food of Andhra Pradesh is known for its chilli heat but the combination of flavours is unique and almost addictive!

karnataka

kerala

goa

Karnataka lies just under Maharashtra and boasts of cites such as Bangalore. The Kannadigas, as the people of this state are called, are artistic and talented. Their arts and crafts, sandalwood sculptures and jewel-like silks are famous all over the country. Karnataka has also given India a classic restaurant style. Udipi, a small temple town famous for its Brahmin cooks, has a beautiful, ancient Krishna temple and the Brahmins will first offer all cooked food to the Gods before serving it to devotees. The best pancakes (dosas), rice cakes (idlis) and luscious chutneys are made in Udipi and tiny cafés that serve such food (called Udipi restaurants) can be seen in every city of India and further abroad as well. They are wholly vegetarian and the food is 'pure' and fragrant. Coconuts, tamarind, beans and kokum, which is a sour purple fruit, are used in the cooking. Coconut is considered the fruit of the Gods and is used in ritual worship. Every home will have a store of fresh coconuts.

My ancestors who are Saraswat Brahmins come from Karnataka and as a child I would spend my summers in a little village called Gokarn just off the coast. There I ate fresh curries flavoured with coriander and cumin, roomfuls of mangoes and many unusual dishes made with jackfruit and breadfruit. We would wait for the breadfruit to fall off the trees and then my aunt would peel and slice them, rub them with chilli and salt and deep-fry the slices. Heaven! Pure jaggery or a slice of star fruit was often the pudding after dinner and some of my best childhood memories are of stoning tamarind trees to get at the sour-sweet fruit.

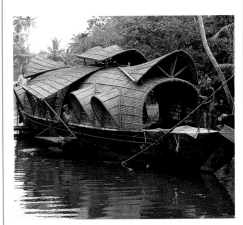

Kerala is the southernmost state and again, it is rich in the arts. The classical dance form of Kathakali comes from here as does a variety of sculpture and craftwork. Kerala is known for its education system and for its matriarchal society where property is handed down from mother to daughter. In this state lies the Periyar wildlife reserve, home to the Indian elephant. The serving of a meal is an art form; traditionally, a banana leaf is used as a plate and all the courses are served at once. Rice, lentils, vegetables, chutneys, crisp accompaniments and sweets, all flavoured with coconut, form a fragrant feast. Curry leaves and mustard seeds are used to temper many dishes. Preparations such as thorans or (vegetable stir-fries), sambhar (lentils with tamarind) and dishes cooked with plantains, yams and cabbage are popular.

Kerala has many communities and therefore there is a great mix of cuisines. The Syrian Christians, Malabar Muslims, Jews from Cochin and the Hindus all live and work peacefully and share a culture that is vibrant and yet gentle.

Goan food is a marvellous blend of the various influences that have been a part of the region's history. The main communities are the Christians and the Hindus. For both the main food is fish, which is natural because Goa is on the coast and has many beautiful beaches. Fishing boats go out early into the Arabian Sea and are back, laden with seafood by dawn.

Goa was a Portuguese colony for many years and its food shows many a Portuguese influence in the Christian cooking. The Hindu fare has more or less been unaffected by them. Goan Christians eat much more meat and their specialities include vindaloos, xacuttis and sorpotels. The exchange of recipes seems mutual. Today, Portuguese cookery boasts of arroz doce, a sweet rice preparation that is not unlike the Goan kheer or pais.

Hindu cookery is mainly from the Saraswat community that uses local produce such as coconuts, cashew nuts and mangoes. Spices such as asafoetida, mustard seeds and tirphal are used to flavour many vegetables like bitter gourds, pumpkins and plantain. Sweets are made of lentils and rice while fruits of the region include pineapples. The special liquor of Goa is feni made with toddy or palm liquor. It is known for its fiery strength and people say that if you have been drinking it you feel its power only when you stand up!

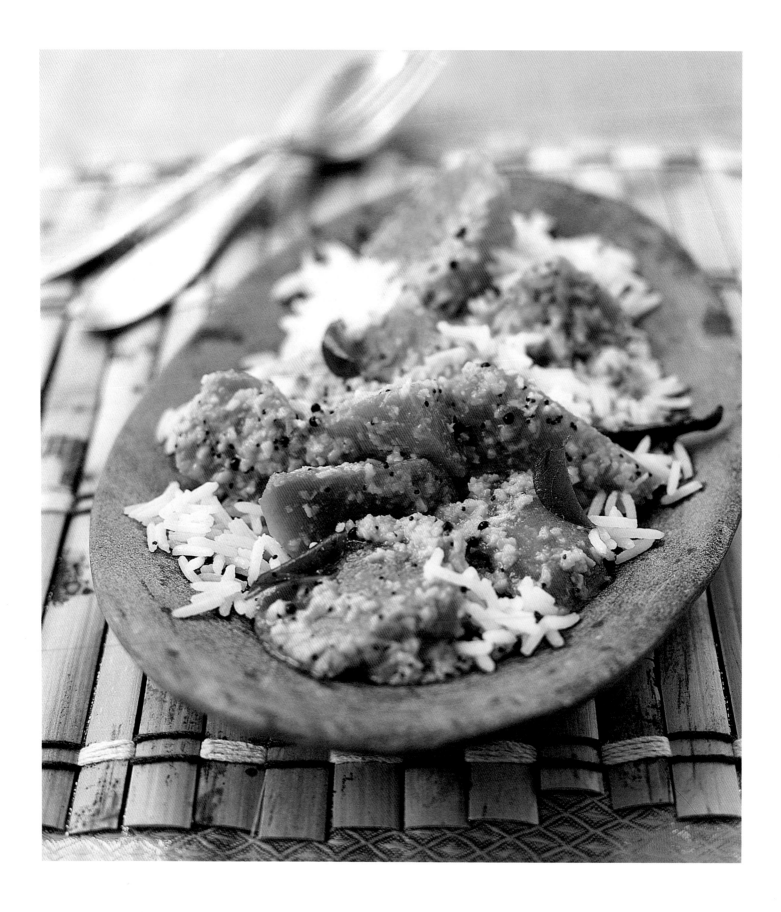

red pumpkin with cashew nuts
tiyya gummadi

Andhra Pradesh has a long coastline along the Bay of Bengal. The cuisine is a rich variety of vegetables cooked in spices and milk. The curry leaves in this recipe add a burst of fresh flavour and, in India, they are often grown at home in pots or in the garden. They are cheap and often a vegetable seller will toss a few stalks into your bag free of charge. They are best used fresh although they can be dried for ease of storage.

Serves: 4
Preparation time: 15 minutes
Cooking time: 30 minutes

150g freshly grated or dessicated coconut
8 cashew nuts
1 tablespoon poppy seeds
2 tablespoons sunflower oil
1/2 teaspoon black mustard seeds
2 dried red chillies, broken in half and seeds shaken out
6 curry leaves
1/2 teaspoon turmeric powder
300g red pumpkin, peeled and chopped into 1cm dice
3 tablespoons soft brown sugar
Salt
150ml milk

1 Put the coconut, cashew nuts, poppy seeds and 4 tablespoons of water in a blender and grind to a paste. Add water as necessary to make a fine paste. Reserve.

2 Heat the oil in a heavy-bottomed saucepan and add the mustard seeds. When they pop, add the chillies and the curry leaves. Sprinkle in the turmeric and pour in the coconut paste at once. Stir to blend.

3 Add the pumpkin and a couple of tablespoons of water.

4 Add the sugar and salt. Pour in the milk and bring to the boil. Reduce the heat and simmer until the pumpkin is just tender but still holds its shape, about 10–12 minutes. Serve hot with rice.

vegetables in yoghurt
avial

This recipe is from palm-fringed Kerala, where it is served as part of a sit-down feast on a fresh green banana leaf that is thrown away after use. Best of biodegradable! The root vegetables taste wonderful in this recipe and you can also add green peas or any kind of green beans.

Serves: 4
Preparation time: 25 minutes
Cooking time: 35 minutes

80g desiccated coconut
2 fresh green chillies
1/4 teaspoon cumin seeds
10 black peppercorns
300g mixed vegetables, peeled, cubed and steamed (potatoes, raw banana, red pumpkin, yam)
150g natural yoghurt, seasoned with salt
10 curry leaves
Salt

1 Grind the coconut, chillies, cumin seeds and peppercorns with some water to a fine paste in a blender.

2 Add this paste to the cooked vegetables and pour in about 150ml of water. Bring to the boil, then simmer for 5 minutes to blend.

3 Beat the yoghurt and the salt and pour it into the pan. Simmer for a couple of minutes, then add the curry leaves and stir. Remove from the heat and serve hot with plain rice.

potatoes with green and black peppercorns
kurumulaku alu

I went to the Periyar elephant reserve in Kerala as a child and I still remember being driven through cool hills where pepper vines curl around trees and fragrance the air. There are more than 24 varieties of pepper grown in south India. Green peppercorns are fresher tasting than the black ones but not as hot. Some Indian shops around the world sell them fresh but they are easier to find bottled in brine.

Serves: 4
Preparation time: 10 minutes
Cooking time: 35 minutes

2 tablespoons sunflower oil
1/2 teaspoon cumin seeds
10 black peppercorns, crushed
1 large onion, finely sliced
1 teaspoon ginger-garlic paste (page 11)
4 dried red chillies
1/2 teaspoon turmeric powder
300g potatoes, peeled and chopped into
  2–3cm dice
Salt
3 tablespoons desiccated coconut
1 tablespoon fresh (or bottled in brine)
  green peppercorns

1 Heat the sunflower oil in a heavy-bottomed saucepan and fry the cumin seeds and crushed pepper for 1 minute. Add the onion and fry until soft, for about 4–5 minutes.

2 Add the ginger-garlic paste and the red chillies and stir a couple of times.

3 Tip in the turmeric powder and the potatoes. Season with salt. Mix well and pour in a few tablespoons of hot water to prevent the potatoes from sticking. Cover and cook until the potatoes hold their shape but are done. Stir in the coconut, heat through and serve at once with the green peppercorns sprinkled on top.

aubergines with tamarind and cashew nuts
bagare baingan

Although this recipe looks a bit complicated, it is possibly one of the first things I learned to make entirely on my own. The results were so successful that it has remained a firm favourite. I sometimes like to add a bit of jaggery for a hint of sweetness. Choose small aubergines that have virtually no seeds for the best flavour.

Serves: 4
Preparation time: 15 minutes
Cooking time: 40 minutes

2 tablespoons sunflower oil
4 dried red chillies, broken in half and
  seeds shaken out
15 cashew nuts
1 tablespoon coriander seeds
1 medium onion, sliced
4 tablespoons freshly grated or
  desiccated coconut
1 tablespoon white sesame seeds
1 tablespoon ginger-garlic paste (page 11)
Salt
1/2 teaspoon turmeric powder
300g small aubergines
1 teaspoon tamarind concentrate, diluted in
  150ml hot water
1 tablespoon soft brown sugar

1 Heat half the oil in a heavy-bottomed saucepan and fry the chillies, cashew nuts and coriander seeds. In a few seconds, add the onion. Stir often and, when the onion turns golden brown, add the coconut and sesame seeds.

2 When the coconut starts to turn brown, add the ginger-garlic paste and mix well. Take off the heat, cool slightly and whizz in a blender with a few tablespoons of water to make a fine paste. Season the paste with salt, stir in the turmeric and reserve.

3 Keeping the stem intact slit the aubergines twice in a cross nearly all the way to the stem. Stuff each aubergine with the reserved spice paste. If there is some left over, reserve this for the sauce.

4 Heat the remaining oil in a heavy-bottomed saucepan or kadhai. Place the aubergines into the pan and fry for a couple of minutes. Add the extra stuffing if available.

5 Pour in the tamarind water, sprinkle in the sugar and bring to the boil. Reduce the heat and simmer until the aubergines are cooked through. Serve hot with Lemon Rice with Cashews and Peanuts (page 120), with a sprinkling of chopped coriander leaves, if desired.

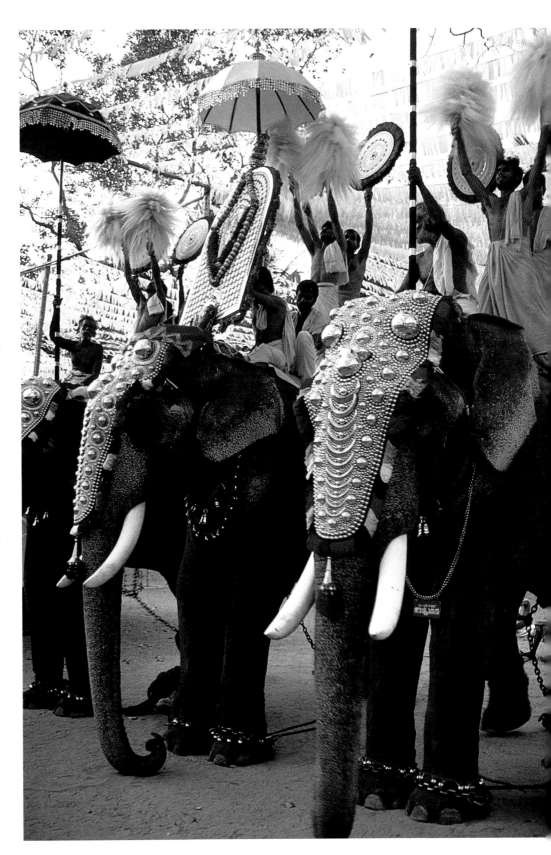

sweet and sour okra
kodel

Okra is a difficult vegetable to cook if you don't know a few tricks. Adding water to it will make it slimier but adding an acid, in this case the tamarind, will help get rid of the slime. The sauce should be thick, almost the consistency of custard. You can substitute the okra for any soft vegetable such as pumpkin or doodhi.

Serves: 4
Preparation time: 15 minutes
Cooking time: 40 minutes

2 tablespoons sunflower oil
3 dried red chillies, broken in half and
  seeds shaken out
1/2 teaspoon cumin seeds
6 black peppercorns
1 teaspoon white poppy seeds
1/2 teaspoon fenugreek seeds
1 medium onion, sliced
5 tablespoons freshly grated or
  desiccated coconut
1/2 teaspoon black mustard seeds
300g okra, washed, dried and sliced into
  long strips
1 tablespoon tamarind concentrate, diluted in
  6 tablespoons water
2 tablespoons soft brown sugar
Salt

1 Heat half the oil in a heavy pan and fry the chillies, cumin seeds, peppercorns, poppy seeds and fenugreek seeds until they start to change colour.

2 Add the onion and fry until slightly brown. Tip in the coconut and continue frying on low heat until the coconut turns brown. Take off the heat, cool slightly and whizz in a blender with a few tablespoons of water to make a fine paste. Reserve.

3 Heat the remaining oil in a kadhai or heavy saucepan and add the mustard seeds. When they pop, add the okra and stir for a couple of minutes.

4 Pour in the tamarind water and add the sugar and salt. Add the reserved paste and bring to the boil. Reduce the heat and simmer for 7–8 minutes until the okra is cooked. Serve hot with rice.

cauliflower with fenugreek
cauliflower sukke

This recipe is from the Saraswat Brahmin community of Karnataka, to which my mother belongs. The final dish should be fairly dry, the vegetables coated with the sauce rather than swimming in it. Jaggery is not easily available everywhere outside India and, although it adds a thicker consistency and a deeper taste, I find that soft brown sugar is acceptable.

Serves: 4
Preparation time: 15 minutes
Cooking time: 40 minutes

2 tablespoons sunflower oil
1 teaspoon split black lentils (urad dal)
1 teaspoon coriander seeds
5 dried red chillies
4 tablespoons freshly grated or
  desiccated coconut
1 teaspoon tamarind concentrate, diluted in
  6 tablespoons water
1/2 teaspoon turmeric powder
1 medium onion, sliced
300g cauliflower, cut into florettes
Salt
1/2 teaspoon jaggery or soft brown sugar

1 Heat half the oil in a heavy pan and fry the lentils, coriander seeds and chillies until they start to change colour.

2 Add the coconut and fry until brown, taking care to stir frequently to prevent it from sticking. Take off the heat, cool slightly and whizz in a blender with a few tablespoons of water and the tamarind, to make a fine paste of pouring consistency. Mix in the turmeric and reserve.

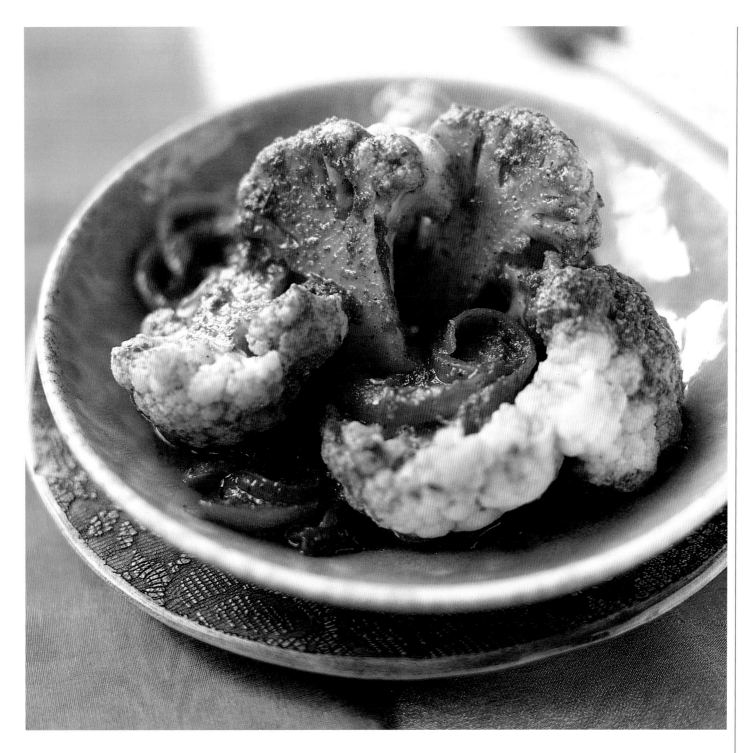

3 Heat the remaining oil in a kadhai or heavy-bottomed saucepan and add the onion. Stir until it browns and add the cauliflower. Season with salt, add the sugar and pour in the reserved spice paste.

4 Bring to the boil, reduce the heat and cook until the cauliflower is just tender. Serve with Coconut-flavoured Rice (page 119).

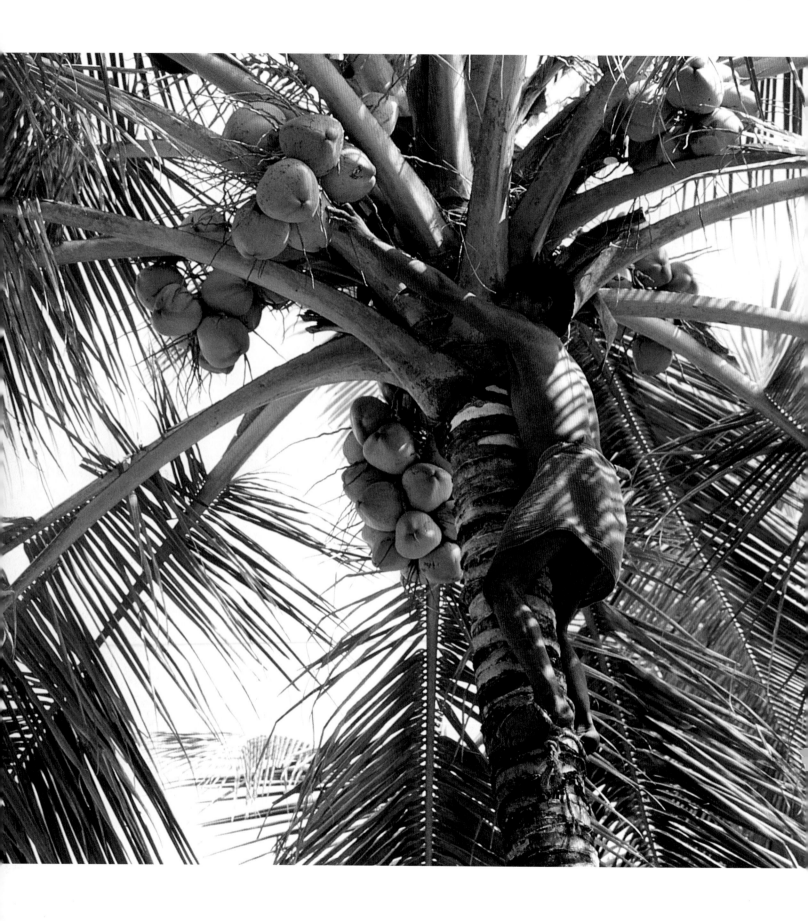

bamboo shoots in coconut milk
kirla ghassi

Mangalore is on the western coast of India and has produced a distinctive coconut-based cuisine that is popular all over India. This is a classic curry with tender bamboo shoots, which are quite common in this region and are cooked on festive days. Fresh bamboo shoots are prepared by peeling off the outer skin and slicing off the tough parts to get to the soft core, which is soaked for 48 hours, changing the water every 12 hours. I prefer to use tinned bamboo shoots!

Serves: 4
Preparation time: 15 minutes
Cooking time: 25 minutes

3 tablespoons sunflower oil
1 teaspoon coriander seeds
150g desiccated coconut
1/2 teaspoon garam masala powder
1 teaspoon tamarind concentrate, diluted in
  4 tablespoons water
1/4 teaspoon chilli powder
1/4 teaspoon turmeric powder
1 x 400g tin bamboo shoots, drained
Salt
150ml coconut milk
7–8 curry leaves

1 Heat half the oil in a heavy saucepan and add the coriander seeds and coconut. Stir until brown.

2 Take off the heat and add the garam masala and the tamarind. Cool slightly and whizz to a fine paste in a blender. Reserve.

3 Heat the remaining oil in a wok and add the chilli and turmeric powders. Add the bamboo shoots and salt.

4 Tip in the reserved coconut mixture, add a little water and bring to the boil. Pour in the coconut milk and add the curry leaves; simmer for 2–3 minutes and take off the heat. Serve hot but without boiling as the coconut milk may curdle.

stir-fried green tomatoes
pacha thakali kari

Firm and tangy green tomatoes are used in south Indian cookery. They are sometimes combined with potatoes or peanuts and used in wedding feasts or on the day of Kerala's favourite festival, Onam. Traditionally a couple of teaspoons of coconut oil are poured onto this dish before serving to add a unique flavour, but I have left this out to make a healthier version of the recipe.

Serves: 4
Preparation time: 10 minutes
Cooking time: 20 minutes

2 tablespoons sunflower oil
2 fresh green chillies, chopped
1 large onion, finely chopped
Large pinch of asafoetida
6 curry leaves
300g green tomatoes, cubed
Salt
2 tablespoons desiccated coconut

1 Heat the oil in a heavy saucepan or kadhai and fry the green chillies and onion until soft.

2 Add the asafoetida, curry leaves and tomatoes. Season with salt and cook on high heat for a couple of minutes. Reduce the heat and add a few tablespoons of water. Simmer for 10 minutes.

3 Take off the heat, stir in the coconut and serve hot with rice and Sambhar (page 138).

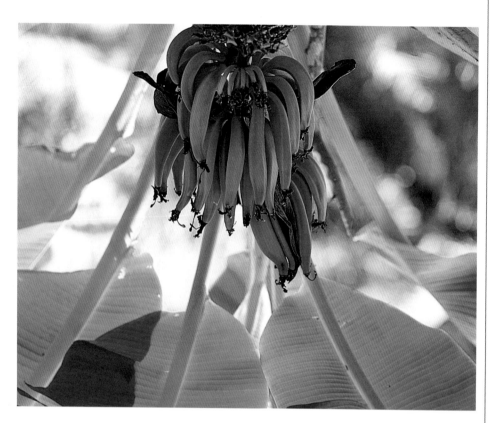

stir-fried plantain with garlic
vazhakai thoran

Plantains are popular in south Indian cookery, especially in Kerala. They are a type of banana with quite firm flesh and a tough skin. They should be cooked. The skin can be easily scraped off with a peeler. The flesh is slightly sticky and tastes like a banana-flavoured potato when cooked. This tastes much better with fresh coconut so do use it if you can.

Serves: 4
Preparation time: 15 minutes
Cooking time: 30 minutes

2 fresh green chillies
6 tablespoons freshly grated or
   desiccated coconut
2 cloves garlic, chopped
300g plantains
Salt
$^1/_2$ teaspoon turmeric powder
7 curry leaves
1 tablespoon sunflower oil
1 medium onion, sliced

1 Put the chillies, coconut and garlic into a blender, add a few tablespoons of water and grind to a fine paste. Reserve.

2 Peel the plantains with a potato peeler and chop into small pieces. Put them into a saucepan with 300ml of water, some salt and the turmeric and bring to the boil. Reduce the heat, add the reserved coconut paste and curry leaves and simmer for 10–12 minutes until the plantains are cooked through and just tender. Heat the oil in a small saucepan and fry the onions until brown. Pour over the plantains and serve hot.

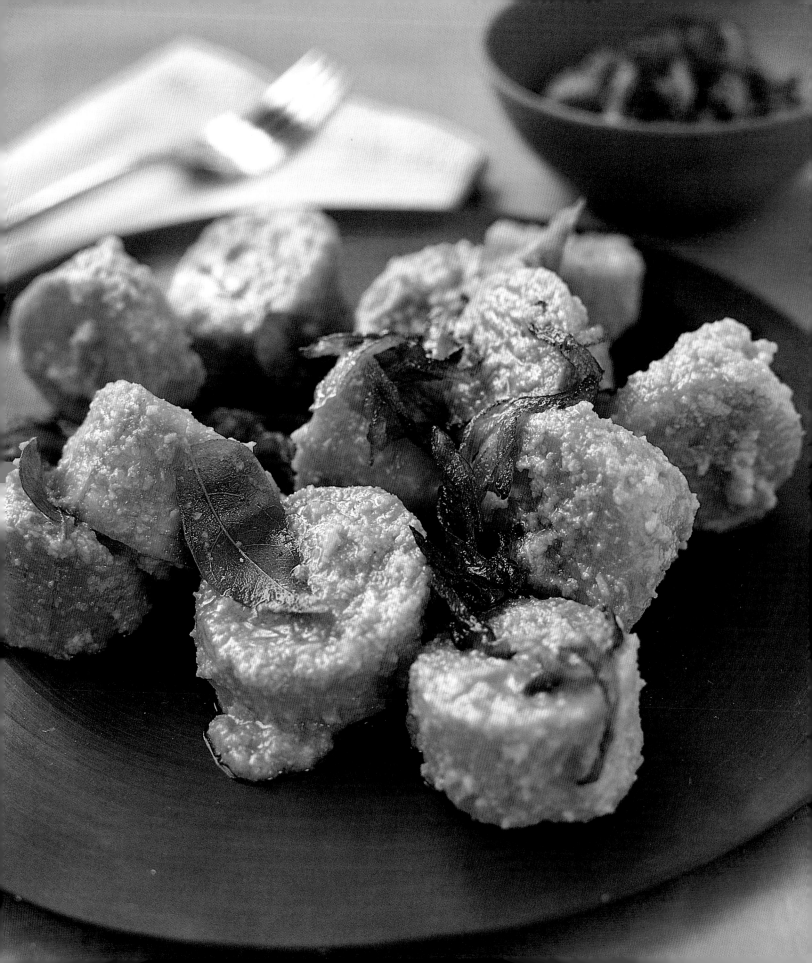

lentil pancakes
dosas

A fabulous dish from south India and one that is served at any time of the day. My own family is part south Indian and I have had dosas for breakfast, as a teatime snack and for dinner. They are served with a variety of chutneys made of coconut, tangy unripe mangoes, red chillies or curry leaves. They can also be served with a spicy potato filling and these are called 'masala dosas'. Please do not be put off by the long preparation time. The final dish is worth it and all it needs is a little bit of pre-planning!

Serves: 4
Preparation time: 15 minutes + overnight
  soaking + 2 hours, fermenting time
Cooking time: 25 minutes

**300g basmati rice or broken basmati rice
  (available at Indian grocery shops and
  cheaper than normal basmati rice), drained
150g skinless split black lentils, washed
  and drained
Salt
Sunflower oil for shallow frying**

1 Soak the rice and the lentils separately in plenty of water, preferably overnight or at least for 4 hours. Drain away the water and grind them separately in a blender, adding a little water as necessary, until you get 2 smooth, thick batters. Combine these batters and season with salt. Leave to ferment in a warm place for a couple of hours.

2 Heat an iron griddle or a non-stick pan and pour in 1 teaspoonful oil.

3 Stir the batter well and pour a ladleful of it into the centre of the pan. Spread the mixture quickly making a neat, small circle.

4 Drizzle a few drops of oil around the edges of the pancake. Reduce the heat, cover the pan and cook for a few seconds. Turn the pancake over with a spatula and cook the other side. You might have to discard the first pancake as it might be sticky and irregular in shape. Not to worry. The first one seems to season the pan for those to follow!

5 Continue similarly for the rest of the pancakes, keeping them warm as you go along, and serve at once.

steamed rice cakes
idlis

Idlis are served for breakfast or teatime over most of south India. These cakes are soft, fluffy and very nutritious. The mixture of lentils and rice means that they have proteins and carbohydrates. My little daughter loves to eat them with a pat of butter. Make variations by adding vegetables or spices to the batter: I love French beans and crushed black pepper.

Serves: 4
Preparation time: 20 minutes + overnight
  soaking + 8 hours fermenting time
Cooking time: 15 minutes

**300g basmati rice or broken basmati rice
  (available at Indian grocery shops
  and cheaper than normal basmati rice),
  washed and drained
100g skinless split black lentils
Salt**

1 Soak the rice and the lentils separately in plenty of water overnight. Drain and grind them separately in a blender, adding fresh water as necessary, to make thick, pouring batter. (If you grind them together the batter will not be smooth enough.) Mix the two batters together and add the salt. Leave to ferment in a warm place for about 8 hours.

2 Pour the batter into little metal bowls (that can be put into a steamer) or an egg poacher and steam the cakes for 15 minutes.

3 To serve, remove each cake by sliding a sharp knife under it and lifting. Set aside and keep warm. Repeat this process until all the batter is used up. Serve warm with Coconut Chutney (page 131) and Sambhar (page 138).

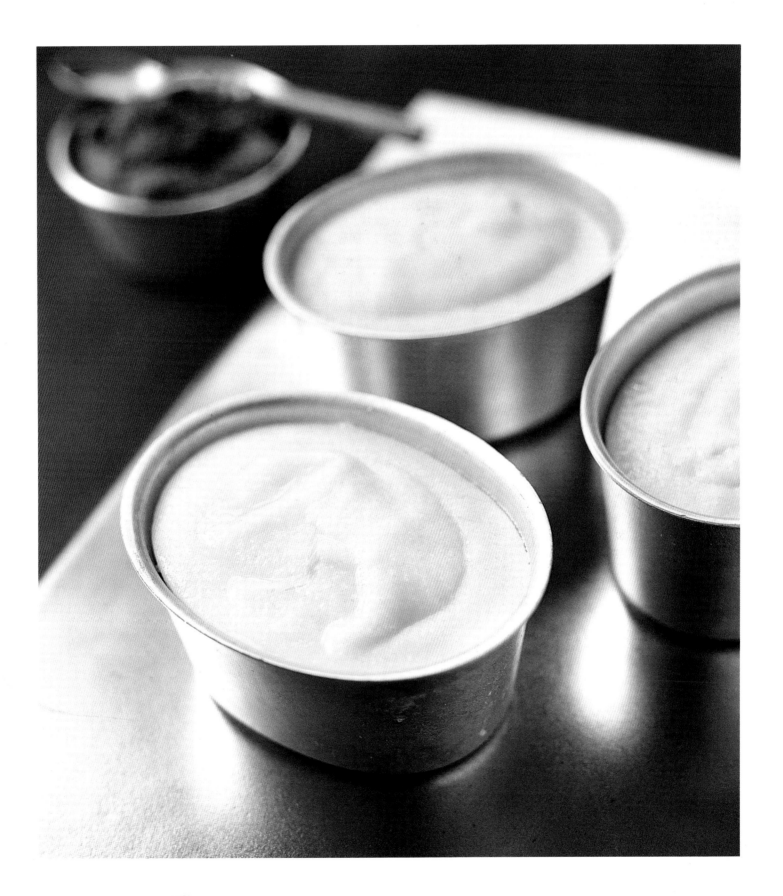

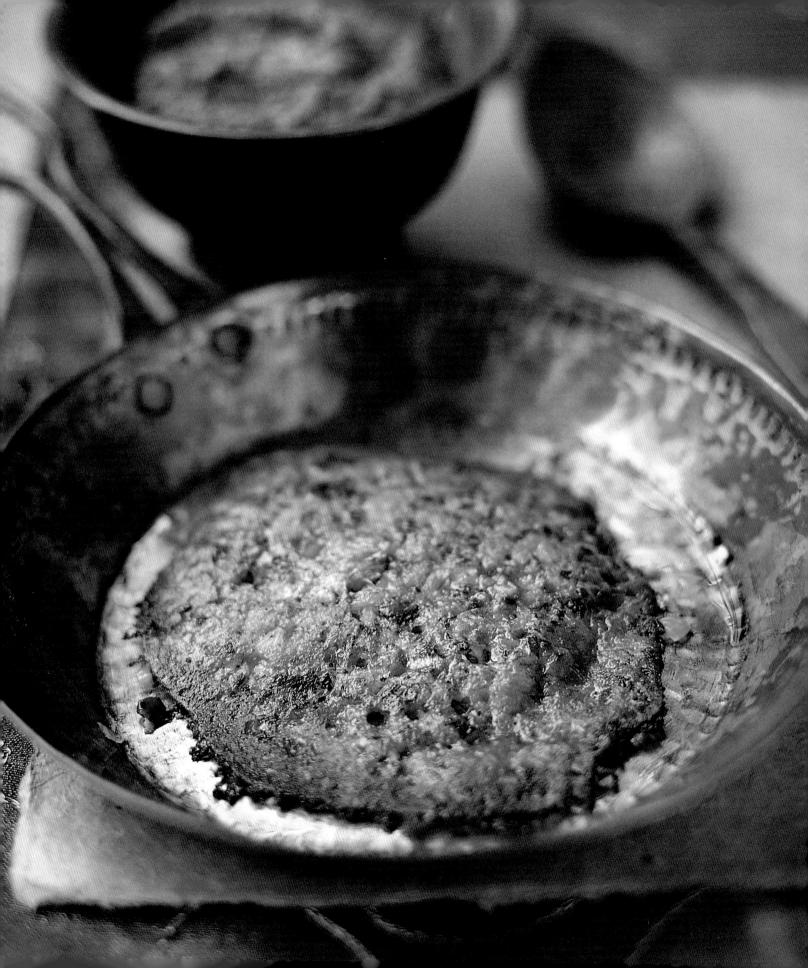

semolina pancake with onion and coriander
rava uttappam

South Indians are skillful at making any number of pancakes. These are eaten with chutneys, sweet preserves or curries. Uttappam is a kind of dosa and can also be flavoured with tomatoes or grated cheese as well as onions. Some dosas like this one, can be made in advance for convenience and reheated, but I always think there is nothing quite like eating pancakes hot from the pan!

Serves: 4
Preparation time: 10 minutes
Cooking time: 25 minutes

1 medium onion, finely chopped
150g coarse semolina
Pinch of turmeric powder
Salt
Handful of coriander leaves, finely chopped
2 fresh green chillies, finely chopped
Sunflower oil for shallow frying

1 Combine the onion, semolina, turmeric, salt, coriander leaves and chillies in a mixing bowl. Pour in enough cold water to make a batter of pouring consistency, almost like thick custard.

2 Heat 1 tablespoon of oil in a large saucepan. Pour a ladleful of the batter into the centre and spread it in quick circles to form a flattish disc about 10cm in diameter. Cover the pan and allow the pancake to cook in its steam.

3 Flip the pancake over when the underside has turned golden and spotty. Cook the other side by dotting the edges with some oil and covering the pan. Keep warm.

4 Make all the pancakes similarly and serve hot with Coconut Chutney (page 131).

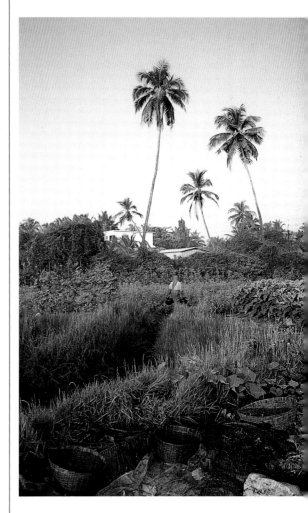

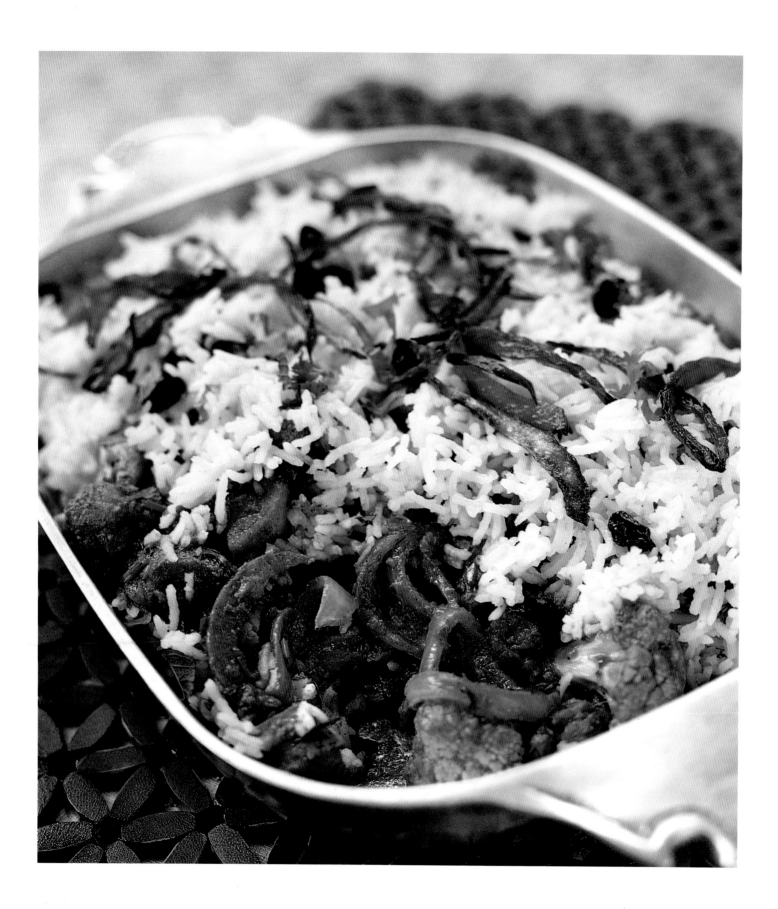

hyderabadi vegetable biryani
tahiri

This is a refined biryani that symbolises the Islamic influence on south Indian food. Built around 1580, the city of Hyderabad in Andhra Pradesh was called Bhagnagar, after the beautiful Bhagmati who was the beloved of the Nawab. She later changed her name to Hyder Mahal and the city was renamed after her. This dish is a festive one that needs time and patience but makes a great Sunday feast!

Serves: 4
Preparation time: 25 minutes
Cooking time: 40 minutes

300g basmati rice, washed and drained
Sunflower oil for deep-frying
300g mixed vegetables (potatoes, aubergine, cauliflower), cut into small pieces
1 large onion, finely sliced
1 teaspoon raisins
2 teaspoons ginger-garlic paste (page 11)
2 fresh green chillies, minced
1/2 teaspoon turmeric powder
1 teaspoon garam masala powder
100g natural yoghurt
Salt
Juice of 1 lemon
Handful of coriander and mint leaves, chopped
2 tablespoons ghee

1 Put the rice with double its volume of hot water in a saucepan and bring to the boil. Reduce the heat, stir, cover and simmer for 10 minutes until done. Reserve.

2 Heat the oil in a deep frying pan and deep-fry the vegetables until cooked, first the cauliflower and potatoes, then the aubergine. Drain and reserve.

3 Fry half the onion until dark brown, drain and reserve. Fry the raisins for 1 minute, drain and reserve them separately.

4 In a clean saucepan, take 2 tablespoons of the same oil and fry the rest of the onion until golden brown. Add the ginger-garlic paste, chillies, turmeric and garam masala. Gently stir in the fried vegetables, yoghurt and salt and simmer for 10 minutes.

5 Now start to assemble the tahiri. In an ovenproof serving dish, put one layer of rice and one of the vegetable mixture. Sprinkle on some lemon juice and some of the coriander and mint leaves.

6 Begin with the next layer of rice and keep going till you have a layer of rice at the top. Drizzle on the ghee and serve hot, garnished with the fried onions, raisins and the remaining coriander and mint leaves.

7 Keep warm in an oven (180°C/gas 4) until you are ready to serve.

coconut-flavoured rice
thengai sadam

A soft and gentle dish, this rice and coconut medley makes a perfect summer meal. The juiciness of fresh coconut is vital to this dish and therefore it cannot be substituted with desiccated coconut. In India, the coconut is given a place of honour at ceremonies such as weddings and rituals. It is also called shriphal or the fruit of the Gods and is sometimes used as a symbol of Divinity.

Serves: 4
Preparation time: 15 minutes
Cooking time: 30 minutes

300g basmati rice, washed and drained
2 tablespoons sunflower oil
1 teaspoon black mustard seeds
2 tablespoons cashew nuts
1 teaspoon chopped fresh green chillies
2 teaspoons split black lentils (urad dal), soaked in water for 15 minutes and drained
Large pinch of asafoetida
7 curry leaves
150g freshly grated coconut
Salt

1 Put the rice with double its volume of hot water in a pan and bring to the boil. Reduce the heat, stir, cover and simmer for 10 minutes until cooked. Reserve.

2 Heat the oil and fry the mustard seeds. When they pop, add the cashew nuts, chillies, lentils, asafoetida and curry leaves. Fry for 1 minute, add the coconut and stir until the colour begins turning golden, then season with salt. Take off the heat and fold in the rice. Serve with Kholombo Powder (page 139) and Plantain Wafers (page 128).

lemon rice with cashew and peanuts
naranga choru

Rice is eaten in every south Indian household every single day. It generally features in two or three courses, first with spiced lentils and lastly with cool yoghurt. I tend to keep lemon rice very lightly spiced although some versions are quite fiery. I like to believe that the rice should be fairly neutral so that it can be enjoyed with stronger dishes.

Serves: 4
Preparation time: 10 minutes
Cooking time: 25 minutes

300g basmati rice, washed and drained
2 tablespoons sunflower oil
1 teaspoon black mustard seeds
6 curry leaves
1 teaspoon gram lentils (channa dal), soaked in water for 15 minutes and drained
10 cashew nuts
2 tablespoons unsalted peanuts
1 teaspoon turmeric powder
3 tablespoons lemon juice
Salt

1 Put the rice and double its volume of hot water in a heavy saucepan. Bring to the boil. Reduce the heat, stir and cover. Simmer for 10 minutes until cooked. Reserve.

2 In a separate pan, heat the oil and fry the mustard seeds until they pop. Then add the curry leaves, lentils, cashew nuts and peanuts. Reduce the heat and, when the cashews are slightly brown, add the turmeric.

3 Take off the heat at once and pour in the lemon juice and season with salt. Gently fold the rice into this mixture and serve hot.

tamarind rice
pulihodara

The tamarind pod is crescent-shaped and brown with a thin, brittle shell. It contains a fleshy pulp held together by a fibrous husk. Within this pulp are squarish, dark brown, shiny seeds. The pulp, used as a flavouring for its sweet, sour, fruity aroma and taste, is dried along with the seeds and husk and sold in the form of little cakes. I use the concentrate for ease.

Serves: 4
Preparation time: 30 minutes
Cooking time: 30 minutes

300g basmati rice, washed and drained
2 tablespoons sunflower oil
1/2 teaspoon black mustard seeds
1/4 teaspoon fenugreek seeds
Large pinch of asafoetida
4 dried red chillies, deseeded and crumbled
1 teaspoon gram lentils (channa dal)
2 teaspoons cashew nuts
10 curry leaves
1 tablespoon tamarind concentrate, diluted in 6 tablespoons water
Salt

1 Put the rice with double its volume of hot water in a saucepan and bring to the boil. Reduce the heat, stir, cover and simmer for 10 minutes until cooked. Reserve.

2 Heat the oil in a heavy saucepan and fry the mustard seeds, fenugreek seeds, asafoetida, chillies, lentils, cashew nuts and curry leaves.

3 Stir in the tamarind and salt, cooking until the tamarind is thick and the paste is well blended. Fold in the rice and serve hot.

flaked rice with potatoes
batate pohe

Serves: 4
Preparation time: 20 minutes
Cooking time: 15 minutes

300g Indian rice flakes (pawa)
1 teaspoon turmeric powder
Salt
1 teaspoon sugar
1 tablespoon sunflower oil
1 teaspoon black mustard seeds
1/2 teaspoon cumin seeds
Large pinch of asafoetida
2 fresh green chillies, minced
12 curry leaves
100g potatoes, peeled, diced and boiled
2 teaspoons lemon juice
Few coriander leaves, chopped
2 tablespoons freshly grated or desiccated coconut

1 Soak the rice flakes in water for 5 minutes and drain. Then mix the rice, turmeric, salt and sugar together gently.

2 Heat the oil in a pan and add the mustard seeds. When they crackle, add the cumin, asafoetida, chillies and curry leaves.

3 Fry for 1 minute and stir in the potatoes. Add the flaked rice. Mix well. Reduce the heat, sprinkle in about 4 tablespoons of water, cover and simmer for about 10 minutes. Drizzle in the lemon juice. The potatoes will become slightly mushy, which will give a creamy texture to the dish.

4 Serve hot, garnished with the coriander and coconut.

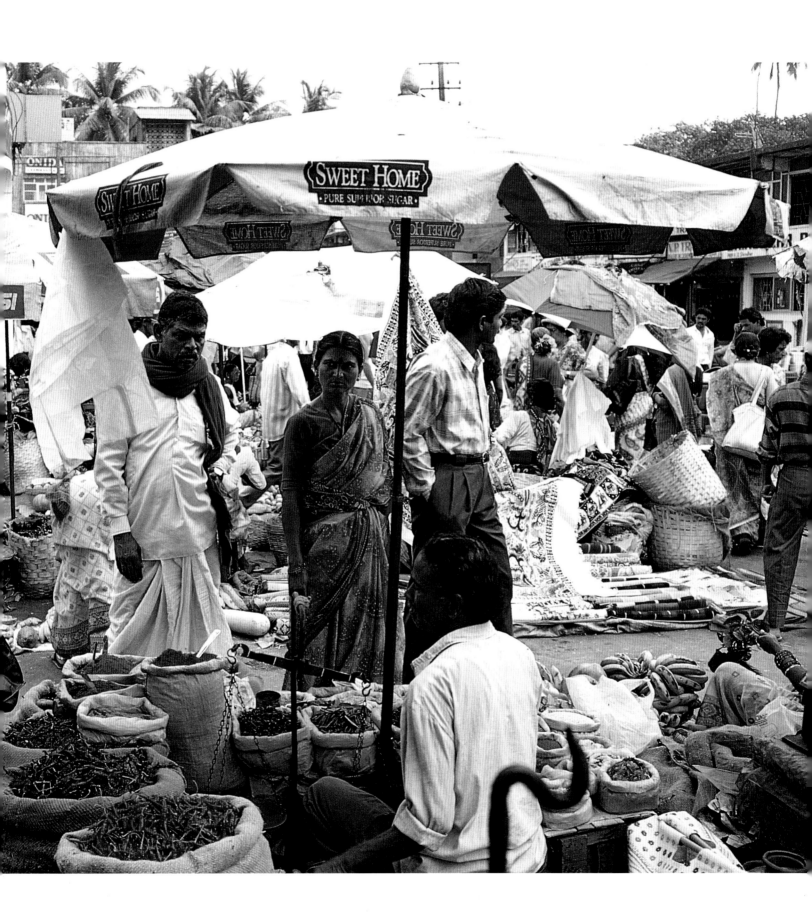

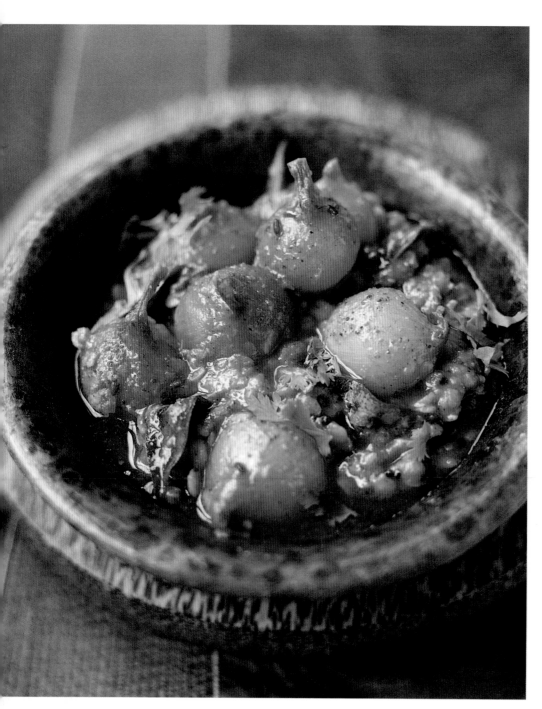

spiced lentils with shallots
vengai sambhar

The aroma of sambhar reminds me of the Temple of Meenakshi, the Goddess with the fish-shaped eyes, in south India. After the ritual worship, streams of devotees are served a simple meal of rice, sambhar, ghee and sweets. Sambhar is made every day in traditional south Indian homes, especially in Tamil Nadu. The recipe for Sambhar Powder, the spice mix that flavours this dish, is given on page 138.

Serves: 4
Preparation time: 15 minutes + 30 minutes
  soaking time
Cooking time: 40 minutes

300g split yellow lentils (toor dal), soaked in
  water for 30 minutes and drained
750ml water
12 shallots, peeled
Salt
1 teaspoon turmeric powder
2 tablespoons sunflower oil
1 teaspoon black mustard seeds
1 teaspoon cumin seeds
12 curry leaves
Large pinch of asafoetida
1 teaspoon tamarind concentrate, diluted in
  6 tablespoons water
2 teaspoons sambhar powder (page 138)
2 tablespoons chopped coriander leaves

lentil soup with tamarind and garlic
rasam

1 Put the lentils and the water in a heavy-bottomed saucepan and bring to the boil. Reduce the heat and simmer, skimming off the scum that rises to the top. When the lentils are nearly tender, add the shallots and simmer until they are just softening. The lentils are done when they get mushy.

2 Add the salt and turmeric powder. Mix well, take off the heat and reserve.

3 Heat the oil in a small pan and add the mustard seeds. When they crackle, add the cumin seeds, curry leaves and asafoetida, then the tamarind and cook on low heat until thick and bubbly.

4 Add the sambhar powder and cook for 1 minute. Pour the mixture over the lentils and stir. Swirl a few tablespoons of water in the pan to gather all the tamarind and spices and pour into the lentils. Serve hot, garnished with the coriander.

Rasam is a close relative of sambhar but it is thinner and is therefore often served as a spicy soup. Try it on cold winter nights! It is also eaten with boiled rice, as a second course after rice and sambhar. You could add lemon juice instead of the tamarind to make lemon rasam, in which case, add the lemon juice at the end, after taking the rasam off the heat (step 3).

Serves: 4
Preparation time: 15 minutes + 15 minutes soaking time
Cooking time: 30 minutes

4 tablespoons split yellow lentils (toor dal), soaked for 15 minutes and drained
750ml water
Salt
1 teaspoon jaggery or soft brown sugar
2 tablespoons sunflower oil
1/2 teaspoon black mustard seeds
1/2 teaspoon cumin seeds
Large pinch of asafoetida
10 curry leaves
4 cloves garlic, peeled and bruised
1 teaspoon tamarind concentrate, diluted in 6 tablespoons water
1 teaspoon sambhar powder (page 138)
1 teaspoon turmeric powder
2 tablespoons chopped coriander leaves

1 Put the lentils and the water in a heavy-bottomed saucepan, bring to the boil and simmer until mushy, skimming the scum off the surface from time to time. Add the salt and the jaggery, mixing until they dissolve.

2 Heat the oil in a separate pan and add the mustard seeds. When they crackle, add the cumin, asafoetida, curry leaves and the whole cloves of garlic. Fry for 1 minute, then add the tamarind and cook until it becomes thick and bubbly. Stir in the spice powders.

3 Pour the lentils into the tamarind mixture, bring to the boil and remove from the heat. Stir gently and serve hot with the coriander.

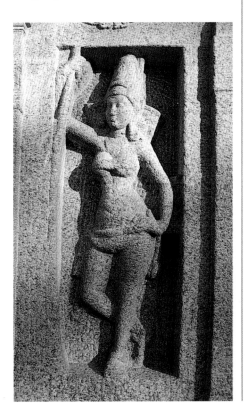

green lentil pancake
pessaratu

This is a speciality of Andhra Pradesh and is not made in other southern states. It is a classic dish and nutritious. There is a story that there was once a great famine in Andhra Pradesh and nothing but chillies could be grown and this is why the cooking here is hot and spicy. Every meal is served with ghee to temper the heat of the chillies, most of which come from a place called Guntur. Soaking the chillies makes them soft enough to blend into a paste.

Serves: 4
Preparation time: 15 minutes + 4 hours soaking time
Cooking time: 30 minutes

150g split green lentils (split mung lentils with the green skin on)
1 teaspoon cumin seeds
2 fresh green chillies, chopped
2 dried red chillies, seeds shaken out, soaked in a little water for 15 minutes and drained
1 medium onion, finely chopped
Few coriander leaves, finely chopped
Salt
Sunflower oil for frying

1 Soak the lentils in plenty of water for 4 hours. Drain and grind them to a smooth paste in a blender, along with the cumin seeds, green and red chillies and enough fresh water to achieve pouring consistency.

2 Stir in the onion and coriander leaves and season with salt.

3 Heat a flat griddle or non-stick frying pan and put a ladleful of the batter at the centre. Spread with the back of a spoon to make a disc about 10cm in diameter and dot the edges with oil. When the underside is cooked, turn it over to cook the other side.

4 Take off the heat and continue similarly with the rest of the batter. Pessaratu are served with butter and jaggery or soft brown sugar.

smoky lentils with tomato
tomato kholombo

This dish is made by the Saraswat community of Karnataka. Diced aubergine or red pumpkin can be substituted for the tomato, in which case, cook the vegetables separately and add to the lentils with the tamarind. This dish tastes better a day after you make it.

Serves: 4
Preparation time: 15 minutes
Cooking time: 50 minutes

225g split red lentils (masoor dal), washed and drained
Salt
1 teaspoon tamarind concentrate, diluted in 4 teaspoons water
3 ripe tomatoes, chopped
1 teaspoon kholombo powder (page 139)
2 tablespoons sunflower oil
1/2 teaspoon black mustard seeds
4 dried red chillies, deseeded and crumbled
Large pinch of asafoetida
12 curry leaves

1 Put the lentils and double their volume of hot water into a pan and bring to the boil. Reduce the heat and simmer until the lentils are mushy, for about 30 minutes.

2 Add the salt, tamarind, tomatoes and kholombo powder and simmer for a couple of minutes, then take off the heat and reserve.

3 Heat the oil in a small saucepan and add the mustard seeds. When they crackle, add the chillies, asafoetida and curry leaves.

4 Pour over the lentils. Mix well and serve with rice and a hot pickle.

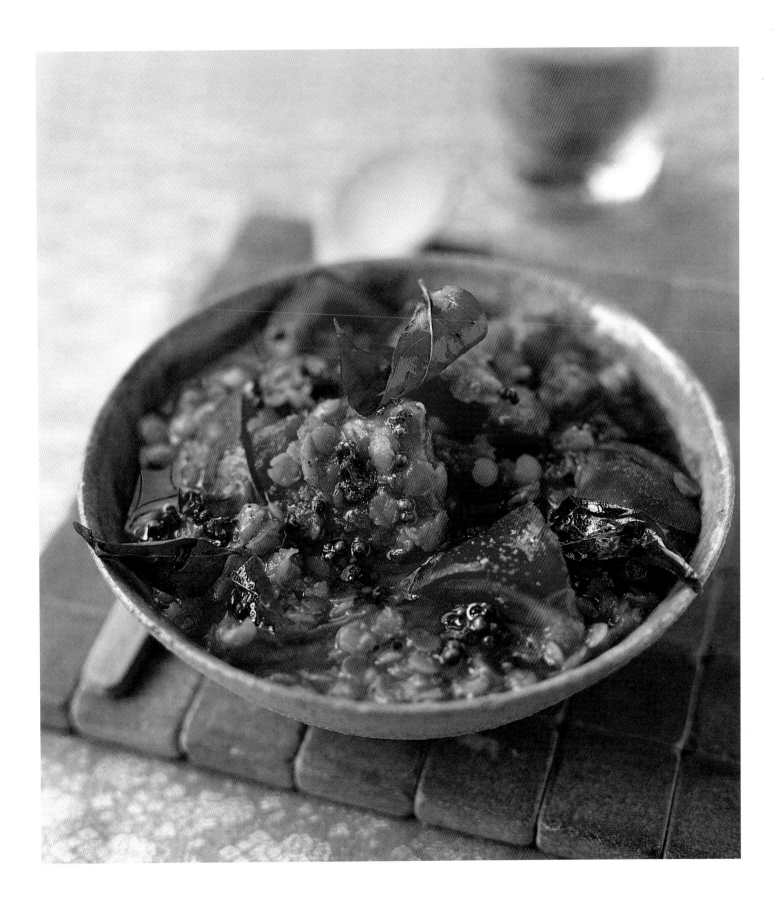

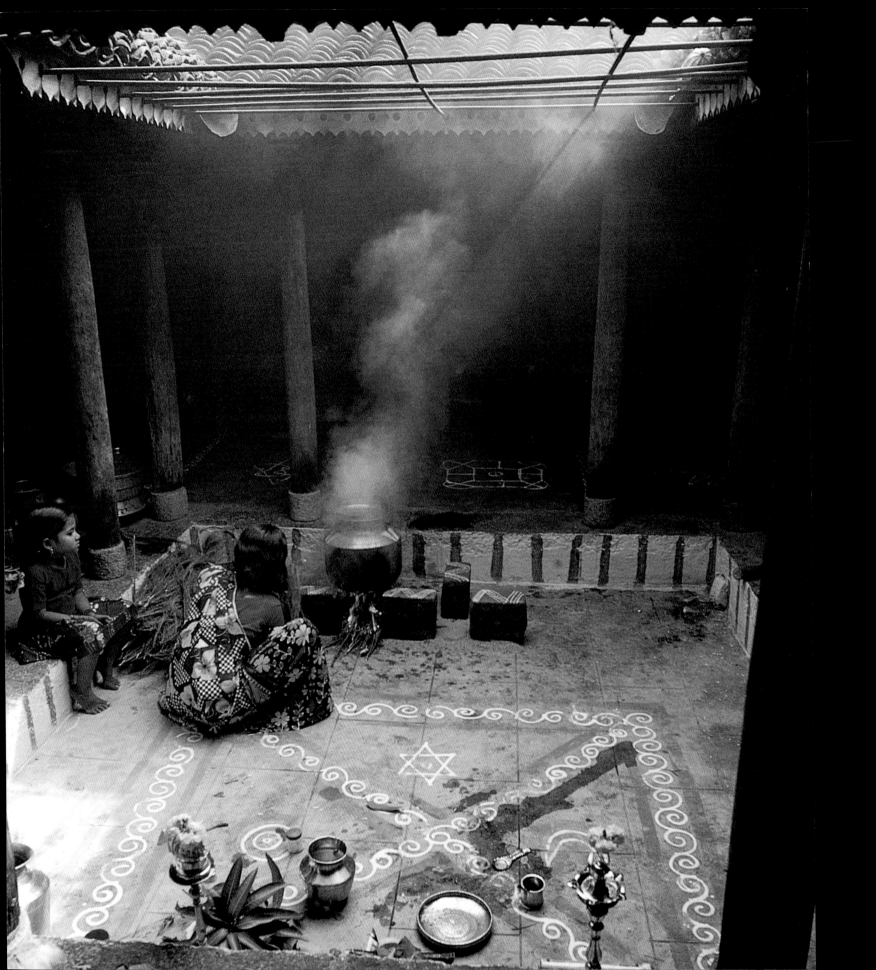

butter beans in garlic and coconut
aurey bendi

This recipe is from the Saraswat community of Goa. It looks quite red and fiery but it is almost creamy and spicy rather than hot. A native spice berry called 'tirphal' which is extremely fragrant and is slightly bitter is used in Goa, when it is not flavoured with this spice, garlic is added as the main flavouring. It is eaten with plain rice. You can use other beans such as black-eyed, which work well in this recipe.

Serves: 4
Preparation time: 15 minutes
Cooking time: 20 minutes

150g freshly grated or desiccated coconut
4 dried red chillies, deseeded, stems removed, soaked in a little water
2 teaspoons tamarind concentrate, diluted in 3 tablespoons water
330g tinned butter beans, drained
Salt
2 teaspoons sunflower oil
2 cloves garlic, sliced

1 Grind the coconut, red chillies and tamarind to a paste in a blender, adding water as needed to make a very fine paste.

2 Combine the beans and the coconut paste, add enough water to make a pouring consistency and bring to the boil. Season with salt. Reduce the heat and simmer for a couple of minutes. Take off the heat and reserve.

3 Heat the oil in a small saucepan. Add the garlic and fry for 1 minute until it just starts to turn golden and a delicious aroma fills the air! Pour over the curry. Stir and serve hot.

lentils with spinach
soppu palya

Serves: 4
Preparation time: 15 minutes
Cooking time: 60 minutes

150g yellow lentils (toor dal), washed
150g spinach, chopped
2 tablespoons sunflower oil
1 teaspoon coriander seeds
3 dried red chillies
4 tablespoons freshly grated coconut
1 teaspoon tamarind concentrate, diluted in 4 tablespoons water
1/2 teaspoon turmeric
Salt
1 medium onion, sliced

1 Put the lentils and double their volume of hot water into a pan and bring to the boil. Reduce the heat and simmer until the lentils are mushy, for about 35 minutes. Reserve.

2 In the meantime, wilt the spinach in a little hot water for a couple of minutes and add to the lentils.

3 Heat half the oil in a saucepan and fry the coriander seeds until they turn dark, then add the chillies and the coconut. Reduce the heat and stir for a couple of minutes. Take off the heat, cool slightly and whizz in a blender along with the tamarind and few tablespoons of water until you get a fine paste.

4 Add this to the lentils, together with the turmeric and salt.

5 Heat the remaining oil in a small saucepan and fry the onions until golden, then add them into the lentils. Reheat thoroughly and serve hot with rice.

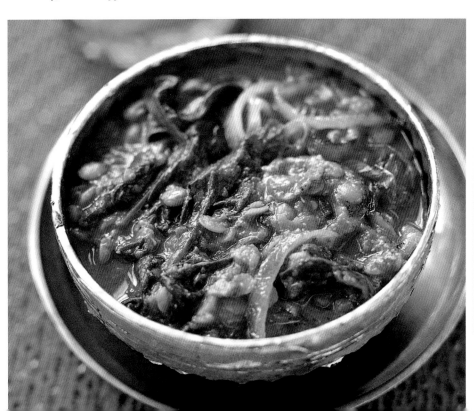

lentil fritters in sweet yoghurt
thayir vadai

The fritters in this recipe can be made with a variety of lentils, but I often choose the split yellow mung ones because they are quick to cook and very easy to digest. They need to be soaked so that they become soft enough to blend into a batter. Versions of this recipe are popular in north India but no sugar is added, and the curry leaves are substituted with coriander leaves.

Serves: 4
Preparation time: 20 minutes + 3 hours soaking time
Cooking time: 25 minutes

150g split yellow mung lentils, washed and drained
Salt
Sunflower oil for deep-frying
300g natural yoghurt
2 teaspoons sugar
1 teaspoon black mustard seeds
1/2 teaspoon cumin seeds
3 large dried red chillies, seeds shaken out
7 curry leaves

1 Soak the mung lentils in plenty of water for at least 3 hours. Drain off the water and grind the lentils in a blender with a few tablespoons of fresh water. The result should be a smooth paste with no grains in it, the consistency of thick custard. Season with salt and reserve.

2 Heat the oil in a deep saucepan or wok. When it is nearly smoking drop in a tiny ball of the lentil batter. It should rise quickly to the top. Reduce the heat slightly and gently drop a few tablespoons of the batter into the oil. Turn them around a few times to brown them evenly. Don't hurry them along as they will brown on the outside but remain uncooked in the middle.

3 When done, remove the fritters on a slotted spoon and drain them on kitchen paper. Do the remaining fritters similarly.

4 In another bowl, whisk together the yoghurt, some salt and the sugar.

5 Heat a tablespoon of oil in a small saucepan and fry the mustard seeds until they pop. Add the cumin seeds, red chillies and curry leaves and pour this tempering along with the oil into the seasoned yoghurt.

6 Just before serving, add the fritters to the yoghurt. Some cooks dip them in water, squeeze them dry and then add them to the yoghurt to soften them and help them absorb the yoghurt, if you like the fritters crisp, add them directly into the yoghurt. Serve cool.

plantain wafers
vazhaikkai varuval

No south Indian meal is complete without some fried accompaniment. Sometimes this might be shop-bought crisps or many kinds of poppadoms made of lentils and rice flour. I love these wafers for their crisp texture and divine taste. In the south, they are often fried in coconut oil. It is easiest to peel the plantain with a potato peeler.

Serves: 4
Preparation time: 15 minutes
Cooking time: 20 minutes

2 plantains, peeled and sliced
1/4 teaspoon turmeric powder
1/4 teaspoon chilli powder
Salt
2 tablespoons rice flour
Sunflower oil for deep-frying

1 Mix the plantains and spice powders together and season with salt. Sprinkle in the rice flour and see that each slice is well coated.

2 Heat the oil in a deep wok and, when nearly smoking, fry a few slices of the plantain at a time until golden. Serve at once or keep warm.

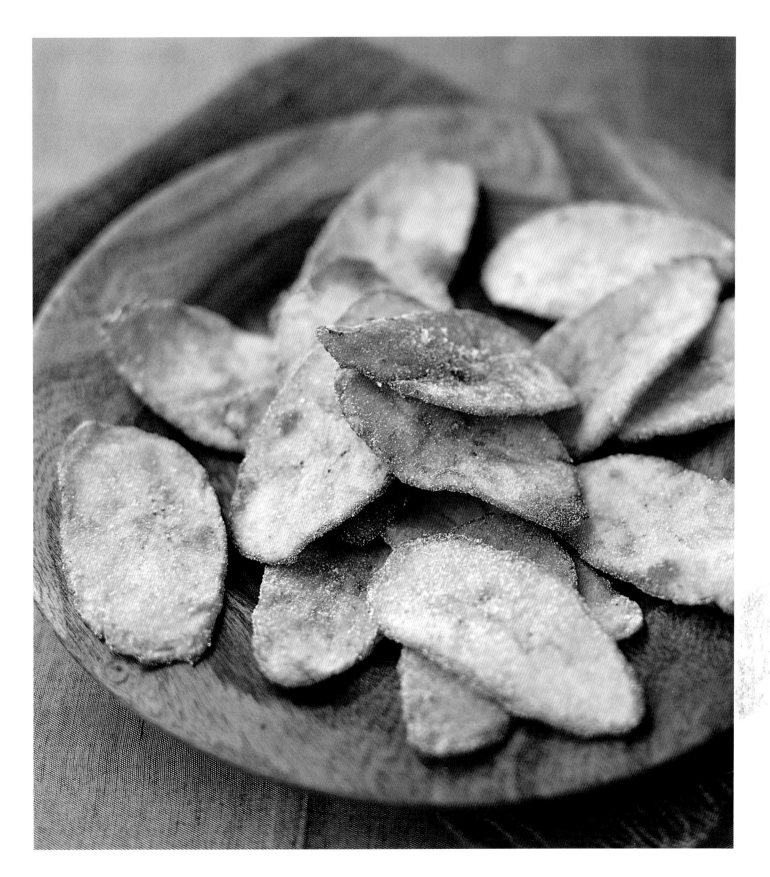

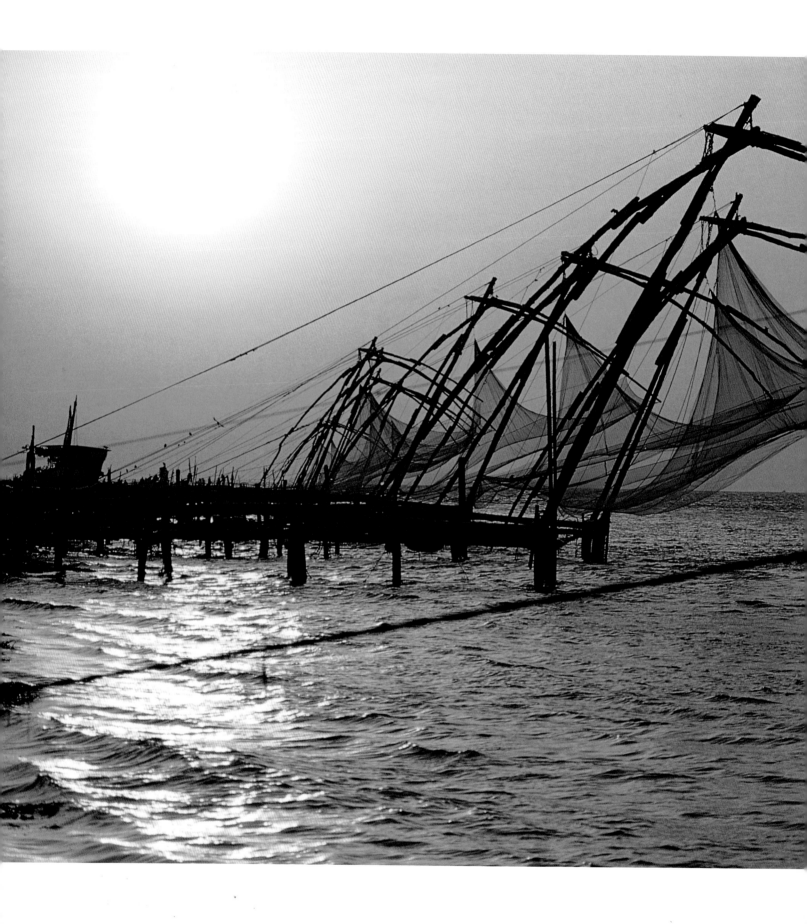

coconut chutney
thengai thuvaiyal

This is the most versatile chutney made throughout south India and is served with pancakes, rice, fried accompaniments or breads. It makes a great sandwich filler too! Desiccated coconut cannot be used here as the chutney must be fragrant with the smell of fresh coconut. Jaggery is unrefined sugar and tastes quite toffee-like. Brown sugar can be substituted.

Serves: 4
Preparation time: 15 minutes
Cooking time: 2 minutes

2 teaspoons sunflower oil
3 dried red chillies
1 teaspoon split black lentils (urad dal)
Pinch of asafoetida
80g freshly grated coconut
1 teaspoon tamarind concentrate, diluted in
 4 tablespoons water
1 teaspoon jaggery or soft brown sugar
Salt
1 teaspoon black mustard seeds

1 Heat half the oil and fry the red chillies, lentils and asafoetida until the lentils turn brown. Remove from the heat and mix in the coconut.

2 Combine with the tamarind, jaggery or sugar and salt in a blender and add enough water to whizz into a thick, smooth paste.

3 Heat the remaining oil in a small saucepan and fry the mustard seeds until they pop, then pour into the chutney. Serve cold.

fresh ginger and yoghurt raita
inji pachadi

Ginger is often seen in festive feasts where the food is first offered to the Gods. Its fragrance is especially prized along with its healing properties in many teas, salads and sweets. Look for shiny, fine skinned ginger when buying it. It should snap easily, which means it is juicy and fresh. As it gets older it turns leathery, dry and fibrous.

Serves: 4
Preparation time: 15 minutes
Cooking time: 2 minutes

1 fresh green chilli, minced
2 tablespoons fresh ginger, chopped
4 tablespoons freshly grated or
 desiccated coconut
Salt
150g natural yoghurt, beaten
1 tablespoon raisins
1 teaspoon sunflower oil
1/2 teaspoon black mustard seeds

1 Whizz the chilli, ginger and coconut in a blender along with some water to make a smooth paste and season with salt.

2 Mix in the yoghurt and raisins and reserve.

3 Heat the oil in a small saucepan and fry the mustard seeds until they pop. Pour into the raita and mix gently. Serve as an accompaniment with Idlis (page 114) or Dosa (page 114).

jewish potatoes
alu mukkadah

The Jews in south India live mainly in Cochin in Kerala though there are few families left now. They follow the rules of their religion but, in deference to local Hindu customs, many of them do not eat beef. This recipe is extremely easy to make. It can be made with roasting potatoes as well but I love the baby ones that cook so quickly.

Serves: 4
Preparation time: 10 minutes
Cooking time: 20 minutes

300g baby potatoes, washed and drained
Salt
1/2 teaspoon turmeric powder
2 tablespoons sunflower oil

1 Prick the potatoes with a fork and drop them into a pan of hot water to which salt and turmeric has been added. Bring to the boil.

2 Reduce the heat and gently simmer the potatoes until they are just tender. Drain.

3 Heat the oil in a shallow pan and add the potatoes. Stir fry on a low heat until golden and slightly crisp. Serve as an accompaniment with lentils and rice.

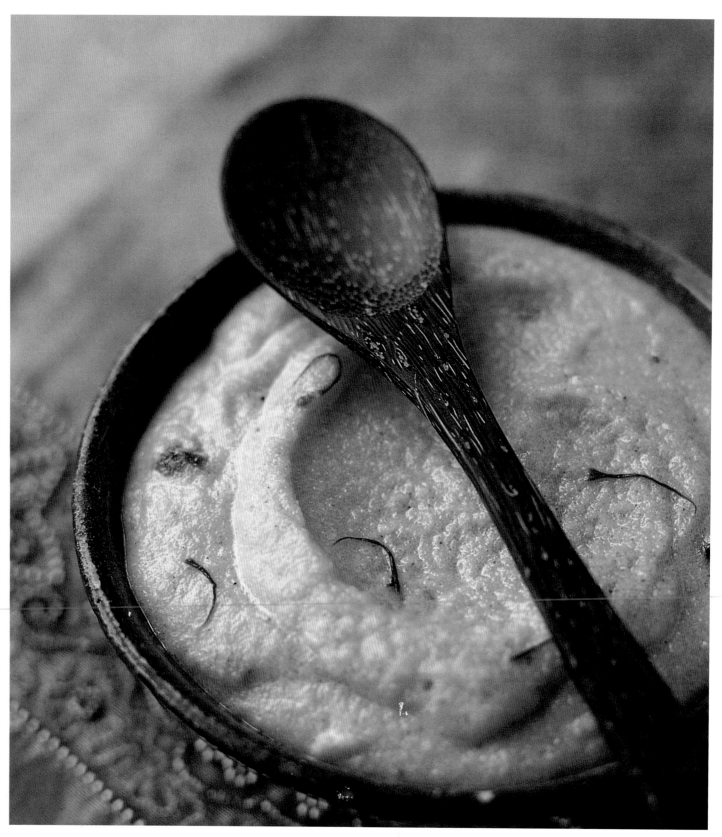

semolina and saffron pudding
rava kesari

This saffron-scented dessert is considered food for the Gods and is often made on festive days. The saffron colours it orange and it is quite soft because of the ghee. Each region of India has its own version – flavoured with pineapples, bananas or nuts and they are all truly delicious.

Serves: 4
Preparation time: 10 minutes
Cooking time: 20 minutes

150ml ghee
150g semolina
150g sugar
Large pinch of saffron
450ml warm milk
Pinch of cardamom powder
2 teaspoons raisins

1 Heat the ghee in a heavy saucepan or kadhai and add the semolina, frying until it becomes pink and fragrant. Reduce the heat and add the sugar and stir until it melts.

2 Mix the saffron into the milk and add it to the kadhai. Stir rapidly to avoid lumps from forming; sometimes I use a whisk to get a smooth consistency.

3 Add the cardamom powder and the raisins and reduce the heat. Cover the pan and cook until the mixture is semi-dry and the semolina is cooked, for about 10–12 minutes. Serve warm.

stewed apricots with cream
qubani ka meetha

This is a very quick and simple party dessert to prepare at short notice. It is believed to have been the favourite of the erstwhile ruler of Hyderabad, the Nizam, who was so rich that he employed servants to wear his collection of pearls in order to keep them lustrous. In fact his pearl collection, it was said, could be spread out on the roof of his palace, from one end to the other.

Serves: 4
Preparation time: 10 minutes
Cooking time: 15 minutes

300g hunza apricots
100g sugar
4 tablespoons double cream
2 tablespoons crushed almonds

1 Soak the apricots for 1 hour in plenty of water and drain. Stone the fruit and discard the seeds.

2 Put the apricots and sugar along with 600ml of water in a heavy saucepan and cook until tender and pulpy.

3 Put half the apricots in a blender and whizz a couple of times until they resemble a jam.

4 Spoon some of the whole apricots and some of the pulp into stemmed serving glasses. Drizzle over the cream, sprinkle the almonds on top and serve chilled. You can also serve the apricots with custard.

rich rice and coconut pudding
thengapal payasam

This dish conjures up rich south Indian feasts served at festivals such as Onam, which is celebrated in Kerala with grand boat races and colourful dances. Coconut grows everywhre along the southern coasts of India and is therefore used in each part of the meal – from soups to chutneys to puddings.

Serves: 4
Preparation time: 10 minutes
Cooking time: 1 hour

6 tablespoons basmati rice, washed
 and drained
600ml tinned coconut milk
Sugar to taste
Pinch of cardamom powder
Pinch of saffron
1 teaspoon ghee or sunflower oil
2 tablespoons cashew nuts
2 tablespoons raisins

1 Put the rice and coconut milk into a heavy-bottomed saucepan and bring to the boil. Reduce the heat and simmer for 40 minutes or so until the rice becomes mushy. Further mash the rice roughly with a whisk while still on the heat.

2 Add the sugar, cardamom powder and saffron and stir well.

3 Heat the ghee or oil in a small saucepan and fry the cashew nuts and raisins briefly. Mix gently into the rice and serve warm or cold.

goan coconut pastries
neureos

Christmas in Goa comes alive with every home cooking up feasts of mains and sweets. Here is a sweet made from fresh coconut and local cashew nuts. The pastries keep for about a week in an airtight container and last longer in the fridge.

Serves: 4
Preparation time: 20 minutes
Cooking time: 1 hour

300g plain flour, plus extra for flouring
4 tablespoons ghee or sunflower oil
Pinch of salt
150g sugar
150g freshly grated or desiccated coconut
2 tablespoons cashew nuts, crushed
2 tablespoons raisins
Large pinch of cardamom powder
Sunflower oil for deep-frying

1 Mix the flour, half the ghee or oil and salt. Add just enough water to knead into a firm dough and reserve.

2 Heat the sugar and an equal quantity of water in a heavy saucepan until a single thread consistency syrup forms. Then add the coconut, cashews and raisins. As the mixture thickens, add the cardamon powder. Remove from the heat when the mixture has turned fairly dry and reserve.

3 Divide the dough into 8 small balls and roll each out into a disc about 1cm thick, flouring the board as necessary.

4 Put a spoonful of the coconut filling in the middle, wet the edges and fold over to form a half-moon shape. Press down the edges and trim with a serrated cutter or knife.

5 Heat the oil in a deep frying pan. When nearly smoking hot, reduce the heat and deep-fry the pastries in batches. Drain and reserve. Serve cold or warm.

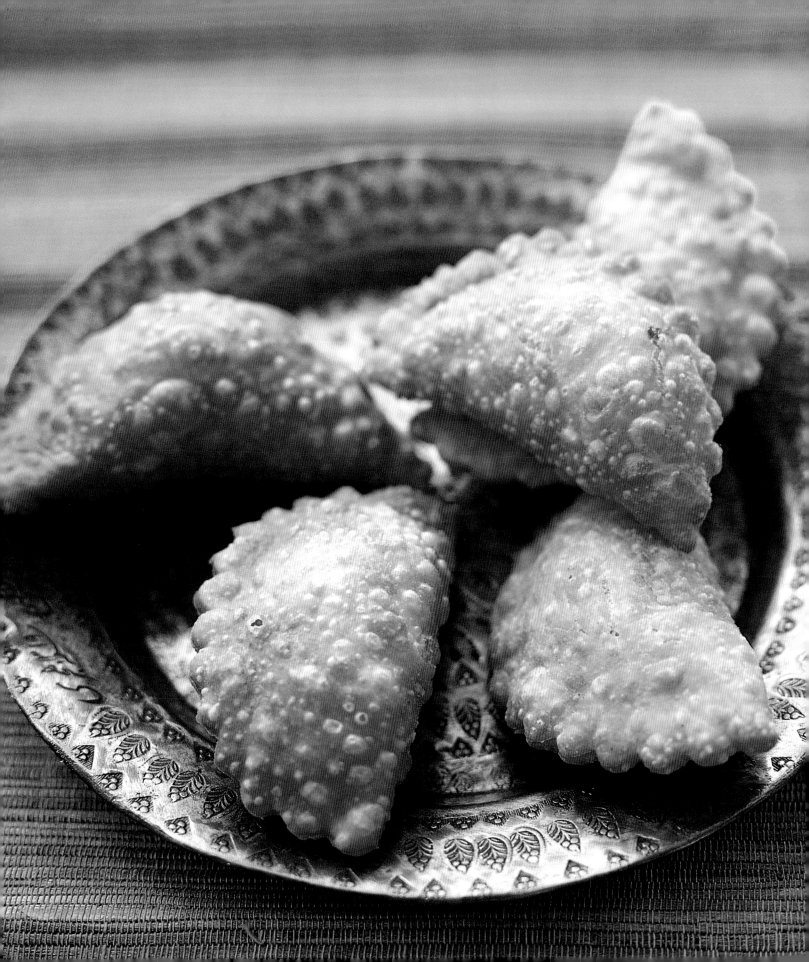

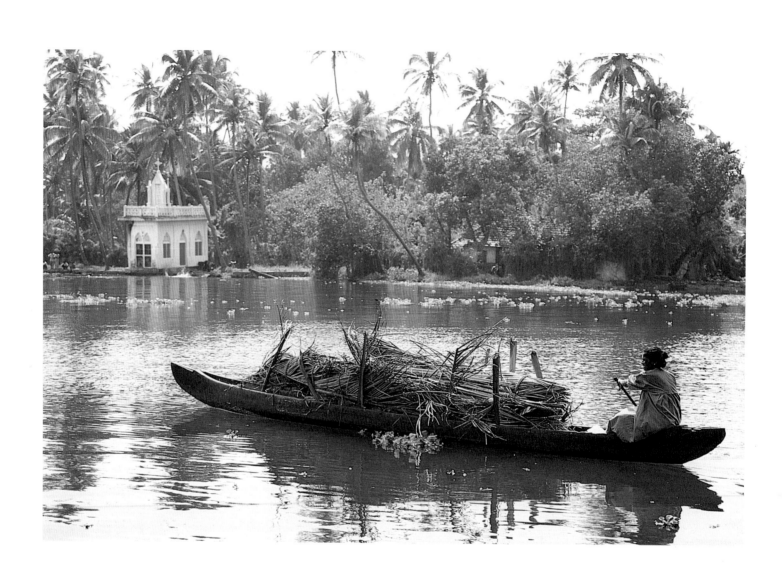

minty yoghurt cooler
boorani

This refreshingly green drink from Hyderabad is a real thirst quencher. It goes well with a spicy main course as it helps neutralise the fiery effect of chillies and hot spices. Traditionally, rock salt is used for this. Indian rock salt has a garlicky aroma which goes well with yoghurt.

Serves: 4
Preparation time: 15 minutes
Cooking time: nil

1 teaspoon cumin seeds
Few mint leaves, chopped
Few coriander leaves, chopped
300g natural yoghurt
300ml water
Salt

1 Roast the cumin on a small griddle and grind to a fine powder in a coffee mill or mortar. Reserve.

2 Grind the mint and coriander leaves to a paste with some water in a blender.

3 Mix this green paste together with the yoghurt, water, salt and cumin powder in a large mixing bowl and pour into individual serving glasses. Serve chilled.

herbal tea
kashaya

South Indians drink this healing tea throughout the day. The spices work to soothe and heal and the warmth of the drink calms the nerves and restores equilibrium. It is especially comforting if you have a cough, cold or the flu but it also makes an exceptional everyday drink to keep the throat well conditioned.

Serves: 4
Preparation time: 5 minutes
Cooking time: 15 minutes

3 tablespoons organic barley
1/2 teaspoon cumin seeds
Pinch of powdered cardamom
0.5cm piece of fresh ginger, bruised
570ml water
Jaggery or raw cane sugar to taste

1 Put the barley, cumin, cardamom powder, ginger and water in a large saucepan and bring to a boil.

2 Reduce the heat and simmer for 5 minutes. Strain and add sugar, if desired. Serve hot.

almond milk
badam doodh

Every Indian festival is associated with certain foods. Sharad Poornima or the full moon night in autumn is considered to be exceptionally beautiful, a night when the Mother Goddess showers her choicest blessings on her devotees. The occasion is celebrated with much feasting, usually on the flat roofs of houses or outdoors in gardens from where the moon can be appreciated. This milk drink is made to serve to visitors and friends.

Serves : 4
Preparation time: 15 minutes
Cooking time: nil

5 tablespoons almonds, soaked in water for
 1 hour
600ml milk
Large pinch of powdered cardamom
Honey or sugar to taste

1 Blend the almonds along with their skins, to a fine paste with a little of the milk in a blender. Don't worry if some nut pieces remain, they will add texture!

2 Stir the paste into the rest of the milk, sprinkle in the cardamom, sweeten to taste and serve at room temperature.

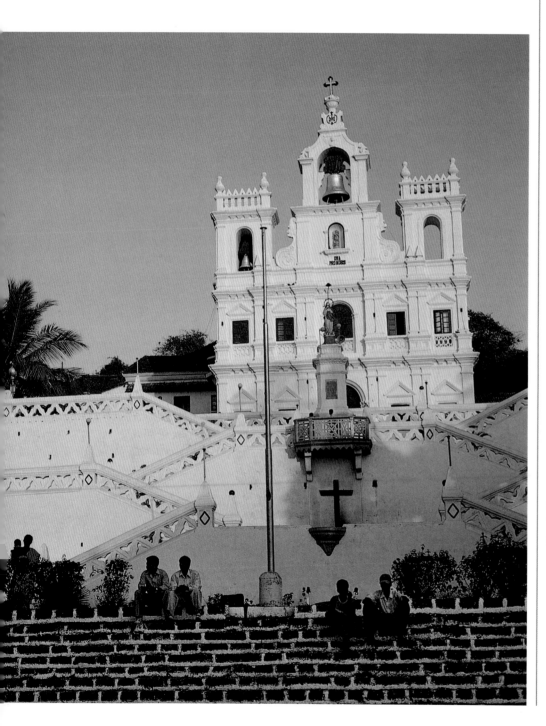

sambhar powder

The special spice blend of south India is sambhar powder. Sambhar is a preparation of lentils and vegetables that is spiked with different spices and laced with coriander. Sambhar is eaten every day in Tamil Nadu as the lentils provide protein in a meat-free diet.

Sambhar powder is fine and has a strong, earthy, dry smell of roasted spices and lentils. Ready-made sambhar powder is available commercially but it is never quite as fragrant as the home-made one. However, if you get an authentic south Indian brand, it is often quite good. Make a small quantity although it will store for up to a year in a dry, airtight jar. There are many recipes for sambhar powder. Here is one:

1 teaspoon black mustard seeds
1 teaspoon fenugreek seeds
2 teaspoons cumin seeds
12 dried red chillies, stalks removed and deseeded
1 teaspoon black peppercorns
1 teaspoon coriander seeds
1 teaspoon turmeric powder
1/4 teaspoon asafoetida
3 teaspoons sunflower oil
3 teaspoons split black lentils (urad dal)
3 teaspoons split yellow lentils (toor dal)

kholombo powder

1 Heat a heavy-bottomed saucepan and dry-roast the mustard, fenugreek and cumin seeds, chillies, peppercorns and coriander seeds. Keep the heat low and stir constantly to prevent burning. The seeds will crackle and fly out so beware!

2 Add the turmeric and asafoetida, give the mixture a good stir and take off the heat. Transfer it to a bowl.

3 In the same pan, heat the oil and fry the lentils. When they turn dark, add to the roasted spices. Cool the mixture and grind in a blender until fine. When the mixture is completely cool, store in an airtight jar.

In the states of Maharashtra, Karnataka and Goa along the western Konkan coast of India lives a community of people called the Konkani Saraswats to which my mother belongs. Saraswat or Konkani food is becoming increasingly popular in restaurants all over India because it is full of flavour and fragrance. As it is still relatively unknown gourmets will have the pleasure of discovering its mysterious secrets.

Kholombo is a lentil dish not unlike sambhar with an aroma reminiscent of wood smoke that enhances the flavour of food, as grilling does meat on a barbecue. The taste is hot with a slightly bitter aftertaste. It is always used in conjunction with tamarind.

Commercially, kholombo powder is only available in very select Konkani shops and there are possibly only a few outside India. Therefore it is necessary to make the blend at home. Make small quantities and store in a dry, airtight container.

One of the best recipes I have found for kholombo powder is:

1 tablespoon sunflower oil
2 tablespoons split gram lentils (channa dal)
2 teaspoons coriander seeds
8 curry leaves
2 teaspoons cumin seeds
4 cloves
1 teaspoon black peppercorns
2cm stick of cinnamon
3 tablespoons desiccated coconut

1 Heat the oil in a heavy saucepan and fry the lentils until they turn slightly dark.

2 Reduce heat and add the coriander seeds, curry leaves, cumin seeds, cloves, peppercorns and cinnamon and fry for 1 minute.

3 Add the coconut and continue frying, stirring until the coconut has turned brown and the aroma is rich.

4 Allow the mixture to cool and grind to a powder in a blender. Store in an airtight jar and use within 3 months.

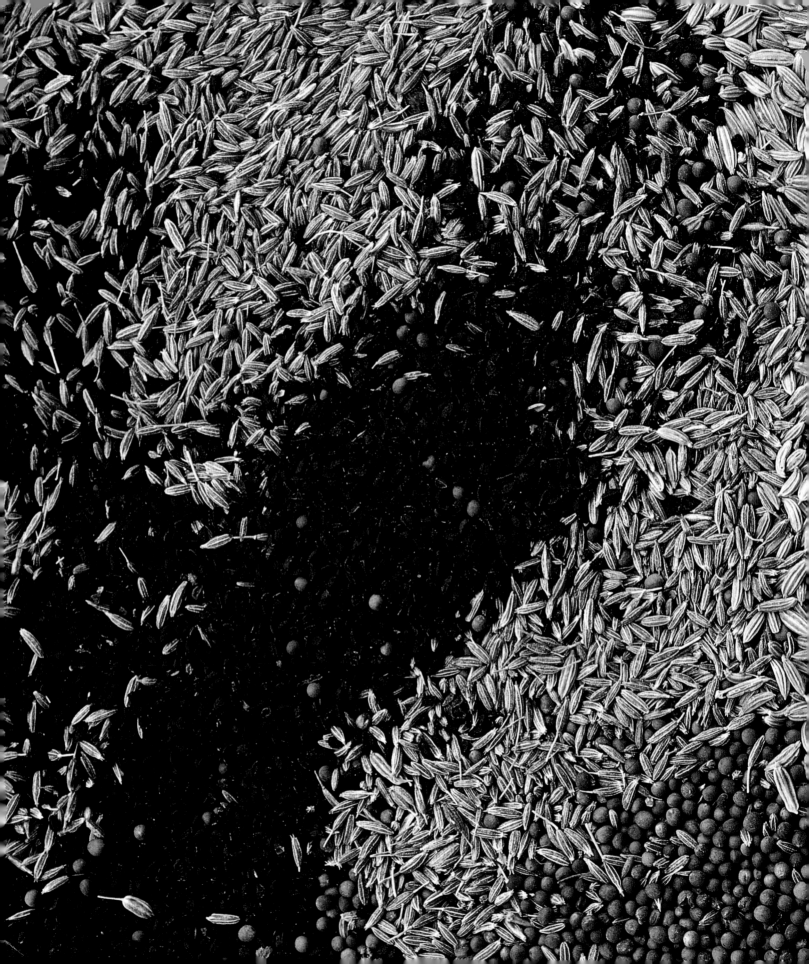

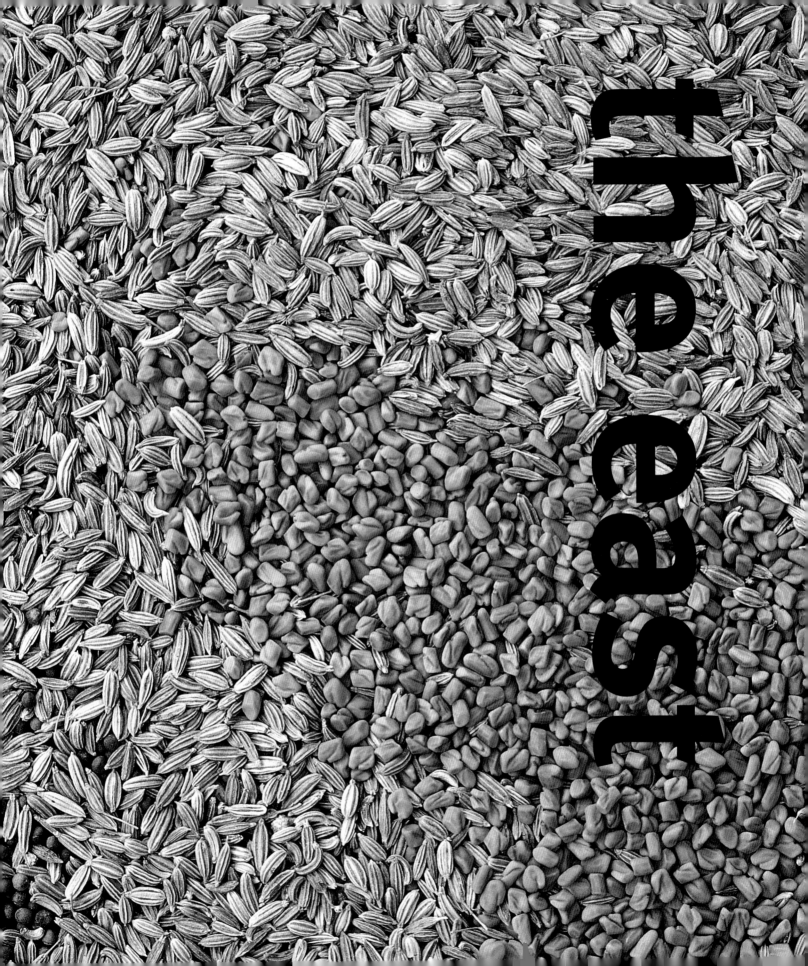

the east

west bengal

The east is predominantly West Bengal and the cooking here is similar to that of the other eastern states such as Orissa. As in other parts of the country, availability of local ingredients has determined the flavour of the region. The many rivers and the fertile soil allow rice, mangoes and coconuts to grow and milk is available in plenty. Yoghurt is spiced and ginger and mustard is used to flavour curries.

Although fish and meat are more popular, many people are, on the basis of their Hindu religion, vegetarian. Strict vegetarians will not eat even onion and garlic, preferring instead a spice called asafoetida that can be said to have a garlic-like aroma. Rice is eaten with all curries and the Bengalis grow one crop a year, leaving enough time to pursue what they love only second to eating – appreciation of the fine arts, namely music, painting and literature.

Due to its proximity to the Mughal-influenced north of India, it is unsurprising that the Bengali Muslims have a cuisine with the best of kebabs and biryanis that are the pride of Mughlai cooking. Kolkatta, or Calcutta as it was formerly known, was the seat of the East India Company and the European traders introduced foods from their part of the world such as potatoes, chillies and tomatoes. Bengali cookery soon adopted these and combined them with native ingredients.

West Bengal has a great vegetarian repertoire although the fish dishes are most famous. They will make ingenious use of parts of vegetables that most people would throw away, thus we have several chutneys made of peels or stalks of vegetables.

The use of spices is unique and a special blend called panch phoron or five spice mixture is used extensively. This is a mixture of cumin, fennel, fenugreek, kalonji (onion seeds) and black mustard. The five spice mixture is fried in a little oil and added to most dishes. Black mustard is ground to a paste to make fiery curries. But the unique feature of Bengali cooking is the repertoire of sweets. A mishti or sweet shop is seen on every street corner in Kolkatta and even in other cities of India. Syrupy rasmalai, milky sandesh and a sweet yoghurt called mishti dhoi all come from here.

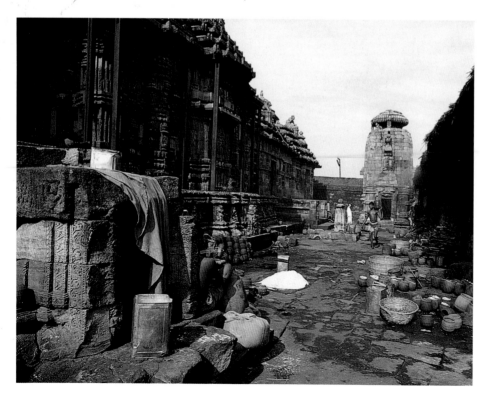

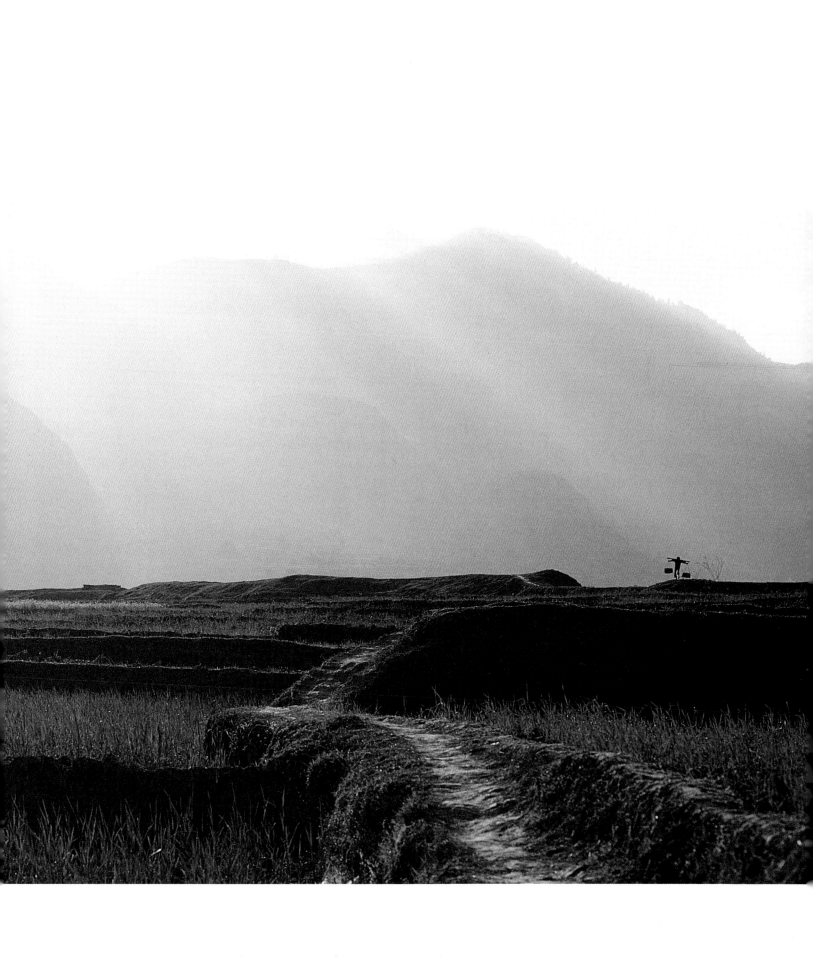

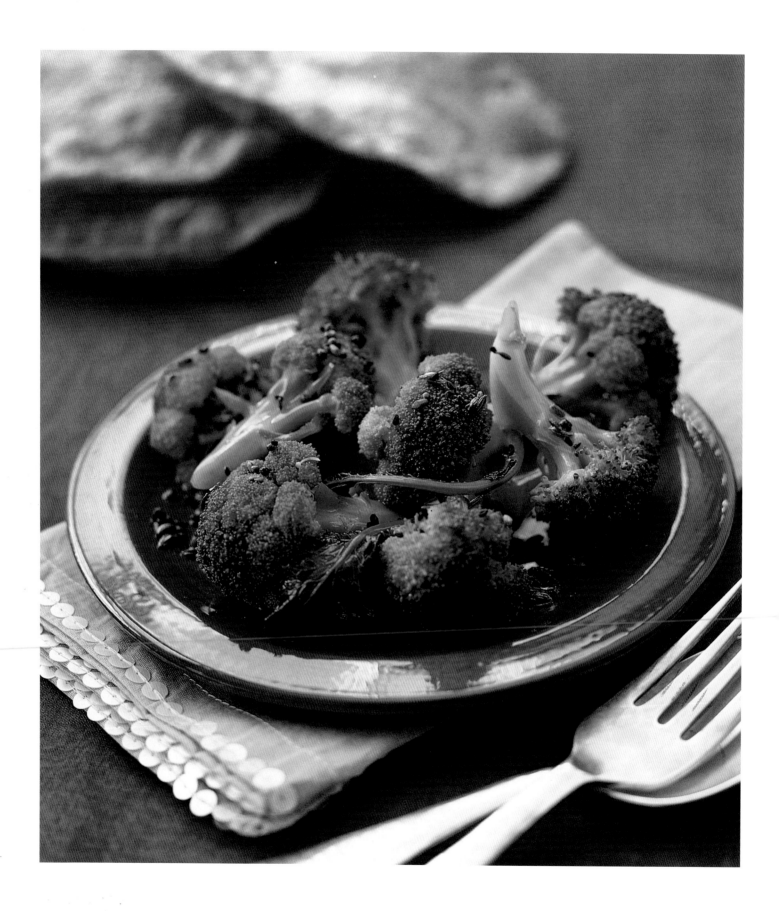

broccoli with five spices
panch phodoner gobi

The Bengalis use this combination of five aromatic spices in many of their recipes. Black onion seeds are sold as 'kalonji' in Indian shops. You can use any vegetable with this spice mixture for a quick stir-fry. I often use cauliflower or red pumpkin.

Serves: 4
Preparation time: 10 minutes
Cooking time: 15 minutes

2 tablespoons sunflower oil
$1/2$ teaspoon cumin seeds
$1/2$ teaspoon fennel seeds
$1/2$ teaspoon fenugreek seeds
$1/2$ teaspoon black mustard seeds
$1/2$ teaspoon black onion seeds
600g broccoli, cut into florettes
1 teaspoon turmeric powder
1 teaspoon chilli powder
Salt
1 teaspoon lemon juice

1 Heat the oil and add all the spice seeds.

2 As they pop and darken, add the broccoli, turmeric and chilli powders and salt. Mix well and pour in a few tablespoons of water. Bring to a sizzle then reduce the heat and cook until the broccoli is tender but still holds its shape.

3 Raise the heat to get rid of any liquid that remains. Drizzle in the lemon juice and serve hot with Luchis (page 151).

baby aubergines in spiced yoghurt
dhoi begun

There are many different kinds of aubergines available today. If you cannot find little ones, slice the large aubergines into discs and fry a few at a time in a shallow frying pan. Aubergines tend to absorb a lot of oil. In order to reduce this, make sure that the oil is very hot.

Serves: 4
Preparation time: 15 minutes
Cooking time: 35 minutes

300g small aubergines, washed and slit
  down the middle
Salt
1 teaspoon turmeric powder
Sunflower oil for deep-frying
1 teaspoon cumin seeds
$1/2$ teaspoon red chilli powder
150g natural yoghurt, beaten
$1/2$ teaspoon sugar

1 Rub the aubergines with the salt and turmeric. Heat the oil in a deep frying pan and deep-fry the aubergines. Drain and reserve.

2 Heat 1 tablespoon of the oil in a small saucepan and add the cumin seeds. As they crackle, add the red chilli powder. Pour this into the yoghurt. Add the sugar and salt and pour the spiced yoghurt over the aubergines. Serve at once.

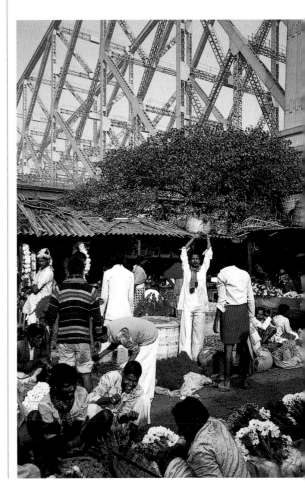

fried bitter gourds and potatoes
alu karela bhaja

Karela or bitter gourd is popular all over India as most people believe in the Ayurvedic advice that bitter tastes are healthy. Karela is also believed to help people who suffer from diabetes. In this recipe, the frying of the karela takes away some of the bitter taste although it is impossible to effectively diminish it by much. Serve this crunchy dish as a side to rice and lentils.

Serves: 4
Preparation time: 20 minutes
Cooking time: 35 minutes

2 tablespoons mustard oil or sunflower oil
1/4 teaspoon nigella seeds
1/2 teaspoon turmeric powder
300g karela or bitter gourd, washed
  and cut into round slices (leave skin on)
300g potatoes, peeled and cut into chips
Salt
2 fresh green chillies, slit

1 Heat the oil in a heavy saucepan or kadhai. When it is quite hot add the nigella seeds.

2 As they start to pop, add the turmeric and the bitter gourd. Stir for 1 minute. Then add the potatoes and stir for another minute.

3 Add salt and the green chillies. Cover the pan with a hollow lid filled with a little water and cook on low heat until the vegetables are done. Serve hot.

bengali-style mixed vegetables
shukto

Every region in India has a recipe for mixed vegetables in spices; in fact many of these dishes are considered festive and offered to the gods. In order for them to be appropriate for this, they have to have a prescribed number of ingredients, especially vegetables. The best of seasonal vegetables are used for this purpose.

Serves: 4
Preparation time: 45 minutes
Cooking time: 45 minutes

3 tablespoons sunflower oil
75g each of:
karela or bitter gourd, sliced
potatoes, peeled and cut into chips
small aubergines, thickly sliced
horseradish, thickly sliced
raw plantain, peeled and sliced
parwal or pointed gourds, peeled and sliced

grind to a fine paste with water as needed:
2.5cm piece of fresh ginger, peeled
1 teaspoon black mustard seeds
2 teaspoons cumin powder
1 teaspoon chilli powder
1 teaspoon turmeric powder

salt
1 teaspoon sugar
1 tablespoon ghee
1 teaspoon panch phoron (page 160)

1 Heat the oil in a heavy saucepan and fry the karela until brown. Add the rest of the vegetables and keep frying until they all start to turn brown.

2 Add the ground ginger and spice mixture, salt and sugar and mix well. Pour in about 100ml of water and simmer until the vegetables are cooked.

3 Heat the ghee in a small pan and add the panch phoron. When it starts to pop, pour the entire mixture into the vegetables and stir gently.

4 Serve hot with Luchis (page 151) or rice.

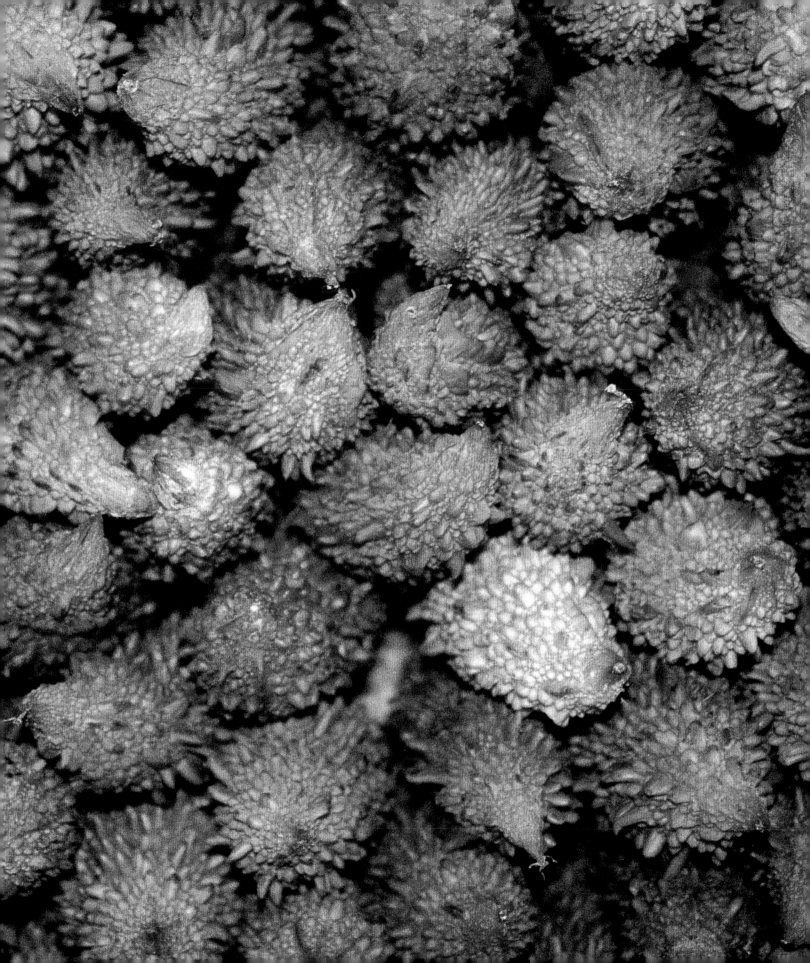

potatoes with tamarind
alurdam

This sort of dish with baby potatoes exists all over north India and has filtered into the east. You can use larger potatoes, peeled and boiled, but these taste better I think. The sauce can be made with other vegetables too – try yams or aubergines.

Serves: 4
Preparation time: 10 minutes
Cooking time: 35 minutes

3 tablespoons sunflower oil
1/2 teaspoon black mustard seeds
Few curry leaves
1 tablespoon freshly grated ginger
300g new potatoes, boiled and drained
3 fresh green chillies, minced
1 teaspoon sugar
Salt
1 teaspoon tamarind concentrate, diluted in
  4 tablespoons water

1 Heat the oil in a heavy saucepan and fry the mustard seeds until they pop, then add the curry leaves and ginger.

2 Add the boiled potatoes and fry for a couple of minutes.

3 Add the chillies, sugar, salt and tamarind. Reduce the heat and cook for about 5 minutes until a thick sauce forms. Serve hot with Luchis (page 151).

cabbage with five spices and ginger
bandhkophir chorchori

This recipe can also be made with cauliflower or red cabbage. I am often asked about which kind of mustard seeds are best to use in Indian cooking. Always use black mustard seeds in curries and stir-fries. Split mustard seeds, without their skin, are creamy in colour and are used in savoury pickles such as hot mango and hot chilli.

Serves: 4
Preparation time: 20 minutes
Cooking time: 30 minutes

1 teaspoon black mustard seeds
2 teaspoons shredded ginger
4 dried red chillies, deseeded, soaked in
  water and drained
3 tablespoons sunflower oil
1 large onion, finely sliced
300g cabbage, finely shredded
Salt
2 teaspoons panch phoron (page 160)

1 Put the mustard seeds, ginger and red chillies in a blender along with 5 tablespoons of water and whizz to a fine paste. Reserve.

2 Heat 2 tablespoons of the oil in a pan and add the onion. Fry until golden, then add the cabbage. Stir-fry for a couple of minutes until just translucent and sprinkle in the ground spice mixture and salt.

3 Add 4 tablespoons of water and cook uncovered until the cabbage is done but still crisp. Take off the heat and reserve.

4 Heat the remaining oil in a separate pan and add the panch phoron. When it crackles, pour the oil and the seeds over the cabbage. Mix well. Serve hot with Luchis (page 151) or with rice and Bengali Dal (page 153)

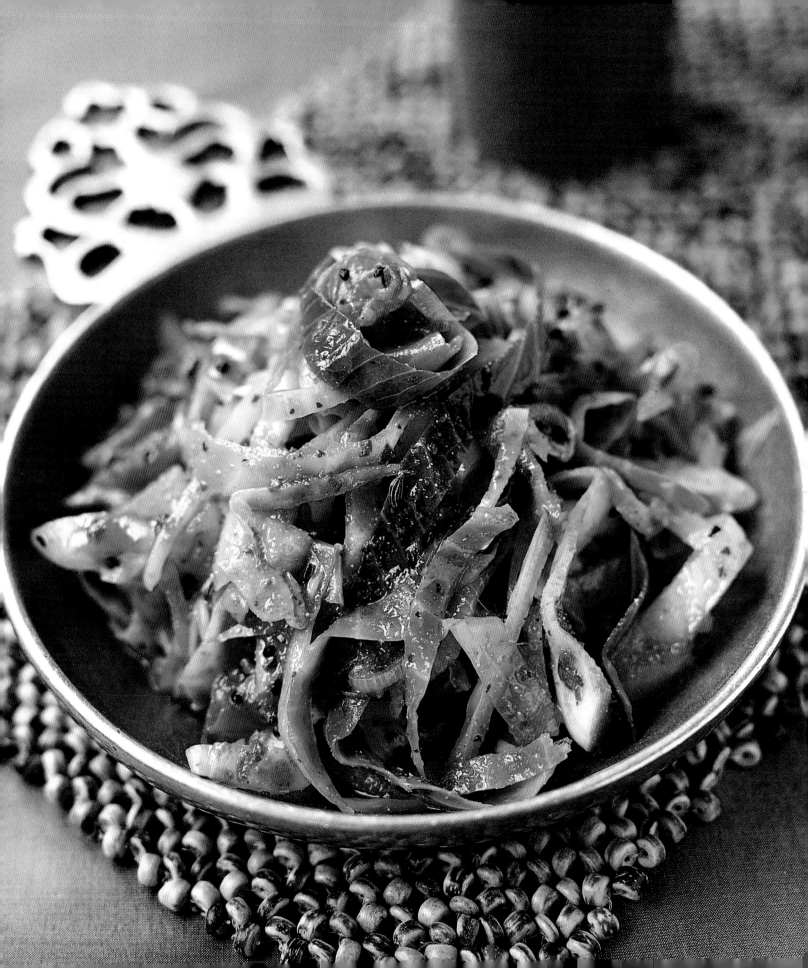

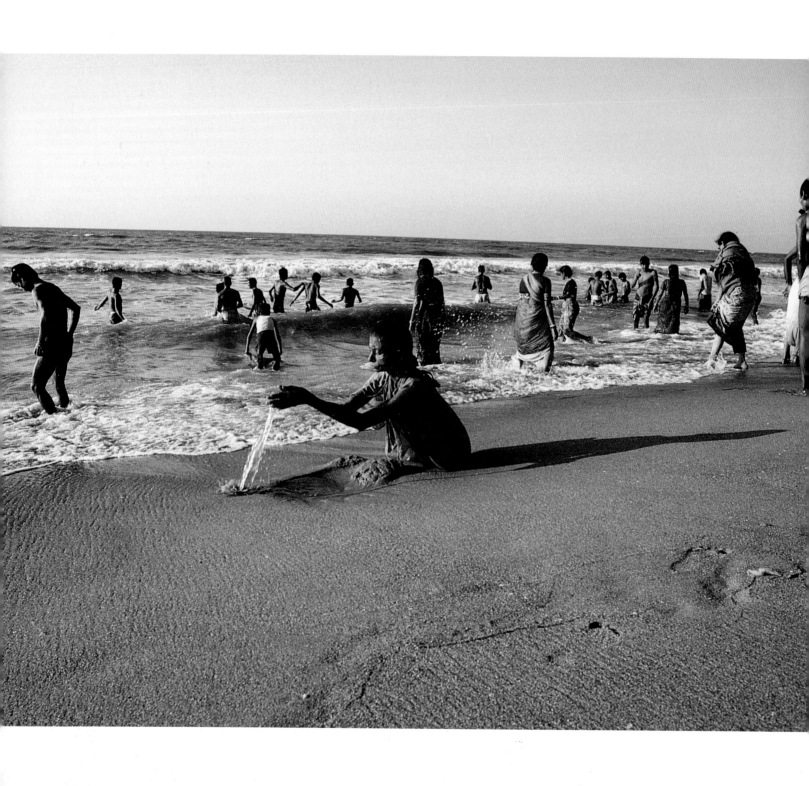

rice with ghee and spices
ghee bhaat

Although this is a simple-sounding recipe, every Bengali I know almost drools at the mention of ghee bhaat. This may be because it is very fragrant and goes well with so many lentils and vegetables. You could add vegetables to the rice such as French beans, carrots or peas.

Serves: 4
Preparation time: 15 minutes
Cooking time: 25 minutes

2 tablespoons ghee
1 medium onion, sliced
4 cloves
3 green cardamom pods
1 small stick of cinnamon
2 bay leaves
1 teaspoon raisins
300g basmati rice, washed and drained
Salt

1 Heat half the ghee in a small saucepan and fry the onion until well browned for about 10 minutes. Stir frequently to prevent them from burning. Drain and reserve.

2 Heat the remaining ghee in a separate pan and fry the spices and bay leaves for 1 minute. Add the raisins and the rice and stir for a couple of minutes. Season with salt and pour in 600ml of hot water.

3 Bring to the boil, stir, reduce the heat and cover. Simmer for 10 minutes and keep covered for a further 10 minutes for the rice to fluff up in the steam.

4 Serve hot, garnished with the fried onions.

fried puffy bread
luchis

These are exactly like the poories of northern and western India and are very popular all over Bengal. In fact a breakfast of luchi and subjee or vegetables is considered special. Luchis are also served as a part of a festive meal. One such time is Durga Puja, the important festival in honour of the Mother Goddess that is especially celebrated in Bengal.

Serves: 4
Preparation time: 15 minutes
Cooking time: 25 minutes

300g plain flour, plus extra for flouring
Sunflower oil for deep-frying
Salt

1 Put the flour in a shallow dish, make a well in the centre and pour in 2 tablespoons of oil. Season with salt. Add enough water to make a stiff dough and knead well. Cover with a wet cloth and keep for 30 minutes.

2 Make 8 equal-sized balls of the dough and roll each one out into a thin disc, flouring the board as necessary.

3 Heat the oil in a deep frying pan. When it is nearly smoking, fry 1 luchi at a time, turning it over until it is puffy and golden on both sides. Serve hot.

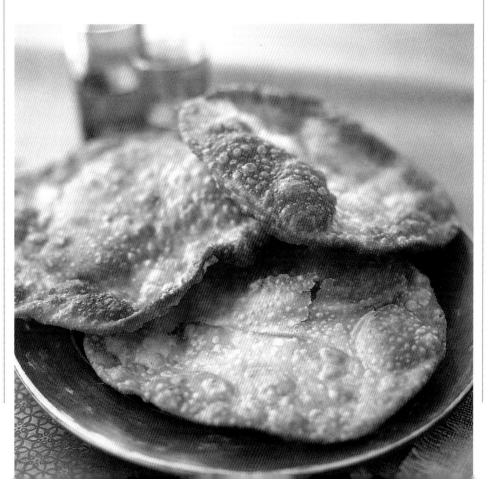

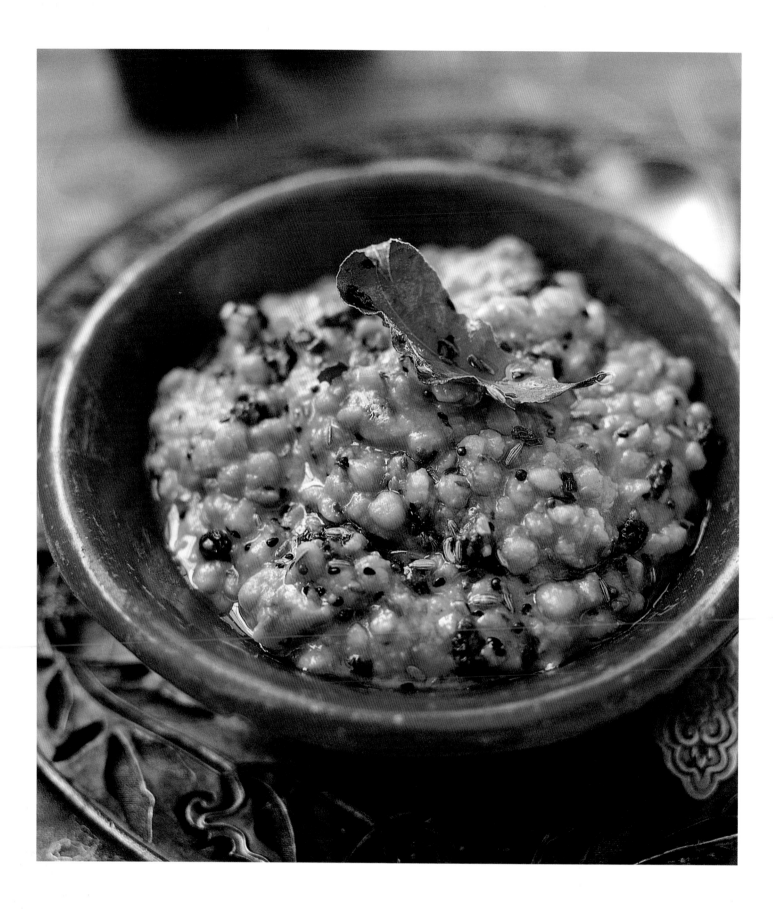

sweet and sour lentils
bengali dal

Enjoy this with luchis for a perfect Bengali meal. If you cannot get hold of mango powder, use 1 teaspoon of tamarind concentrate diluted in a few tablespoons of water. Channa dal takes a long time to cook. If you have the time to soak it overnight, do so as this will drastically reduce cooking times.

Serves: 4
Preparation time: 20 minutes + at least 1 hour soaking time
Cooking time: 1 hour

300g split gram lentils (channa dal)
1 teaspoon turmeric powder
Salt
2 teaspoons sugar
3 tablespoons sunflower oil
2 tablespoons panch phoron (page 160)
4 dried red chillies, deseeded and crumbled
2 bay leaves
2 teaspoons mango powder (amchoor)

1 Simmer the lentils in about 600ml of hot water until soft and mushy. Add water as necessary to get a thick consistency, then stir in the turmeric, salt and sugar. Blend well.

2 Heat the oil in a small pan and add the panch phoron. When it crackles, add the red chillies, bay leaves, mango powder and raisins. Reduce the heat and pour the oil and the spices over the lentils.

3 Add water if required to adjust the consistency which should be that of a thick soup. Bring to the boil once and serve hot.

spiced red lentils
mushur dal

Red lentils are available as whole or split. The whole ones are brown like puy lentils while the split ones are orangey-red. These cook very easily and do not need to be soaked. The consistency of the dal should be quite thick and soupy.

Serves: 4
Preparation time: 10 minutes
Cooking time: 30 minutes

150g red lentils (masoor dal), washed and drained
Salt
1/2 teaspoon turmeric powder
2 fresh green chillies, minced
2 tablespoons sunflower oil
2 dried red chillies
1 teaspoon panch phoron (page 160)
1 medium onion, chopped

1 Put the red lentils along with the salt, turmeric and green chillies into a heavy saucepan with about 600ml of hot water and bring to the boil. Reduce the heat and cook for about 15 minutes until the lentils are mushy. Take off the heat and reserve.

2 Heat the oil in a saucepan and add the red chillies and the panch phoran. As it turns dark, add the onion and fry until soft.

3 Add the cooked lentils and bring to the boil. Take off the heat and serve hot with plain rice.

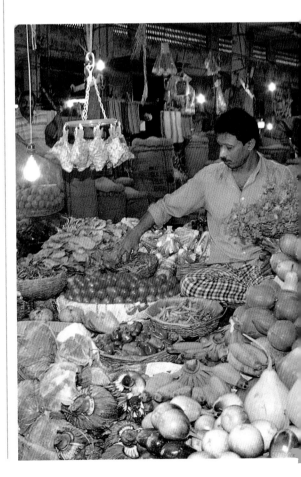

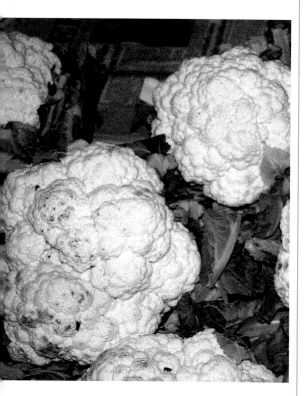

cauliflower fritters
phoolkopir bhaja

Vegetable fritters are found not just all over India but around the world. The onion bhaji has become a popular snack everywhere. Spices make the fritters easy to digest.`

Serves: 4
Preparation time: 20 minutes
Cooking time: 25 minutes

For the batter:
150g gram flour
1/2 teaspoon chilli powder
1 teaspoon turmeric powder
1 teaspoon cumin seeds
1/2 teaspoon ajowan seeds
Salt
Sunflower oil for deep-frying

300g cauliflower, cut into medium-sized
  florettes

1 Make a thick batter of all the batter ingredients and water as needed to achieve the consistency of thick custard.

2 Heat the oil in a deep kadhai or frying pan until it is nearly smoking.

3 Dip each cauliflower florette in the batter and gently add to the hot oil. Reduce the heat to allow the cauliflower to cook through. Do this in batches, a few at a time, frying until golden, then drain on absorbent paper.

4 Serve hot with Pineapple Chutney (right) or tomato ketchup.

pineapple chutney
ananas chutney

Each year my grandmother would prepare a seasonal pineapple chutney that would make the house smell like a tropical paradise. I loved to eat this sweet confection with rotis at teatime when I got home from school. This is the Bengali version, rich with dried fruit and spices. It can be stored in the fridge, in an airtight container or jar, for up to 10 days.

Serves: 4
Preparation time: 25 minutes if using
  fresh pineapple
Cooking time: 15 minutes

1 tablespoon sunflower oil
1/2 teaspoon panch phoron (page 160)
2 dried red chillies
1 teaspoon raisins
2 dates, stoned and chopped
1 teaspoon peeled and freshly grated ginger
150g fresh or tinned pineapple, chopped
  (drained if using tinned)
1 tablespoon lemon juice
Salt
Sugar

1 Heat the oil in a heavy-bottomed saucepan and add the panch phoron. When it crackles, add the chillies, then the raisins, dates and ginger, and stir a couple of times.

2 Add the pineapple and 5–6 tablespoons of water if using fresh pineapple, or juice if using tinned pineapple. Cook over low heat for 5 minutes until the pineapple is quite mushy. Sprinkle in the lemon juice, season with salt and add sugar. Cook for a further 2 minutes and take off the heat. Cool and serve with any main meal.

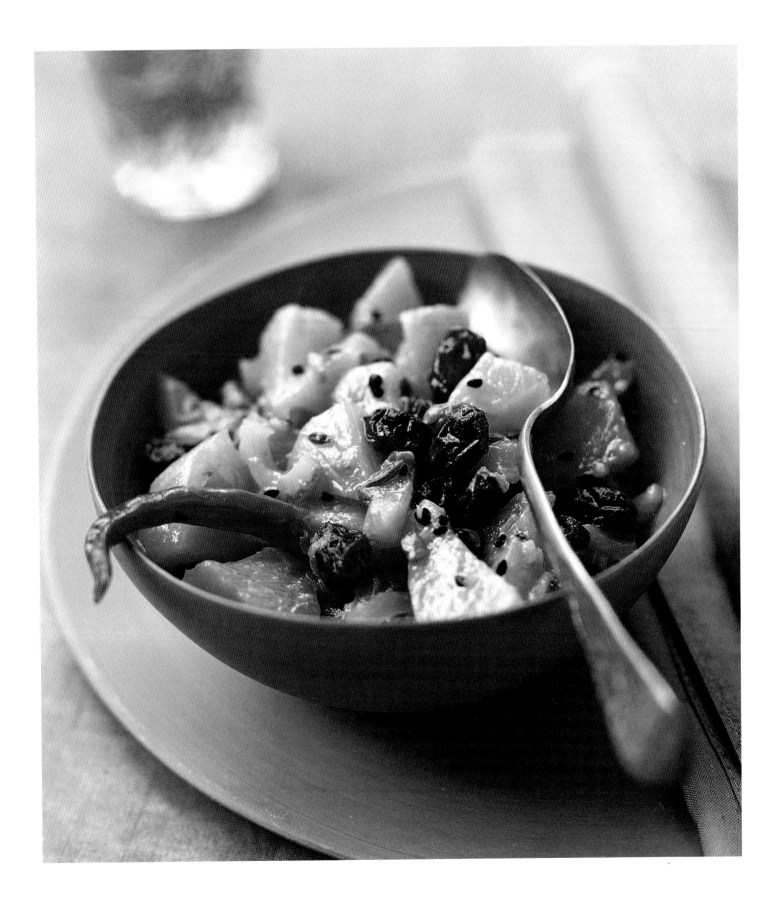

cottage cheese in spiced sweet milk
rasmalai

Rasmalai is one of the most famous Indian desserts known outside of India. The one you eat in restaurants is usually commercially mass-made and this home-made version is more crumbly and delicate. I hang up the paneer for quite a long time to make sure that it does not crumble up too much during the cooking. Sometimes I serve the rasmalai in mango-flavoured milk – just add a little mango purée to the milk before serving.

Serves: 4
Preparation time: 10 minutes + 1 hour draining time
Cooking time: 45 minutes

1.8 litres milk
Few drops of lemon juice
150g sugar
1/2 teaspoon powdered cardamom seeds
Pinch of saffron
2 teaspoons sliced almonds and pistachios

1 Put 1.2 litres of the milk into a pan and bring it to the boil. Add the lemon juice and let the milk curdle. Hang up the curdled milk in a clean piece of muslin and allow the whey to drain off for about 30 minutes.

2 In the meantime set 1.3 litres of water to boil in a large, shallow saucepan and add a couple of tablespoons of the sugar to it.

3 Take the paneer out of the muslin and knead it lightly for about 1 minute. Shape it into balls the size of a small lime and flatten them slightly. You should get about 8 balls.

4 Reduce the heat under the boiling water and slip the balls in gently.

5 Drain and remove them after about 10 minutes. The water will go milky and bits will break away from the paneer balls but this is normal. Keep the drained paneer balls flat on a plate. They should be quite spongy.

6 In a separate pan, heat the rest of the milk and sugar. Reduce it until it is quite thick, for about 30 minutes, taking care not to let it burn or spill over. This is done on fairly low heat. Add the cardamom powder and the saffron.

7 Take off the heat, cool and gently add the paneer balls to the milk. Chill well and serve sprinkled with the sliced nuts.

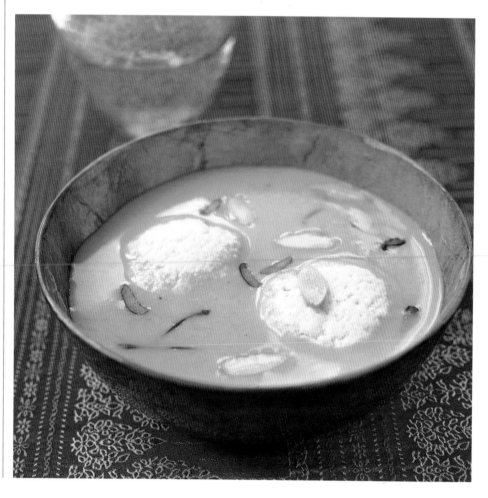

yoghurt balls in saffron syrup
ledikini

Bengali sweets are usually made with sugar syrup and therefore taste quite rich and sweet. Many Bengalis will take a leisurely stroll after dinner to the nearest sweet shop for a spot of pudding! There is a huge variety of sweets to tempt the eye and the palate.

Serves: 4
Preparation time: 10 minutes + 12 hours draining time
Cooking time: 45 minutes + 30 minutes steeping time

600g full fat yoghurt
80g fine semolina
1/2 teaspoon powdered cardamom
300g sugar
Pinch of saffron
Sunflower oil for deep-frying

1 Hang up the yoghurt in a clean cheesecloth or muslin for at least 12 hours until it is quite dry and flaky.

2 Scoop out the hung yoghurt into a mixing bowl and beat it to loosen it. Knead in the semolina and cardamom. Mix well to form a dough and reserve.

3 Now make the sugar syrup. Combine the sugar with 450ml of water in a heavy-bottomed saucepan. Add the saffron. Bring to the boil and reduce the heat to simmer until a single thread consistency forms. To check this, put a drop of the syrup onto a cold plate. Cool slightly and dab with your finger. When you lift your finger, a single thread of syrup should be seen. Take off the heat and reserve.

4 Shape the dough into equal-sized balls the size of a large cherry. Heat the oil in a deep frying pan or kadhai. When it is nearly smoking hot, gently slip a few balls at a time into the hot oil. Fry them on low heat to prevent them from splitting and to cook them evenly, turning from time to time.

5 When they are brown, drain and remove onto absorbent paper. When all the balls are fried, add them to the cool sugar syrup and let them steep for 30 minutes.

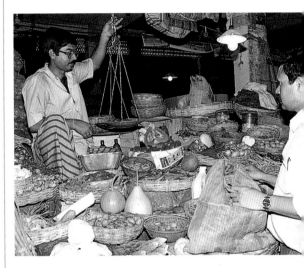

baby milk dumplings in rose syrup
rossogulla

In 1866, Nobin Chandra Das set up a small sweet shop in Calcutta and, being from a sugar trading family, conjured up a new sweet dipped in sugar syrup. This was the rossogulla. The story goes that a wealthy businessman's carriage stopped for some water at Das's shop. Das offered a rossogulla with the water and the businessman loved it, creating fabulous opportunities for the young shopkeeper. Rossogullas keep very well in the fridge so you could make them in advance if cooking for a party.

Serves: 4
Preparation time: 1 day
Cooking time: 30 minutes

600ml full fat milk
Juice of 2 lemons
1 tablespoon plain flour
150g sugar
2 tablespoons rose water

1 Bring the milk to boiling point in a heavy saucepan and add the lemon juice to the pan. The milk will begin to split. Reduce the heat and keep simmering until all the milk solids have separated. Line a large bowl with cheesecloth or muslin and pour the split milk into it. Lift the cloth out and drain off the whey. Hang it up over the sink to continue the draining. (I tie the muslin cloth to my kitchen tap!)

2 When the milk solids are almost dry, put the bundle into a colander, press down with a weight and leave to drain for a further 3–4 hours.

3 Once the solid cheese (paneer) has been formed, knead it with the flour to form a soft dough. Make small balls the size of large cherries from this dough. Reserve.

4 Now make the rose syrup. Boil the sugar and double its volume of water in a heavy-bottomed saucepan. Reduce the heat and simmer until the syrup thickens and you get a single thread consistency. (Check by putting a drop on a cool plate and dabbing it carefully with your finger. If a thin thread of syrup rises with your finger, it is ready.)

5 Add the cheese balls and the rose water to the syrup. Cook on low heat for 10 minutes. Cool and serve.

frosted pastries
malpua

These sweet, crisp discs should be soft at the centre and crispy at the edges. I like to serve them with a spoonful of cream and some fresh fruit. They are quite easy to make and keep quite well. Street stalls in some cities sell them freshly made, hot and fragrant. I think they taste good when cold as well.

Serves: 4
Preparation time: 20 minutes + 2 hours resting time
Cooking time: 30 minutes

300g self-raising flour
3 tablespoons semolina
150g natural yoghurt
Pinch of bicarbonate of soda
Ghee or sunflower oil for frying
Few crushed pistachios

For the syrup:
150g sugar
150ml water
1 teaspoon fennel seeds
1 teaspoon cardamom powder

1 Mix the flour, semolina, yoghurt and bicarbonate of soda, adding a little water to make a thick batter. Then cover and leave in a warm place for about 2 hours.

2 In the meantime, make the syrup by mixing the sugar, water and fennel seeds. Cook on high heat until a light syrup forms. Take off the heat, add the cardamom powder and reserve.

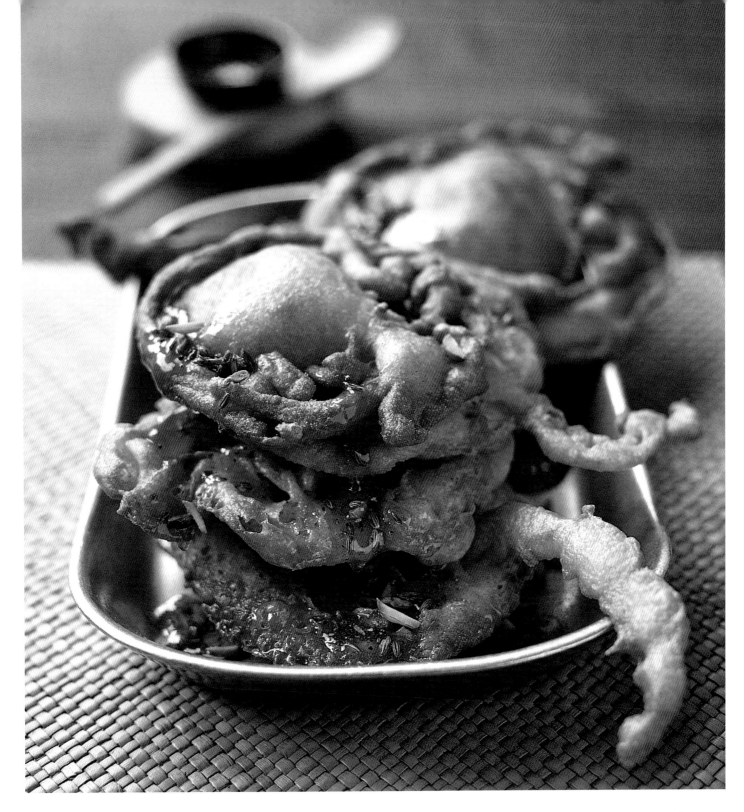

3 Heat the ghee or oil in a kadhai or deep frying pan. When it begins to smoke, lower the heat and pour in a ladleful of the batter. It will spread so shape it into a thick disc.

Fry, turning over once, until golden. Drain and arrange on a platter. Continue with the rest of the batter.

4 When all the discs are fried, pour the warm fennel syrup over. Serve sprinkled with the pistachios.

sweet coconut pancakes
patishapta

My mother used to make these for Sunday breakfast and they always remind me of indulgent days when all one needs to think of is relaxation. The cardamom and nutmeg give these pancakes a real lift and you can add your favourite nuts for a bit of texture. The pancake should be white and fine and, if you find it breaking up, add a couple of teaspoons of plain flour to bind the batter.

Serves: 4
Preparation time: 30 minutes
Cooking time: 30 minutes

300g rice flour
Salt
150g jaggery or soft brown sugar
220g freshly grated or desiccated coconut
80ml milk
1/2 teaspoon cardamom powder
1/2 teaspoon nutmeg powder
4 tablespoons ghee or sunflower oil

1 Make a batter with the flour, salt and as much water as necessary to create a pouring consistency.

2 Heat a heavy pan and melt the sugar or jaggery. Add the coconut and cook until the mixture thickens.

3 Pour in the milk and continue cooking until the mixture is thick. Then take off the heat and stir in the spices.

4 Heat a few drops of the ghee or oil in a shallow frying pan. Reduce the heat and pour a ladleful of batter in the centre, spreading it with the back of the ladle to make a thin disc. Cover and cook for 1 minute on low heat.

5 When the edges start to curl up, turn the pancake and cook on the other side for 1 minute. Arrange some of the coconut mixture along the centre of pancake and roll it up into a cylindrical shape. Serve warm.

panch phoron

Bengal lies in the north-east of India. Art, literature, food and festivals are all an inseparable part of every Bengali person's life. The people are known for their passion for rice and sweets made of clotted or burnt milk, flavoured with rose water or saffron and soaked in sugar syrup or cold, sweet milk. The most popular blend of spices here is panch phoron – Bengal's equivalent of the Chinese five-spice powder. This mixture too has five different spices which are used either in their whole form or ground to a powder and this is used to flavour lentils, pulses or vegetables. Its unique aroma is bittersweet and powerful. Panch phoron is added to hot oil first before adding vegetables, lentils or pulses. As it begins to splutter, the rest of the ingredients are dropped into the pan. Alternatively, it is fried in oil or ghee which is poured on top of a dish to flavour it. As with other blends, you can vary the ingredients according to taste.

My recipe for panch phoron is to mix equal quantities of:

Cumin seeds
Fennel seeds
Fenugreek seeds
Black mustard seeds
Nigella seeds

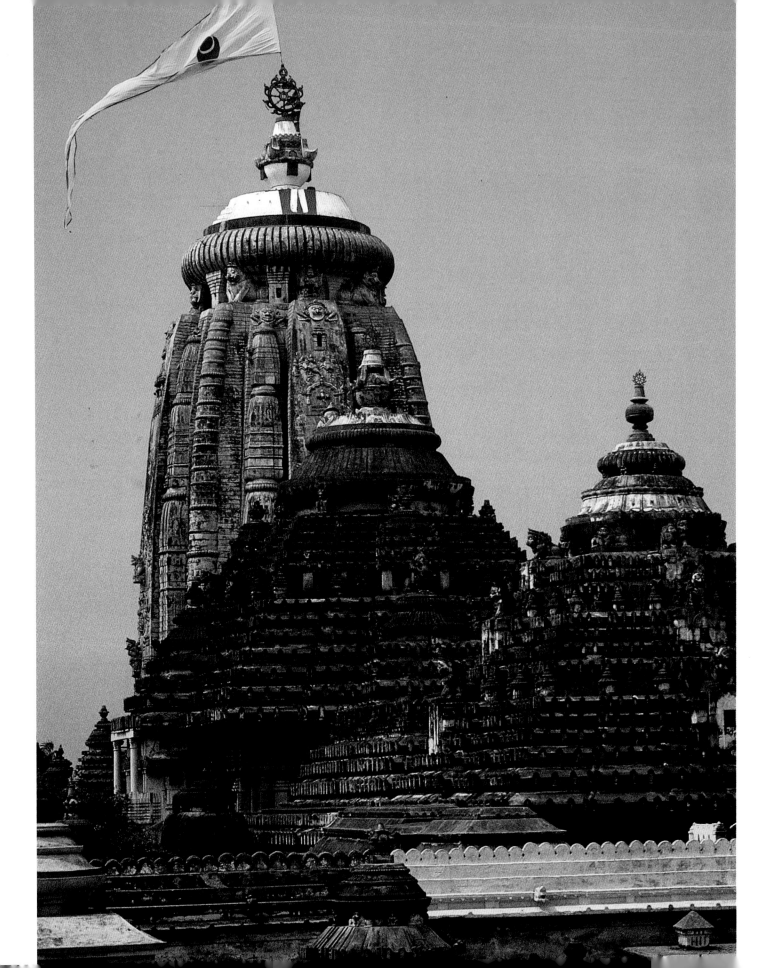

orange/red lentils
masoor dal

yellow lentils
toor dal

gram lentils
channa dal

Orange lentils are the seeds of a bushy plant that grows in cold climates. When mature, the long pods in which the lentils are contained are plucked, dried and threshed.

When left whole the lentils are dark brown to greenish-black in colour, round and flattish. The fairly thick skin conceals a pinkish-orange centre. Split lentils are the familiar orange ones found in shops. These lentils are delicate in flavour and have a nutty, fresh taste. The whole lentils are chewy, muskier and coarser.

Whole red lentils and split lentils have quite different qualities so when buying make sure you buy what is asked for in the recipe. Split red lentils are useful as they are fast cooking and make a quick, nutritious meal. Both the varieties store well for up to 6 months in a dry, airtight container.

The yellow lentils plant is a deep-rooted shrubby perennial which is grown from seed. The pods are dried in the sun or mechanically, and husked to separate the seeds, which are the lentils. In some parts of India, yellow lentils are slightly oiled to increase shelf-life, more so when the lentils are exported, and therefore Indian shops outside India usually stock the oily variety of yellow lentils.

These lentils are yellow and sold split into 2 round halves. The oily variety is sticky and glossy, the unoily one is matte. They are very easy to digest and have a pleasant, subtle, nutty flavour.

If you buy oily yellow lentils, soak them in hot water for a while and throw away the resulting cloudy, white liquid. Then wash the lentils several times to get rid of most of the oil. Yellow lentils store well for up to 6 months in clean, dry containers.

Gram, or Bengal gram as it is also known, is the most widely grown lentil in India. The bushy shrub bears seed-filled pods, each containing 2 or 3 lentils. They are picked in early winter when they turn ripe and brown. Then they are husked and left whole, split or ground into a flour called besan. This flour is used to make batter (as in fritters), as a thickening in curries or is cooked with sugar to make many different sweets.

Matte and yellow, gram lentils resemble yellow lentils but are slightly bigger and coarser. They are stronger in taste than most other lentils with a nutty sweet aroma and flavour.

Good gram lentils should be plump and bright. Store in an airtight container for about 4 months.

mung beans
moong

Mung beans, or green gram, are the most versatile of all the lentils. Bean sprouts, commonly available everywhere, are actually sprouted mung beans.

The small mung bean plant grows all over India as a rain fed crop. The beans, which grow inside pods, are threshed out after the pods are dried – either on the plant or in the sun. Mung beans are left in their skin or split. There is also a variety which is split but left in the skin.

Whole mung beans, or green gram, are small, oval, and olive-green in colour. When split, they are small, flattish and yellow. Whole mung beans have a stronger flavour than the split ones. They are rather chewy and musky. The yellow, split mung beans are extremely easy to cook, need no soaking and are easy to digest.

The whole beans and the split ones are quite different and are seldom interchangeable so you will need to get both, depending on what you plan to make. Store in an airtight container for up to 4 months.

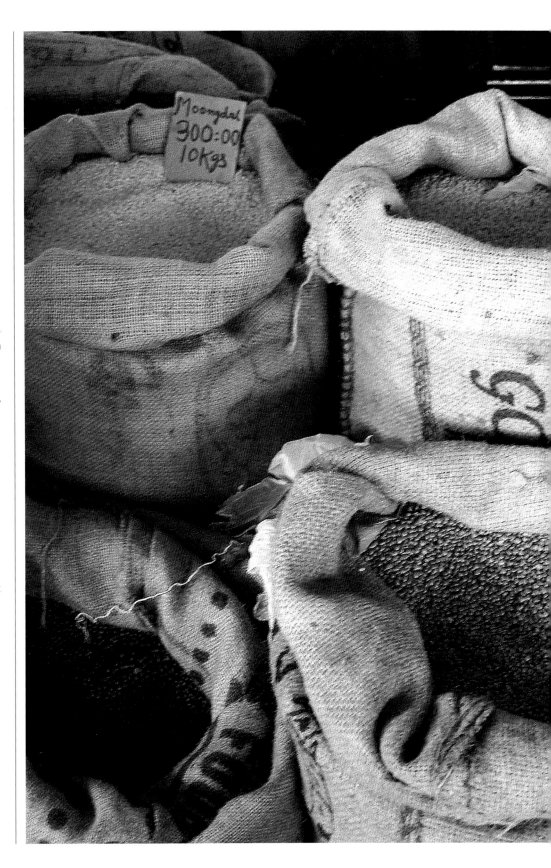

jaggery
gur

Sugar cane grows in abundance in the tropical heat of central India. During the manufacture of sugar from sugar cane, as the cane turns to crystal, several bi-products are formed: molasses, alcohol and jaggery. Jaggery is dehydrated sugar cane juice and is produced mostly by small cultivators in huge crushers run by bullocks. The jaggery is not purified and therefore has all the quality of the juice itself. Jaggery is as important as sugar in Indian cookery. It has a special flavour that cannot really be substituted by sugar, although brown or demerara sugar is the closest equivalent.

Jaggery ranges from mustard yellow to deep amber in colour, depending on the quality of the sugar cane juice. It is sticky but crumbles easily. Jaggery has a heavy, caramel-like aroma which is slightly alcoholic, like sweet sherry or port. The taste is very sweet and musky. It goes well with lentils and tamarind. You will find that jaggery is available in various sizes and wrapped in plastic or in jute cloth. Use within 6 months.

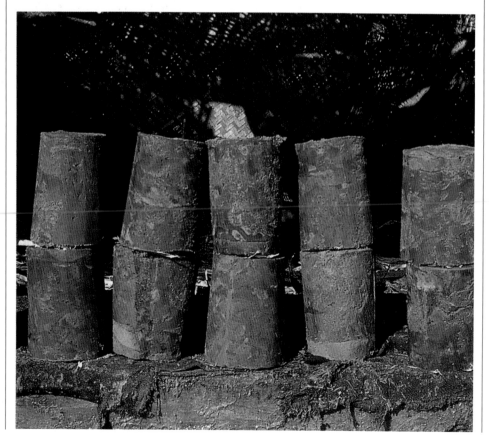

asafoetida
hing

Although not native to India, asafoetida has been an essential part of Indian cookery and medicine for ages. Due to its offensive smell it is also sometimes referred to as 'devil's dung'.

Asafoetida is the dried latex from the rhizomes of several species of ferula or giant fennel. It is grown chiefly in Iran and Afghanistan from where it is exported to the rest of the world. In India it is cultivated in Kashmir. Asafoetida is the product of a tall, smelly, perennial herb, with strong, carrot-shaped roots. In March or April, just before flowering, the stalks are cut close to the root. A milky liquid oozes out, which dries to form asafoetida. This is collected and a fresh cut is made. This procedure continues for about 3 months, by which time the plant has yielded up to 1kg (2¼lb) of resin and the root has dried up.

Fresh asafoetida is whitish and solid and gradually turns pink to reddish-brown on exposure to oxygen. It is ochre when sold commercially and the most widely used form is the fine yellow powder or granules. Asafoetida has a pungent, unpleasant smell quite like that of pickled eggs, due to the presence of sulphur compounds. On its own it tastes awful but its powerful aroma complements lentils, vegetables and pickles, completing the flavour of the dish. It is always used in small quantities – a tiny pinch added to hot oil before the other ingredients is enough to flavour a dish for 4.

Most commonly available boxed as powder or as granules, asafoetida is also sold as a hard lump that needs to be crushed. It keeps well for up to a year.

fenugreek
methi

Ancient herbalists believed that fenugreek aided digestion. Even today the seeds are eaten to relieve flatulence, chronic cough and diarrhoea. Fenugreek the spice consists of small, hard, ochre, oblong seeds. The leaves of the plant are also eaten as a popular vegetable all over India. The whole plant has a pronounced, aromatic odour and the seeds smell of curry. Fenugreek is one of the most powerful Indian spices known for its aroma and lingering taste. It is an essential ingredient of curry powder.

The seeds are available whole, crushed or powdered. The fresh stalks with leaves are sold in every Indian food shop and the dried leaves, called kasuri methi are sold in packs, either whole or powdered. It is well worth buying kasuri methi – it is used as a flavouring and adds a very wholesome touch to meats, vegetables and onion-based curries. Store the seeds as well as kasuri methi in dry jars. Use the seeds in 6 months, the dried leaves in 4.

nigella
(black onion seeds)
kalonji

The nigella plant is a relative of the delicate 'love-in-a-mist' which decorates many gardens worldwide. In India, nigella is also known as black onion seed although the seeds have nothing to do with onions.

Nigella is the dried seed-like fruit of a small herb with wispy sage-coloured leaves and graceful flowers which ripen into seed capsules. These are collected when ripe. They are then dried, crushed whole and sieved to separate the seeds.

Nigella seeds are jet black with a matte finish like tiny chips of coal. They have a faint nutty, but bitter taste due to the presence of nigellin. Nigella goes beautifully with fish, in naan bread and in salads. In west Bengal the most prolific spice blend is panch phoron, a mixture of five spices including nigella.

indian cottage cheese
paneer

Paneer is Indian cottage cheese and is neutral in taste. Unlike cottage cheese eaten in the west, commercially made paneer is firm, dry and can be cleanly cut. It tastes delicious both fried or au naturel.

In India, the people of Punjab make the most wonderful paneer. The milk is first heated and then lemon juice is added to split it. The result is clotted milk and this is hung in muslin until all the liquid or whey has drained away, usually overnight. This home-made paneer is softer, wetter and more like the cottage cheese we see in the West. This is because factory-made paneer is pressed down with heavier weights and so more of the liquid is squeezed out.

grains

The Indian kitchen uses a variety of grains. Rice is as common as wheat and is eaten whole or is milled into flour used for making batter and doughs, especially for festive sweets. Wheatflour is used daily. In most places in India, people still buy wholewheat, clean it and take it to the nearest chakki or mill to make sure they get the freshest, purest flour possible. This wholewheat flour or 'atta' is brownish and coarser than refined flour because it contains more bran and is used for making a number of rotis, parathas and poories. The finer the wholewheat flour, the softer the rotis will be. Refined wheat flour, which is used for making certain breads, is fine, white and soft.

Semolina is made by processing wheat into tiny grains. The wheat is cleaned, the wheatgerm is separated and the remainder is coarsely milled into semolina. You can buy fine or coarse semolina. Fine semolina is used for recipes that require a smoother finish such as a south Indian snack called upma, a kind of savoury cake sprinkled with fresh coconut and fragrant coriander. Coarse semolina is often made into a pudding with sugar, raisins and ghee called halwa. Fish or vegetable patties are rolled in semolina before frying to give a crisp coating. Babies are fed a porridge made with semolina as a first weaning food.

In India corn is commonly called maize and is grown as a vegetable or for grinding into flour.

Coarse milling produces cornmeal and cornflour, which are rich in fats and carbohydrates. Cornflour is fine, white and soft whereas cornmeal is coarse, grainy and pale yellow. When fried, both the flours become very crisp. Cornmeal is added to batters and vegetable stir-fries. Corn rotis or bread called 'makke ki roti' are popular in Punjab and are traditionally served hot with spiced mustard greens during the cold winter months.

Other grains that are used include bajra and jowar, which are milled into a flour for thick rotis. Bajra and jowar flours are often combined to make bhakri or other breads. They are pounded together with spices, rolled out into thin discs and dried to make poppadoms.

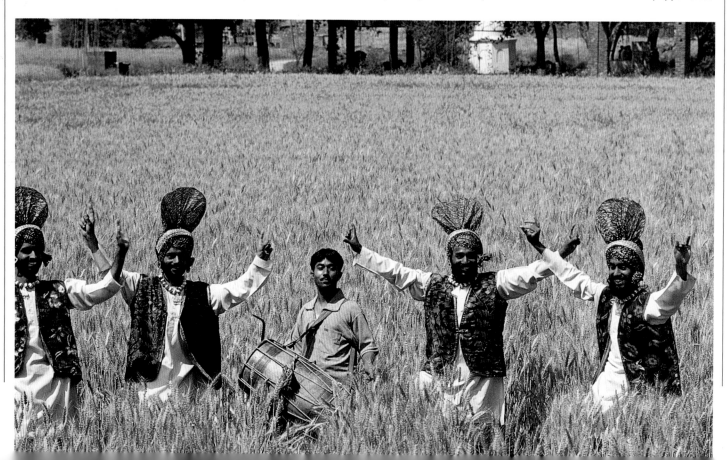

gourds

The gourd family has about 800 species and many of these are grown in India and some are available in the West. Historians claim that cultivation of these tropical plants began in Africa or India several thousand years ago. Gourds vary in size, shape and colour, but almost all have a distinctive skin and a multitude of seeds embedded in the inner flesh. Many gourds are hollowed out and dried to store water and food or used as musical instruments.

Some Indian gourds include 'turai' or ridged gourd. The fruit has raised ridges along its length. As the fruits mature these, as well as the seeds within, harden and make the fruit dry and lifeless. The young fruits are cooked in stir-fries much like a zucchini. When preparing, peel the ridges thinly, but the remaining skin can be eaten. In some places in India, these discarded ridges are soaked in water and ground up into a delicious chutney with coconut and spices.

Karela or bitter melons are popular in spite of their intense bitter flavour and are often combined with onions and tomatoes. Their skin is bright green and knobbly when fresh and, as they mature, the skin turns yellow and the seeds start to turn orange. The flesh is white and cottony but can dry out in over-ripe fruits. There is a Chinese variety of bitter melon which is lighter in colour and fatter, and a Thai variety, which is white. To prepare karela, slice thinly and soak in salted water for a couple of hours. Some people drink this bitter water as a tonic. It is a good vegetable to hollow out and fill with spiced mashed potatoes and can also be used in curries.

Dudhi or doodhi is also called bottle gourd. There are many varieties of different shapes and sizes and these grow on climbers in many domestic gardens. They have a smooth pale green skin and the inner flesh is white, spongy and a bit like cucumber in taste. It is quite a bland watery vegetable and cannot be eaten raw. Dudhi is very versatile and can be made into curries, pancakes or sweets such as halwa.

Petha or fuzzy melon looks like an uneven-skinned version of bottle gourd. It has a nipped centre. It is made into a sweet called 'petha' which is very sweet and translucent. Agra is most famous for this sweet.

Snake gourds are long and thin and can measure over 1.8m in length! They are plucked when very tender and flexible and weights are often placed on them while growing to keep them straight. If left to grow naturally, they end up curling around themselves like huge green snakes. This strange looking vegetable is chopped up and sold in manageable lengths. It cooks easily and is combined with lentils for texture and nutritional value.

Tindora, tendli or Ivy gourds are long oval fruits measuring only about 5cm in length. They taste crunchy and cucumber like and are quite fresh and juicy. Over-ripe tindora are red on the inside and can be bitter, in which case they need to be discarded. They are sliced lengthways or in small discs and are used in stir-fries or pickles. They go very well with cashew nuts, coconut and garlic.

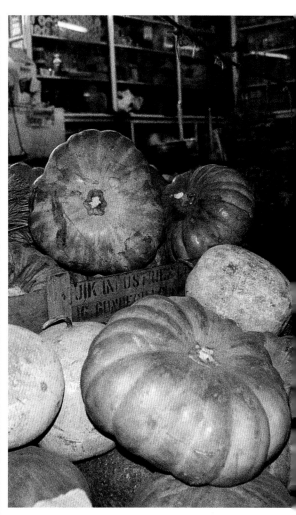

Tinda are smooth-skinned lemon-sized round gourds that are cooked with garlic and tomatoes and are quite popular in north Indian cookery.

Parwal or pointed gourds have a dark green striped skin and large seeds. The skin is quite coarse but edible. They taste wonderful when dusted with rice or wheat flour and deep-fried.

garlic and onions

There are 325 varieties of onion, all belonging to the lily family. Indian onions are white, pink or purple and range from small to about the size of a tennis ball. There are also the small pearl onions that are used in south Indian 'sambhar' or lentils. In Gujarat and Maharashtra they are combined with stuffed aubergines to add a hint of sweetness. Spring onions are white with green leaves and have to be eaten fresh. They are cooked with gram flour to make a traditional Maharashtrian dish called zunka. The onions called for in most Indian recipes can be substituted with Spanish onions in the west. These are mild and juicy and add bulk as well as moisture to curries.

Onion is perhaps the most widely eaten vegetable in India and is grown on farms and in kitchen gardens. It contains an essential oil and organic sulphides which gives it a peculiar, sulphurous smell. This smell is released when the tissues of the onion are cut. The taste of raw onions is quite pungent with a hint of sweetness. When cooked, onions have a wholesome aroma and sweetish taste.

It is best to store onions in a cool, dry, airy place as any moisture will cause them to rot. In India, white onions are woven onto ropes quite like the way garlic can be sold in the West. Some onions seem to keep for weeks, while others become mouldy and soft rather quickly. The reason lies in the moisture content. A firm dry onion will keep quite a bit longer than one that is soft and springy. Many people assume that it is good practice to store onions and potatoes together but this is not so. Potatoes have a lot of moisture and can give off a gas that causes onions to spoil more rapidly.

Peeling or chopping onions is never easy. In my many cookery classes and demos, this is the task that draws all the moans from participants because Indian cookery seems to need so many onions! When I was studying at the Catering College in Mumbai, we all had to work for a part of the week in the Quantity Kitchen producing about 500 meals a day. You can imagine the tears generated by bags and bags of onions! I have found that the best way to lessen the crying is to put onions into the fridge for a little while before chopping them. This seems to make the sulphur oils a bit more stable.

Onions are available all year round. They have diuretic properties and are often used to relieve catarrh in the bronchial tubes. A teaspoon of onion juice mixed with honey is even given to babies for this purpose.

Onions are used in every kind of Indian cookery to flavour, thicken, colour, garnish or accompany dishes. They can be boiled or fried and ground to a paste as a base for curries, fried until dark brown as a garnish or simply sliced, drizzled with lemon juice and served as a side salad. They go well with tomatoes, ginger, garlic, meat and potatoes.

Hailed as the 'bulb of life', garlic was known to ancient physicians as an incomparable medicine. Garlic is a bulbous perennial herb of the onion family consisting of 6–30 individual bulbs called cloves. Several varieties of Indian garlic such as Poona, Nasik and Madurai are popular all over the world. What one sees in the West is an oriental variety called elephant garlic which is larger and milder than the small variety sold in India. Fresh garlic or garlic greens are grown in many household kitchens. They are wonderfully aromatic, more herb-like in aroma than bulbs of garlic and in the winter they are combined with a mixture of vegetables to make a Gujarati delicacy called Undhiyoon. Garlic powder or flakes are also sold but do not have the power and potency of fresh garlic.

Garlic has an unmistakable and pungent aroma. It has a flavour that is much stronger than that of onion. The smell has an undernote of sulphur which is either loved or hated, as some people find its lingering smell distasteful. The taste can be quite sharp and biting and can increase the heat of a dish so do take this into account when adding the other spices to the pan.

Garlic is one of the most widely used ingredients in the world. In India it is used in curries, marinades, chutneys, vegetable dishes, barbecued meats, pickles and countless other preparations. Each clove of garlic is first peeled, and then the flesh can be chopped, grated or made into paste. Garlic can be eaten raw or cooked; when frying make sure that the oil is not too hot or the garlic will burn and taste acrid. A few cloves of garlic, roughly bruised, fried in a little hot oil and poured into a curry can give it a real lift. Garlic and ginger complement each other and are often used together. Ginger-garlic paste (page 11) uses equal quantities of each and can be stored successfully in the freezer in an airtight box for a couple of months. If you find that your curry is too mild and insipid, a teaspoonful of ginger-garlic paste is sure to give it a bit of life.

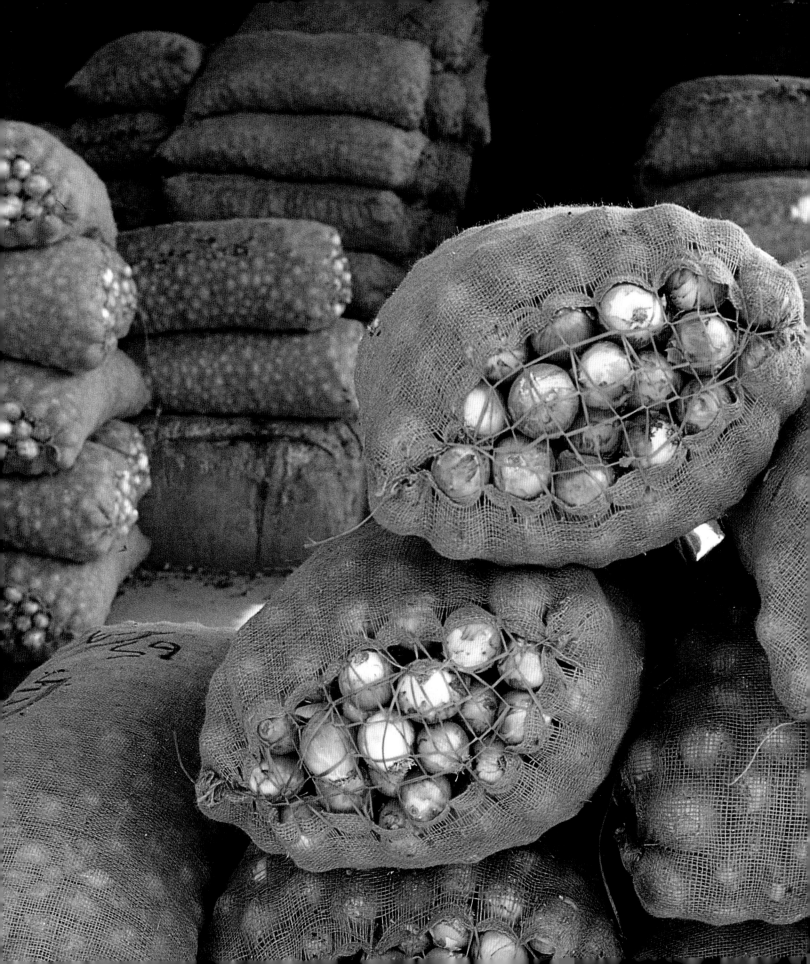

chillies

Given that they are used in almost every savoury recipe from any part of the country, it is surprising that until about 400 years ago, chillies were unknown in India. They were introduced by the Portuguese at the end of the 15th century. Commercially, chillies, which are fruits of the capsicum species, are classified on the basis of their colour, shape and pungency, and over a hundred varieties are grown and eaten all over the world. Chillies have a strong, smarting aroma and their taste ranges from mild to dynamite. The level of heat is dependent on the amount of capsaicin present in the seeds, veins and skin of the chillies and is not diminished by cooking, storing, or freezing. This is why generally, the smaller the chilli, the seeds and veins being more concentrated, the hotter it is.

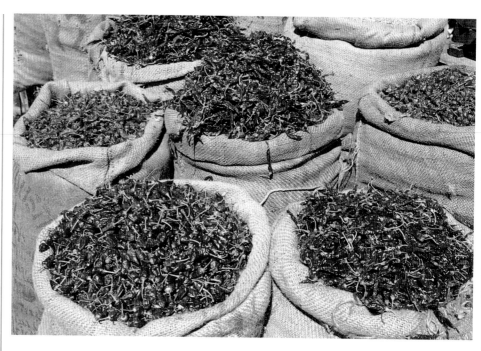

Chillies bring heat as well as fragrance to a dish. Contrary to expectation, many of India's hottest places boast of a fiery cuisine because chillies actually cool down the system in hot weather. The capsaicin dilates blood vessels to increase circulation and encourage perspiration. However, if you ever bite into a chilli unexpectedly, don't reach for a jug of water – capsaicin is insoluble in water (like oil). Dairy products have the power to neutralise capsaicin so try yoghurt or milk to calm the fire.

India is the largest producer of chillies today, contributing 25 per cent of the total world production. They are available fresh, dried, powdered, flaked, in oil, in sauce, bottled and pickled. When buying fresh chillies, look for crisp, unwrinkled and glossy ones. Red chillies are often dried for the purpose of better storage although varieties such as the ivory white, hot

Kanthari chilli are also used. The pungency can vary from the mild Kashmir chilli and some dried south Indian varieties such as Tomato chillies and Byadagi chillies that give more colour than heat, to the fiery birds eye chillies from the north-east and the dried Guntur chillies which have a dark red, thick skin and incredible firepower. As with all ground spices, chilli powder loses its strength and sparkle after a few months. Whole dried chillies will keep for up to a year if stored in a dry, dark place. When they are to be used in curry pastes, they are first soaked in some warm water to soften them. I like to shake out the seeds before grinding them up as the seeds are hard and often stay whole.

Chillies are very high in vitamins A and C and have more vitamin C per gram than many

oranges. However, an inordinate intake of chillies can burn the lining of the stomach, so beware of overindulgence. I have seen many people in England eat more chillies than most Indians I know!

All chillies need to be treated with respect. The capsaicin in chillies is highly irritating to skin, so be careful when preparing them. Try to avoid contact with the inside of the fruit and wash your hands with soap and water immediately after use. To reduce the pungency of chillies, discard the seeds and soak the rest in cold salted water. For maximum fire, slice the chillies and leave the seeds in. To prepare dried chillies, remove the stems and shake out the seeds. They can also be torn into bits, soaked in warm water and ground to a paste for curries and sauces.

rice

Although India grows hundreds of varieties of rice such as the mango-perfumed ambemohur or the short-grained kolum, the flavour of basmati rice is celebrated the world over. Its name conjures up visions of lush, green paddy fields being watered by the snow-fed rivers of the Himalayas. Basmati is considered to be the king of rice and as such, in India, it is reserved for special occasions or particular dishes. India was one of the earliest countries to grow rice. From here it travelled first to Egypt, then via Greece, Portugal and Italy, to America. Historians estimate that it was first cultivated at least 3000 years ago. Rice has always been a symbol of plenty in Hindu tradition. According to custom, married women in India are honoured and wished a life of plenty by presenting them with a coconut, a handful of rice and a length of fabric on festive occasions. The throwing of rice is associated with all weddings, whether Hindu, Christian or Islamic.

Rice is gluten free, making it an ideal food for babies or those with wheat or gluten allergies. It is also cholesterol free and low in sodium unless you add salt to the cooking water (I never do this). It is rich in protein and contains all eight amino acids but it is poor in the amino acid lysine, which is found in beans, making the combination highly nutritious.

The grains of basmati rice are white, long and very silky to touch. They are even in size and clean looking. The fragrance is unmistakable. Rich and wholesome, it has a pure scent and a fresh, uncluttered taste. It is available whole or as broken grains which are much cheaper.

Broken basmati is used in dishes that require a sticky texture such as rice pudding or for recipes that require the grinding up of rice as in batters. Rice flour is also used for batters or to coat vegetables when deep-frying them. It is made with cheaper varieties of rice. Rice is like wine – it gets better with age. Good basmati is left to mature in controlled conditions for up to 10 years. Old rice cooks better and remains fluffy whereas new rice becomes sticky when cooked. The only way to know whether the rice is old is to ask, but most brands of packaged rice in the West are suitable. Store in the package that the rice comes in or remove to an airtight container and store for up 3 months.

Although there are as many ways of cooking perfect rice as there are rice eaters, one way is to wash the rice thoroughly until the water runs clear. Put it with double the quantity of fresh water into a heavy saucepan, bring to the boil and stir well. Reduce the heat, cover and simmer for 10 minutes. Turn off the heat and allow it to sit in its steam for a further 5 minutes. There is a saying in India that perfectly cooked rice should be like two brothers, close but not stuck together. Indians always serve rice piping hot and most often with lentils, beans or a curry. Dal and rice is a staple meal in most of India. Basmati rice is made into rich biryanis, pulaos, sweets, stuffings and snacks.

It is important to store cooked rice properly. It must be refrigerated soon after it has cooled down as it is easily contaminated. Also, I like to cook only the amount needed for each meal because once refrigerated, the starch amylase present in cooked long grain rice tends to toughen up and make the rice hard.

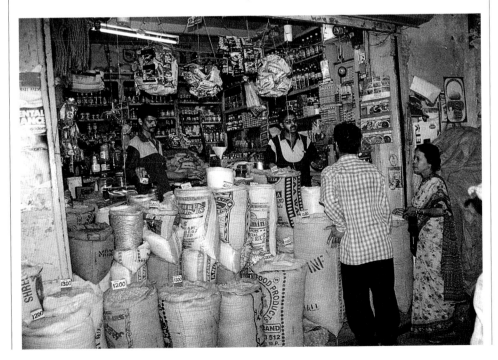

turmeric

One of the most traditional and versatile of spices used in Indian cooking, turmeric is the very heart and soul of any curry. This key ingredient is used daily in every part of India as its unique colour, due to the presence of the pigment curcumin, and flavour enriches every regional cuisine. Turmeric is used prolifically in a host of Indian dishes ranging from starters, lentils, meats and vegetables. It has also been used for centuries as a curative and cleansing agent. Since early times, it has been associated with purification so that even today, an Indian bride and groom are ritually anointed with turmeric as part of a cleansing ceremony, after which they do not leave the house until the wedding.

Turmeric has an earthy, sensual fragrance reminiscent of the aridness of vast fields parched in a hot Indian summer. On its own, it has a musky, dry taste, but it is used wholeheartedly in Indian cooking for its wonderful quality of enhancing and balancing the flavours of all the other ingredients. However, be careful not to use turmeric when cooking green vegetables as they will turn dull and taste bitter.

Store turmeric in a dry jar and use within 4 months or it may lose its vibrancy. Be careful while storing and using turmeric; it will stain hands and clothes quite quickly. Only cured turmeric has the aroma and colour (chiefly due to the presence of the pigment curcumin) necessary for cooking.

cumin

Cumin the spice has been known to man since Biblical times. Sometimes confused with caraway or nigella, cumin is an important spice in its own right and one that makes a happy addition to almost every Indian savoury.

Cumin seeds are really the fruits of the herb. They are elongated, oval and long. They range from sage green to tobacco brown in colour and have longitudinal ridges. During the drying process, some fine stalks invariably get left on, so cumin appears slightly bristly. Another variety of cumin is black cumin or kala jeera, shahi jeera or siya jeera. The seeds are dark brown to black and are smaller and finer than cumin. The smell of cumin is distinctive. It can be described as peculiar, strong and bitter and is usually loved or hated. Cumin has a warm, somewhat bitter taste.

It is available whole as seeds or crushed to a powder which is often blended with coriander powder to form a widely used mixture called dhana-jeera. This combination is one of the essential spice blends used in Indian cookery.

Toasted cumin powder gives a lift to many curries and yoghurt-based raitas. It is not at all difficult to make this at home. Roast the seeds on a griddle until they change colour and crush them into a fine toasty powder in a mortar. Roasting the cumin releases and enriches its earthy flavour. As with all other spices, store cumin in a dry place away from light. The powder is best used within 3 months.

coriander

Most Indian cooks will not allow a curry to leave their kitchen without a good sprinkling of fresh, fragrant coriander leaves. This pretty herb is the most commonly used garnish in the northern and western parts of India, and adds a dewy green touch to red or brown curries. Seeds of the coriander plant are the spice. Coriander is perhaps one of the first spices known to man and has been around for over 3,000 years. It finds mention in ancient Sanskrit texts and in the Bible where the colour of manna is likened to that of coriander seeds.

Coriander leaves and the seeds are completely different from one another with regard to aroma and flavour. The leaves taste and smell fresh and fruity with a hint of ginger. The seeds, on the other hand, have a sweet, heady aroma with a subtle whiff of pine and pepper.

Little bunches of fresh coriander are commonly available at greengrocers. It looks quite like parsley but the test lies in the aroma – parsley has a more delicate smell than coriander.

Coriander seeds have many healing properties. An infusion of the seeds is cooling and helps reduce fever. Suited to almost every savoury Indian dish, coriander (the spice and the herb) is used daily in curries, chutneys, soups and drinks. The fresh green chutney made by grinding coriander leaves, coconut, ginger, garlic and spices is a popular sandwich spread or meal accompaniment. It is also served in Indian restaurants all over the world.

captions to photographs

Page 1 Golkonda Fort, Hyderabad, Andra Pradesh.

2/3 Rann of Kutch, Rabari woman (nomad) carrying water to her village.

6 a woman carries leafy branches she uses for animal feed

7 Vegetables for sale in Southern Indian market.

8 Dakshineswar Kali Temple, near Kolkata (Calcutta), built in 1847 on the banks of the river Hoogly.

9 roadside stalls in Dacres Lane, Calcutta. Famous for tasty but basic lunches visited by office workers.

10 a group of cooks prepare chapattis which will feed visitors for Baisakhi Day (Harvest Festival in Punjab)

11 Udaipur City Palace. The bedroom of the Maharana Bhopal Singh born 1884, crowned 1930, died 1958. He was disabled from polio, you can see his wheelchair and bed. He tried to live a simple life with simple possesions.

12 At a water well near the town of Alkalkot in Maharashtra

15 Dakshineswar Kali Temple, near Kolkata (Calcutta), built 1847, on the banks of the river Hoogly.The temple is dedicated to the goddess Bhavatarini (Kali). This Temple is where the famous 19th century Hindu saint Ramakrishna attained his spiritual vision of the unity of all religions.

16 Irrigating plants on a plantation near Panaji, Goa

17 Harvesting coconuts in Kerala. The men climb up using a rope around their ankles and the tree.

20 The central Pillar of the Diwan-i-Khas (assembly hall) in Fatehpur Sikri, Rajasthan. The Emperor Akbar (ruled 1556-1605) sat above the pillar and his ministers on the balconies, with spectators standing below.

21 Pounding of turmeric in a granite bowl. Bhatoli Village, in the Yamuna Valley.

28 Bhatoli Village, women cook rice and dahl over the 'chula' under the verandah of their house

33 Presenting jaggery 'cakes' made from sugar cane.

36 Jaggery 'gur' making from sugar cane. Cottage industry. Three large concrete vats are heated from underneath. Sugar cane juice is boiled to extract sugar and in the purification process thickening liquid is scooped from vat to vat.

40 Harvesting rice by cutting it with a scythe and laying the cut grain in the field to dry.

49 Rann of Kutch, Rabari woman (nomad) carrying water and crossing an irrigation channel.

53 Worker in a vegetable market carrying sacks of potatoes.

56 Dried Basmati rice stalks with the grain attached are collected and bundled into sheafs.

59 New Delhi, Lodi Gardens, a monument from the Lodi Dynasly (1451-1526).

62 Udaipur, Rajasthan, view from City Palace to the luxury Lake Palace Hotel in Lake Pichola.

68 The last corn of the season is being de-husked for the cooking of rotis.

77 Two farm workers cut the ripe basmati rice.

81 Rann of Kutch, Jambouri viallage. A herder returns.

92 Rann of Kutch. Nomadic Rabari children in traditional costumes at their campsite.

95 Creative display of fruits for juicing. Chowpatti Beach, Mumbai.

96 Pouring milk into urns. Village near Anand, Gujarat.

98/99 Men carrying water on their way to Pushkar, Rajasthan.

102 Qutb Shahi Tomb near Hyderabad, Andhra Pradesh.

103 Backwaters of Kerala near Alleppy. Converted rice-(transport) boats, now luxury houseboats 'kettuvalla', operated by long bamboo poles, take tourists through the canals to view backwater life.

107 Kerala Temple, the elephant festival, Maradu Village, north of Cochin. The goddess Badhrakalan is symbolised by the golden shield on the biggest and tallest elephant, to the tune of drums and trumpets. Brahmins rise peacock feather fans and sheep's tail whisks.

110 Harvesting coconuts in Kerala. The men climb up using a rope around their ankles and the tree.

112 Banana tree in Kerala

117 Vegetable plantation, Goa.

121 Friday market in Mapusa, Goa.

123 Figure along one of the four Ratha Temples in Mamallampuram (7th century), 45km south of Chennai.

126 In the courtyard of a private house near Pondicherry, Tamil Nadu. Cooking of Pongal rice, during the Pongal Harvest Festival.

130 Chinese fishing nets at the northern tip of Fort Cochin, Cochin, Kerala.

136 Backwaters near Allepy, Kerala. A boat load of dried palm fronds is paddled past an old Catholic Church.

138 Catholic Church 'Our Lady of the Immaculate Conception', Panaji, Goa.

142 Preparations for a temple festival in Bhubaneshwar, Orissa.

143 Rice fields along the foothills of the Himalayas.

145 Morning flower market close to the entrance of the Howrah Bridge, Kolkata (Calcutta), West Bengal.

150 Woman pilgrim performing a water ritual at the seaside of Puri, Orissa.

153 Vegetable market in Kolkata (Calcutta).

157 Kolkata (Calcutta), Javardpore Municiple Market. Shopping for vegetables.

161 View of the Jagannath Temple in Puri, Orissa, which is inaccessible for non-Hindus.

166 Baisakhi harvest festival. Bhangra dancers perform in wheat fields, wearing tradional Punjabi folk dress. Baisakhi, on 13th April, also celebrates the beginning of the New Year in Punjab.

171 Rice and spice emporium, southern India

173 Vegetable plantation, Panaji, Goa

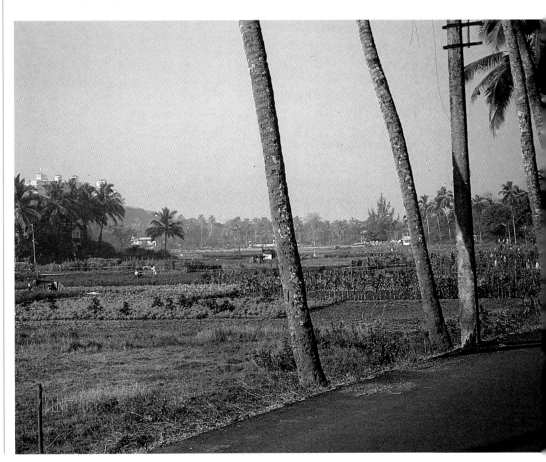

index

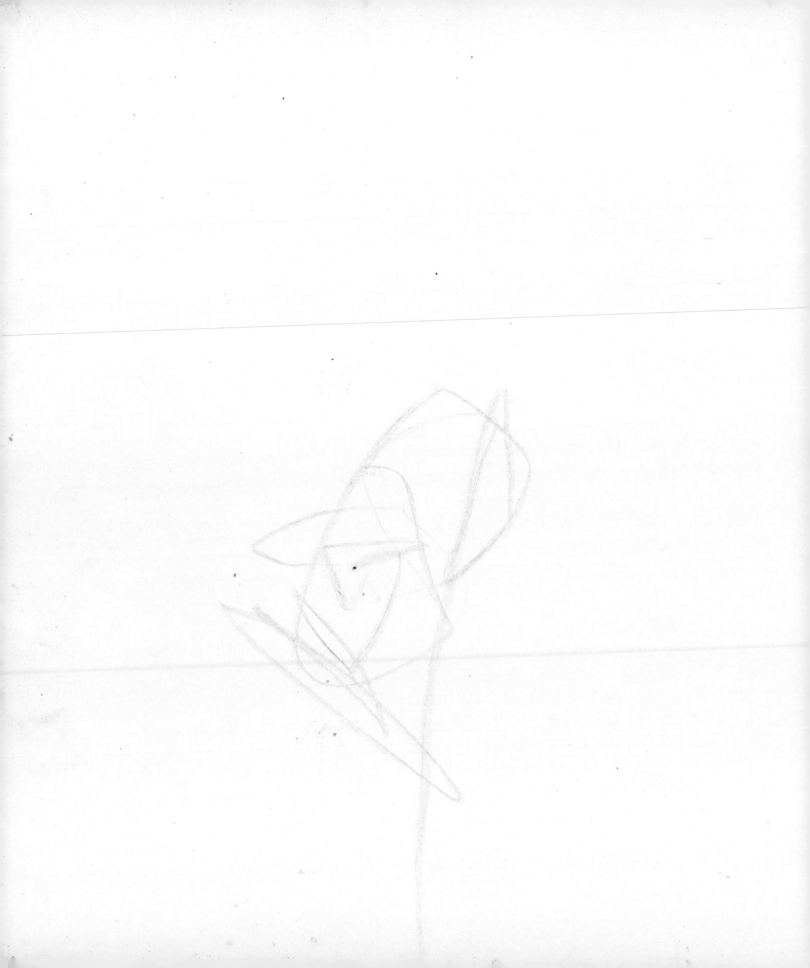